T0265163

Melanoma

TRANSLATIONAL MEDICINE SERIES

Melanoma

Translational Research and Emerging Therapies

Edited by

Sanjiv S. Agarwala
St. Luke's Cancer Center
St. Luke's Hospital & Health Network
Bethlehem, Pennsylvania, USA

Vernon K. Sondak
H. Lee Moffitt Cancer Center
Tampa, Florida, USA

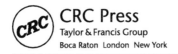

CRC Press
Taylor & Francis Group
Boca Raton London New York

CRC Press is an imprint of the
Taylor & Francis Group, an **informa** business

First published 2008 by Informa Healthcare, Inc.

Published 2019 by CRC Press
Taylor & Francis Group
6000 Broken Sound Parkway NW, Suite 300
Boca Raton, FL 33487-2742

© 2008 by Taylor & Francis Group, LLC
CRC Press is an imprint of Taylor & Francis Group, an Informa business

First issued in paperback 2019

No claim to original U.S. Government works

ISBN 13: 978-0-367-45262-9 (pbk)
ISBN 13: 978-0-8493-9018-0 (hbk)

This book contains information obtained from authentic and highly regarded sources. Reasonable efforts have been made to publish reliable data and information, but the author and publisher cannot assume responsibility for the validity of all materials or the consequences of their use. The authors and publishers have attempted to trace the copyright holders of all material reproduced in this publication and apologize to copyright holders if permission to publish in this form has not been obtained. If any copyright material has not been acknowledged please write and let us know so we may rectify in any future reprint.

Except as permitted under U.S. Copyright Law, no part of this book may be reprinted, reproduced, transmitted, or utilized in any form by any electronic, mechanical, or other means, now known or hereafter invented, including photocopying, microfilming, and recording, or in any information storage or retrieval system, without written permission from the publishers.

For permission to photocopy or use material electronically from this work, please access www.copyright.com (http://www.copyright.com/) or contact the Copyright Clearance Center, Inc. (CCC), 222 Rosewood Drive, Danvers, MA 01923, 978-750-8400. CCC is a not-for-profit organization that provides licenses and registration for a variety of users. For organizations that have been granted a photocopy license by the CCC, a separate system of payment has been arranged.

Trademark Notice: Product or corporate names may be trademarks or registered trademarks, and are used only for identification and explanation without intent to infringe.

Visit the Taylor & Francis Web site at
http://www.taylorandfrancis.com

and the CRC Press Web site at
http://www.crcpress.com

Library of Congress Cataloging-in-Publication Data

Melanoma : translational research and emerging therapies / edited by
Sanjiv S. Agarwala, Vernon K. Sondak.
    p. ; cm. — (Translational medicine series ; 8)
  Includes bibliographical references and index.
  ISBN-13: 978-0-8493-9018-0 (hardcover : alk. paper)
  ISBN-10: 0-8493-9018-4 (hardcover : alk. paper)

1. Melanoma. 2. Melanoma—Treatment. I. Agarwala, Sanjiv S. II. Sondak, Vernon K.,
1957- III. Series.
  [DNLM: 1. Melanoma—physiopathology. 2. Melanoma—drug therapy.
QZ 200 M5179 2008]
  RC280.M37M52 2008
  616.99′477—dc22

                                                                            2008015015

Foreword

The official National Cancer Institute's definition for translational research is as follows: "Translational research uses knowledge of human biology to develop and test the feasibility of cancer-relevant interventions in humans and/or determines the biological basis for observations made in individuals with cancer or in populations at risk for cancer. The term 'interventions' is used in its broadest sense to include molecular assays, imaging techniques, drugs, biological agents, and/or other methodologies applicable to the prevention, early detection, diagnosis, prognosis, and/or treatment of cancer." Said more simply, translational research involves all types of investigations from bench-to-bedside or bedside-to-bench, but the best examples are more complete by bridging bench-to-bedside-to-bench or bedside-to-bench-to-bedside. The melanoma field has many examples of out-standing translational research over the last few decades with immunotherapy of melanoma being the frontrunner. This book discusses in superb chapters the current state of the art in translational science of melanoma.

The discovery of mutations in the *BRAF* oncogene in July of 2002 has given the field a major boost because suddenly there was a bona fide gene whose constitutive activation could explain many properties of melanoma cells, par-ticularly their exuberant growth and invasive capacity. When combined with mutations in *NRAS* and *c-KIT,* the MAPK signaling pathway appears to be activated in almost all melanomas. Mutations in *BRAF* (or *RAS* or *c-KIT*) alone are not sufficient to transform melanocytes, suggesting that we need at least one more genetic hit. This may be in any of the cell cycle–related genes, among DNA repair genes, or in pathways unrelated to the most obvious candidates. Thus, a broad analysis of the melanoma genome is highly welcome for discovering additional nonrandom mutations that could be the target for new therapies. As the list for transforming genes in melanoma is further enlarged, experimental therapists have not waited and have begun to target mutant BRAF with small molecules. The very first inhibitor, sorafenib, made it very quickly into the clinics and was greeted with exuberant enthusiasm. However, sorafenib as monotherapy does not appear to be efficacious. Therefore, combination therapies with classical chemotherapeutic drugs are the order of the day. Every major drug company and many smaller biotechnology companies have generated inhibitors with ever more specificity for the mutant kinase of BRAF. The major question that is vexing the field is whether kinase inhibitors should be less or more specific. Since melanoma cells show constitutive activation of many kinases, it is appealing to try to inhibit them all with one drug, and sorafenib is such an example. On the other hand, more focused "scalpels" should be more effective, particularly when used in combination with inhibitors that specifically block other pathways. Finding those additional drugs that block alternative/synergistic pathways to the MAPK pathway will be the challenge for the next few years.

Melanoma cells have managed to find several ways to activate the MAPK pathway by either mutating *BRAF, NRAS* or *c-KIT,* or by amplifying genes including *BRAF* or adaptor proteins to the MAPK pathway. This book provides chapters dealing with the highly diverse strategies that melanoma cells use to grow, invade, and avoid death. Our therapies of the future will have to accommodate the diversity of melanoma cells to become growth autonomous and to survive in a harsh environment, as it exists in hypoxia or when the cells circulate in the bloodstream. We can no longer afford treating melanoma as one disease, even the genetic signature of superficial spreading melanoma is diverse and will require individualized therapies, because each tumor will respond to drugs on the basis of its specific mutations and/or specific epigenetic changes that are yet to be discovered. Its fate, dormancy and survival, growth and invasion, protection by the stroma or attack by the innate and specific immune system resulting in destruction will depend on who the driver for the malignancy is. We need to find those drivers, and they will not be the same for every tumor. Thus, melanoma therapy, particularly targeted therapy, will need to be individualized on the basis of the genetic, epigenetic, and microenvironmental signature of a given tumor. We need to screen for mutations of the most obvious candidates to also prevent unnecessary therapies for those patients who will likely not benefit.

As we can no longer afford to treat all melanomas as equal, we may face the added challenge that within each tumor not all cells are equal and respond in the same manner to the same drugs. Tumor heterogeneity may be seen not as a random collection of cells in which each is equal, but instead there may be a hierarchy in which the melanoma stem cells are on top of this pyramid. Any therapy that such cancer stem cells can escape would rapidly lead to not only regrowth of a tumor with the same diversity but even more aggressiveness. The next few years will determine whether and how we need to develop two therapies for each tumor: one for the major population, the so-called "transient amplifying cells" that can still be tumorigenic and that rapidly proliferate, and another approach for the slowly proliferating and highly drug-resistant cancer stem cells. Should the cancer stem cell hypothesis not survive further scrutiny, we would still have to deal with the infamous heterogeneity in melanoma that is likely the cause of much of the drug resistance. Potentially, immunotherapies will find an important role for cancer stem cell therapy, because tumor destruction by immune cells occurs independent of the proliferation cycle of the tumor cells.

Immunotherapy of melanoma has gone through several phases. Each raised considerable excitement in all of cancer research because each began with promising early clinical results. The first phase involved active immunization using crude cell extracts or secreted cell products. Some of these vaccine studies are still going on; particularly, defined antigens or peptides loaded onto dendritic cells have shown promise, as had tumor antigens when combined with ever better adjuvants. When cytokines were discovered in the mid-eighties, we all thought that they were the key to melanoma therapy because they could either directly target the melanoma cells or stimulate the immune response against the tumor. Several cytokines, including interleukin 2, interferon alpha, and granulocyte macrophage colony–stimulating factor, are still being given to patients, but there is no general consensus on their usage. Adoptive immunotherapy was a novel approach to boost those immune cells that had antitumor activities, and the research waves went from lymphokine-activated killer cells to tumor-infiltrating lymphocytes to the genetically engineered T cells that are currently in clinical trials. Then, inhibitory (regulatory) lymphocytes were discovered and their targeting with monoclonal antibodies resulted in exciting clinical responses that continue to stimulate new clinical investigations.

Several chapters in this book discuss the different strategies for immunotherapy in melanoma. Where will immunotherapy in melanoma carry us in the future? Will the next phase be a matter of better fine-tuning? Each approach has given us *some* responses. Can we apply what we learned in the last two decades to stimulate the "right" T cells, eliminate the "bad" lymphocytes, and guide the patients to elicit a strong immune response against the "best" tumor antigens? What are the best immunological targets? Mutated proteins such as mutated BRAF are optimal targets, and clinical applications in the future will likely favor these. Like in other human malignancies, immunotherapy of melanoma will find its niche among the many other options that patients and their oncologists have.

Much of our future progress depends on technology-related science. Biomarkers are becoming indispensable not only for early detection but also for prognostication and prediction disease outcome. If therapy is dictated by biomarker analyses, then therapy outcome will be determined not just by survival analyses but in a faster way by biomarker analyses. Much is still in the experimental phase, but the use of biomarkers will penetrate every step in translational melanoma research. Such technology-driven approaches make it difficult to conduct research in a conventional laboratory of a handful of postdocs and technicians. Technology-driven translational research of the future will be highly interactive because no single laboratory will be capable of being in the forefront of all technologies that are becoming an essential part of bench-to-bedside-to-bench research. The technology and preclinical models are ever improving and enormous amounts of knowledge and data are being produced, and melanoma researchers must take full advantage of such improvements. This can only be achieved through solid collaborations between experts in different fields (melanoma- and non-melanoma-related), through the integration of knowledge gained from all institutions (big and small alike), through lobbying for improved funding, and through nurturing and promoting young melanoma researchers to take on future challenges. Some institutions have heavily invested in genomics, proteomics, imaging, or computational biology that provide the foundation for biomarker investigations in translational research, but those investments are unevenly distributed among institutions, leaving many investigators to wonder how they can meet the future demands of our competitive science environment, i.e., how they will get their grants. Another potential threat is the institutional support of translational scientists. While clinical investigators doing clinically related research have historically been well nurtured (if they survive the double demands on time and energy), there are very few career paths for Ph.D.-type translational researchers. Such highly trained individuals are required for maintaining competitiveness in cutting-edge technologies. The melanoma field has far too few translational researchers and needs a continuous influx for the growing demand. Equally important will be for basic scientists to communicate with clinicians to fine-tune preclinical therapeutic models and understand the strengths and weaknesses of particular treatments in order to improve them. Developing synergies between multidisciplinary investigators will be the key for the future success of all translational investigations, which also include the important areas of tissue storage, annotation, and analyses as described in this book.

We are currently at an exciting time in translational melanoma research. We can build on a tremendous foundation of outstanding work done by the many scientists in the field. We are not at a crossroads but can drive along a well-paved road that should bring us each day, each week, and each month closer to solving the many puzzles that have prevented us from seeing more cures. They will come, but we have to work together to be faster and more efficient. We owe it to the patients.

Meenhard Herlyn
The Wistar Institute, Philadelphia, PA

Preface

There are an estimated 160,000 patients newly diagnosed with melanoma annually worldwide. The lifetime risk of developing this disease in the United States is estimated at 1 in 49 for men and 1 in 73 for women. While the majority of patients diagnosed in early stages have a good outlook for cure, the prognosis of patients diagnosed after the disease has spread to distant sites remains grim.

The treatment of melanoma is truly multidisciplinary and involves input from diverse specialties including dermatology, surgical, medical and radiation oncology, nursing, and supportive care. The crucial and often-forgotten "unsung heroes" in the battle against this disease are the laboratory scientists who silently carry on the crusade to find newer therapies for clinicians to offer their patients. In this regard, this book attempts to bring together the clinician and the researcher in a format that addresses several important aspects of melanoma research and therapy, spanning the spectrum from prevention and etiology of the disease to the genetic makeup of advanced metastatic melanoma. Hence the name "Translational and Emerging Therapies."

Dr. Berwick addresses the controversies and difficulty in understanding the role of ultraviolet radiation in the pathogenesis of melanoma, including the potential role of tanning parlors in melanoma etiology, in chapter 1.

No translational text on melanoma would be complete without a discussion on molecular pathways, and in the next chapter, Dr. Fecher provides a comprehensive overview, with particular focus on signal transduction pathways as potential therapeutic targets.

Pediatric melanoma is fortunately a relative rare event, but is increasing in incidence and attracting greater attention. Diagnosis of melanomas in childhood poses inherent challenges, and several areas of controversy exist in terms of classifying melanocytic lesions in childhood. Drs. Celebi and Messina tackle the difficult topic of Spitzoid melanomas in chapter 3.

Drs. Daud, Sondak, and Weeraratna provide a comprehensive overview of melanoma genomics and implications for therapy. This is a burgeoning field and is likely to be the platform on which many new and exciting therapeutic targets will be identified.

Chemoprevention of melanoma is an attractive concept and is being explored in diseases such as breast cancer and familial adenomatous polyposis. Dr. Demierre provides an up-to-date review of the current status of chemoprevention strategies in melanoma, with emphasis on targeting Ras signaling. The molecular pathway in melanoma that has received the most therapeutic attention is the BRAF pathway downstream of Ras. Indeed, several agents targeting BRAF either singly or in combination with chemotherapy are in clinical trials for advanced melanoma patients. Drs. Smalley and Flaherty outline the rationale for the exploitation of this pathway as a paradigm for melanoma therapy.

The role that stem cells play in cancer development, progression and metastasis is receiving increasing attention. Drs. Smalley, Desai and Herlyn tackle this important topic in chapter 7, making the argument that therapies for melanoma are not likely to be successful unless they affect and modify the stem cell population.

The importance of skin pigmentation and the role of micropthalmia-associated transcription factor is an exciting area of current research with potentially druggable targets. Drs. Haq and Fisher discuss the current state-of-the-art in this area.

Recombinant interferon alfa is an agent that is widely used in melanoma and is approved for use in the adjuvant setting. Although clinically effective, the mechanisms by which this agent exerts its therapeutic effect are still unclear. The chapter by Drs. Lesinski and Carson provides an overview of the topic and places into context what is known about mechanisms of interferon activity. Drs. Gogas and Kirkwood address a very important area of research with interferon: How can we target this toxic agent to individuals most likely to benefit? The exciting findings as related to autoimmunity and their potential impact on interferon effectiveness are discussed.

Clinical data with the use of vaccines in melanoma has been disappointing despite apparent potential in the laboratory. Dr. Vohra and colleagues provide a timely review of this topic, with emphasis on potential approaches to optimizing vaccine therapy and selecting appropriate patients for future clinical trials. Finally, Drs. Tsai and Chang provide an update on the role of adoptive immunotherapy, an approach that has been shown to be clinically effective in selective patients as far back as the 1960s.

The difficult issues surrounding procurement of melanoma tumor tissue for research purposes in the face of providing adequate tissue for diagnosis are elegantly addressed by Dr. Hoover and colleagues from the Moffitt Cancer Center, where a very successful melanoma tissue procurement program is in place. The fact that most melanomas are diagnosed in the primary physician's or dermatologist's office, removed entirely and therefore not often available for academic study, makes this a particularly challenging problem.

Finally, we have attempted to provide a glossary of technical terms for easy reference as they appear in the text. This should facilitate the reader with quick definitions of sometimes confusing terminology.

The explosion of revolutionary basic science methodologies and the ability to probe the tumor down to the molecular level have enabled us to understand disease at a basic level and potentially devise therapeutic choices based on real information. It is only a matter of time before the elusive breakthrough is here.

Sanjiv S. Agarwala
Vernon K. Sondak

Contents

Contributors

Marianne Berwick   Department of Internal Medicine and University of New Mexico Cancer Center, University of New Mexico, Albuquerque, New Mexico, U.S.A.

William E. Carson III   Department of Surgery, The Ohio State University, Columbus, Ohio, U.S.A.

Julide T. Celebi   Department of Dermatology, Columbia University, New York, New York, U.S.A.

Alfred E. Chang   Department of Surgery, University of Michigan, Ann Arbor, Michigan, U.S.A.

Adil I. Daud   Department of Medicine, University of California San Francisco, San Francisco, California, U.S.A.

Marie-France Demierre   Boston University School of Medicine, Boston University Medical Center, Boston, Massachusetts, U.S.A.

Brijal Desai   The Wistar Institute, Philadelphia, Pennsylvania, U.S.A.

Leslie A. Fecher   Abramson Cancer Center of the University of Pennsylvania, Philadelphia, Pennsylvania, U.S.A.

David E. Fisher   Melanoma Program, Dana-Farber Cancer Institute, Boston, Massachusetts, U.S.A.

Keith T. Flaherty   Abramson Cancer Center of the University of Pennsylvania, Philadelphia, Pennsylvania, U.S.A.

Helen Gogas   First Department of Internal Medicine, University of Athens, Athens, Greece

Rizwan Haq   Department of Medical Oncology, Dana-Farber Cancer Institute, Boston, Massachusetts, U.S.A.

Meenhard Herlyn   The Wistar Institute, Philadelphia, Pennsylvania, U.S.A.

Tyron C. Hoover   World BioBank, Accelerated Community Oncology Research Network, Inc., Memphis, Tennessee, U.S.A.

Shane A. Huntsman   H. Lee Moffitt Cancer Center, Tampa, Florida, U.S.A.

John M. Kirkwood   University of Pittsburgh Cancer Institute, Hillman Cancer Center, Pittsburgh, Pennsylvania, U.S.A.

Gregory B. Lesinski   Department of Molecular Virology, Immunology and Medical Genetics, The Ohio State University, Columbus, Ohio, U.S.A.

Jane L. Messina   H. Lee Moffitt Cancer Center and the Department of Pathology and Cell Biology, University of South Florida College of Medicine, Tampa, Florida, U.S.A.

James J. Mulé   H. Lee Moffitt Cancer Center, Tampa, Florida, U.S.A.

Shari Pilon-Thomas   H. Lee Moffitt Cancer Center, Tampa, Florida, U.S.A.

Keiran S.M. Smalley   H. Lee Moffitt Cancer Center & Research Institute, Tampa, Florida, U.S.A.

Vernon K. Sondak   H. Lee Moffitt Cancer Center and the Departments of Oncologic Sciences and Surgery, University of South Florida College of Medicine, Tampa, Florida, U.S.A.

Susan Tsai   Department of Surgery, University of Michigan, Ann Arbor, Michigan, U.S.A.

Nasreen Vohra   H. Lee Moffitt Cancer Center and Department of Surgery, University of South Florida College of Medicine, Tampa, Florida, U.S.A.

Jeffrey Weber   H. Lee Moffitt Cancer Center and the Department of Oncologic Sciences, University of South Florida College of Medicine, Tampa, Florida, U.S.A.

Ashani Weeraratna   Laboratory of Immunology, National Institute on Aging, National Institutes of Health, Baltimore, Maryland, U.S.A.

UV Radiation in Melanoma Development and Pathogenesis

Marianne Berwick

Department of Internal Medicine and University of New Mexico Cancer Center, University of New Mexico, Albuquerque, New Mexico, U.S.A.

INTRODUCTION

There is not a direct dose-response relationship between ultraviolet radiation (UVR) and the development of squamous cell carcinoma, basal cell carcinoma, and cutaneous melanoma. In fact, the likelihood of developing any of these skin cancers probably differs on the basis of the *type* of UVR, the *pattern* of UVR, and the particular characteristics of the *individual*, mainly pigmentation. This overview will only briefly address the role of UVR received from suntan parlors. The epidemiologic studies that underlie the association between UVR and melanoma have multiple issues that need to be evaluated to clarify the role of UVR: the representativeness of the population studied, the study design used, the variables collected, and the inherent biases associated with each type of study.

UV RADIATION

Solar UVR consists of two broad types of wavelengths, UV-B (280–320 nm) and UV-A (320–400 nm). UV-B at ground level is reduced by the thin stratospheric ozone shield around the earth at 10 to 16 km above the earth's surface and by factors in the atmosphere, such as cloud cover, pollution, and water vapor. UV-A is not substantially modified by stratospheric or atmospheric conditions and accounts for approximately 90% of UVR reaching the earth's surface. A common measure utilized is erythemal UV irradiance, a measure of spectral irradiance between 250 and 400 nm "weighted" for UV by erythema-inducing capacity in human skin.

Objective Measurement of UVR

Measurement of UVR is characterized by satellite, ground-level meters, self-reported outdoor behavior, or some combination thereof. Satellite measurements calculate *potential* exposure of individuals at specific latitude, longitude, and altitude and do not take into account a particular individual's characteristics, such as pigmentation, or exposure behavior. Ground-level meters include such devices as the Robertson-Berger meter and Dobson ozone column meters as well as a variety of other spectral meters, none of which have been globally calibrated. The Robertson-Berger meters have been placed at ground level at various weather stations throughout the world and give readings for the erythemal action spectrum. Unfortunately, these are not often calibrated and so the accuracy of these readings is somewhat suspect. Currently, there is no international network of ground-level measurement for UV and so it is somewhat difficult to compare UV between hemispheres.

Several algorithms using satellite measures (TOMS, or total ozone mapping spectrometer) have been developed and are generally considered more accurate than the Robertson-Berger meter readings. Satellite measures and mathematical algorithms have advantages in that they can take into account variations in the Earth-Sun distance, cloud cover, ozone column, and surface elevation. Each "objective measure" of UVR has limitations, and the most severe limitation applies to all. All measures evaluate potential exposure to the individual as if a person is lying flat on the ground for all daylight hours. Actual exposure is based on individual behavior.

Self-Reported Outdoor Activities as a Proxy for UVR Exposure

As the potential exposures cannot capture individual behavior, UVR measurement should take into account the idiosyncrasy of individuals. Generally, UV activities are reported as "chronic" for people who are outdoors because of occupational activities or "intermittent" for those who tend to remain indoors through most weekdays and spend time outdoors sporadically on weekends or during holidays.

Combination of Satellite Measures and Self-Reported Outdoor Activities

Perhaps the most rigorous estimation of individual level UVR exposure has been published by Kricker et al. (1), where a number of types of exposures are presented in relation to the risk of melanoma, including potential lifetime and early life ambient erythemal UV exposure, estimated using a combination of a satellite-based model, lifetime residential history, and history of sunburns, holiday hours in sunnier climates, and hours in outdoor beach and waterside recreational activities. Less rigorous algorithms often use latitude of current residence as a proxy for ambient UVR exposure combined with beach activities, or another similar combination.

THE EFFECTS OF UV-A AND UV-B IN MELANOMA INDUCTION

Most research on the effects of specific wavelengths of UV and melanoma has focused on the role of UV-B. UV-B has important deleterious effects directly on DNA—by creating cyclobutane pyrimidine dimers that alter the conformation of the DNA. However, in relation to melanoma development, it may be that UV-A exposure is more important (2). UV-A appears to induce reactive oxygen species (ROS) by means of a melanin redox reaction, so that UV interaction with melanin leads ROS to damage DNA. Specific mutations have often been associated with both UV-B (C→T transitions) and UV-A exposure (G→T transversions) (3); it is of interest that the common induced BRAF V600E mutation is not a UV-B mutation, although Thomas et al. (4) have posited a mechanism by which UV-B could actually lead to that specific mutation.

MEASUREMENT OF HUMAN EXPOSURE

The association of UV and melanoma is based on epidemiologic studies that infer "doses" of UV from objective measurements, such as satellite and ground level meters, and from recalled behavior from individuals. Sunlight exposure depends on multiple variables—length of time outdoors, type of dose (intermittent or continuous), time of year, time of day, amount of cloud cover, individual skin type, clothing, and other protection, and thus it is difficult to calculate in vivo.

Type of Exposure—Intermittent or Continuous

While there is no standard measure, sun exposure can be generally classified as intermittent or chronic, and the effects may be considered as acute or cumulative. Intermittent sun exposure is that obtained sporadically, usually during recreational activities and particularly by indoor workers who have only weekends or vacations to be outdoors and whose skin has not adapted to the sun. Chronic sun exposure is incurred by consistent sun exposure, usually by outdoor work, but also among those people who are outdoors a great deal. Acute sun exposure is that obtained over a short time period on skin that has not adapted to the sun. Depending on the time of day and the skin type of the individual, acute sun exposure may result in sunburn. Sunburn in epidemiology studies is usually defined as burn with pain and/or blistering for two or more days.

Occupationally associated UV exposure is generally determined by a combination of an individual's self-reported occupation—either as a lifetime

Table 1 Results of Meta-Analyses of Intermittent and Chronic Sun Exposure

Author/s, yr	Intermittent sun exposure, odds ratio, 95% CI	Chronic sun exposure, odds ratio, 95% CI	Comments
Nelemans, 1995	1.6 (1.3–1.9)	0.7 (0.6–0.9)	Lack of standardized measures an issue
Elwood and Jopson, 1997	1.7 (1.5–1.9)	0.9 (0.8–0.9)	Need to understand the mechanisms for the differences in types of exposure
Gandini, 2005	1.6 (1.3–1.9)	0.9 (0.7–1.0)	

Abbreviation: CI, confidence interval.

history or as the occupation engaged in for the longest period. This information is then often converted by an occupational hygienist into an exposure matrix, and a summary variable of exposure is generated. Recreational UVR exposure is also determined from numerous self-reported activities, time outdoors, and combinations thereof.

It is surprising that analytic epidemiologic studies have shown only modest risks at best for the role of sun exposure in the development of melanoma incidence, and three systematic reviews have demonstrated very similar estimates of effect for the role of intermittent sun exposure, an odds ratio of 1.6 to 1.7 (5–7). It is important to note that chronic sun exposure, as in those occupationally exposed to sunlight, is either protective or without increased risk for the development of melanoma, with an odds ratio of 0.70, or shows no increased risk (Table 1). The mechanisms for the difference in risk for melanoma by the type of sun exposure have not been fully elucidated.

Cumulative sun exposure is the additive amount of sun exposure that one receives over a lifetime. Cumulative sun exposure may reflect the additive effects of intermittent sun exposure or chronic sun exposure or both.

As chronic exposure seems to have no effect on increasing risk, one explanation for the rise in melanoma incidence that takes into account the different effects of chronic and intermittent sun exposure, proposed by Gallagher et al. (8), is that as people have replaced outdoor occupations with indoor ones, they have engaged in more intermittent sun exposure. Data from very different settings seem to suggest that intermittent sun exposure is critical to the risk for developing melanoma.

EPIDEMIOLOGIC STUDIES OF UVR AND MELANOMA DEVELOPMENT

Ecologic Studies

An analysis, typical of ecologic studies (9), evaluated all cancer sites in the United States over a 32-state area during 1998–2002 for incidence and 1992–2002 for mortality in relation to daily satellite measures of UV-B with control for cloud conditions, ozone column, and length of day. Such measurements, as stated above, reflect potential exposure. Boscoe and Schymura found a positive association for UV-B levels and the development and mortality from melanoma. This ecologic study attempted to control for confounders using proxy variables for a county and not individuals. Of note, the UV values are estimated for the time of diagnosis or death and do not take into account lifetime exposures. As multiple studies of melanoma have implicated childhood sun exposure as the critical period for UV exposure, the inability to measure lifetime behavior is a serious omission in what is an otherwise highly creative and informative study.

Analytic Studies

Analytic studies, on the other hand, are able to assess exposures for individuals—past, present, potential—and measure covariates that may "confound" associations. Important covariates include skin pigmentation (skin color, nevus phenotype, ability to tan), behavior, and family history. Sometimes individual genetic characteristics are measured as well. Numerous studies evaluating sun exposure as a risk factor for melanoma have been published for over 50 years. Meta-analyses give the most succinct insights. The most recent and thorough meta-analysis of sun exposure and melanoma has been published by Gandini et al. (7), where 57 papers published up to 2002 were analyzed. The major findings complement those of Elwood and Jopson (6) and Nelemans et al. (5) (Table 1).

The importance of the type of sun exposure and, potentially, the age at exposure has been repeatedly shown. Although many studies demonstrate that intense sun exposure among adolescents and young children is an important risk factor (1), there are a number of studies that indicate that sun exposure prior to diagnosis is also important (8,9). Therefore, excessive intermittent sun exposure throughout life is associated with the development of melanoma.

The Role of Tanning Bed Exposures

UVR exposure from suntan parlors and tanning beds has been the subject of intense interest recently. The International Agency for Research on Cancer (10) published an analysis suggesting that the "added" risk of UV exposure from tanning parlors is on the order of 1.75 (95% CI, 1.35–2.26). A number of meta-analyses have also been published and show a similar effect of suntan parlor use on the risk of melanoma. Perhaps the most compelling evidence comes from a very large cohort study conducted in Sweden and Norway (11), which showed that, in addition to sun exposure, "ever use" of a tanning salon more than once a month at a young age (10–40 years) increased melanoma risk 1.6-fold (95% CI, 1.04–2.32).

RISKS AND BENEFITS OF UV EXPOSURE IN RELATION TO MELANOMA

Precision in the estimation of the relationship between solar exposure and melanoma is critical if one is to understand the biology of melanoma and to create effective prevention programs. Melanoma is heterogeneous, and an important feature of melanoma is the differential growth rates (12), with the suggestion by Lemish (13) and Burton and Armstrong (14) that most of the sun-induced melanomas were "indolent" and unlikely to lead to death. Dennis (15), among others, has demonstrated that the increased incidence of melanoma is almost entirely due to an increase in thin lesions, that is, lesions with a Breslow thickness less than 1 mm. Whether there is a "true" increase in melanoma incidence, and how greatly that incidence may have increased, is confounded by heavier detection pressure and modified histopathologic criteria in the wake of medicolegal pressure. Controversy was stimulated by Welch et al. (16) who suggested that the increased rate of biopsy might entirely account for the increased incidence of melanoma. The major critique of this work was that Welch and his colleagues were measuring all skin lesions biopsied and not only those suspected of melanoma. Regardless, they have demonstrated that biopsy rates have increased overall during the same period as the "epidemic" of melanoma has increased.

The idea that sun-induced melanomas could be more indolent than those not associated with increased solar exposure is further supported by papers in the literature showing that individuals with more sun exposure prior to the development of melanoma also had better survival (17–19). Therefore, it is possible that the risk factors invoked for "most" melanomas do not actually address those that are more aggressive, such as the nodular melanomas, and that some find are not associated with increased sun exposure. For example, this class of melanomas accounts for 10% of diagnosed melanomas, but is associated with 50% of all deaths from melanoma in the United States.

Vitamin D in Relation to Benefits and Risks of UV Exposure

In 2005, the Australian and New Zealand Bone and Mineral Society, Osteoporosis Australia, Australasian College of Dermatologists, and the Cancer Council Australia published a position statement indicating that "sun exposure is the cause of around 95% of melanomas in Australia, however, ultraviolet radiation B exposure in small amounts is essential to good health. In Australia, where ultraviolet radiation levels are in the high to extreme range for much of the year, sun protective measures to reduce the incidence of skin cancer must continue as a high public health priority."

There has been controversy about whether sun exposure has benefits and how to differentiate between beneficial effects and harmful effects. Diffey (20) delineates between "adventitious, or low dose" sun exposure, which does not necessarily require protective measures, and "elective, or high dose" which is likely to lead to skin cancer. Thus, he argues for sun protection when sun exposure is at its peak, but allows for regular low levels of sun exposure, that are, it seems, likely to increase DNA repair capacity and serum vitamin D levels.

An important caveat regarding UV exposure and serum vitamin D levels is that there are few data, and those that exist have multiple problems. The relationship of UV exposure to serum vitamin D levels depends on multiple factors: latitude, time of year, amount of skin exposed, pigmentation, sunscreen use, and individual genetic factors. There are natural feedback inhibitory mechanisms to prevent vitamin D overdose from UV. Furthermore, the measurement of serum vitamin D is somewhat variable, depending on the laboratory conducting the analyses. Finally, optimal levels of serum vitamin D have been changing and a clear consensus of "optimal" levels has not yet been established.

In addition to the creation of vitamin D, UV light can be a positive regulator of DNA repair capacity. DNA repair capacity has been shown for many years to be upregulated by exposure to UV light (21–23), both nucleotide excision repair (24) and base excision repair (25). Thus, it could be that Gallagher was more accurate than he may have thought when he suggested that the large increase in melanoma might be due to a decline in outdoor occupations and an increase in indoor ones (with a concomitant increase in leisure time spent *sporadically* under intense sun conditions).

SUMMARY AND CONCLUSION

In sum, UVR has shown a clear and consistent association with melanoma; however, there are multiple issues that make it difficult to determine the precise role of UVR: the accuracy of measurement of UVR, the specific effects of each wavelength and their relationship to the development of melanoma (UV-A, UV-B, or their interaction), and the growth rate of the melanoma—indolent or aggressive—and how that may relate to genetic characteristics of the individual as well as the type and pattern of UVR received. The positive view is that we are close to learning more about these issues and are likely to have more precise answers in the near future.

REFERENCES

1. Kricker A, Armstrong BK, Goumas C, et al. Ambient UV, personal sun exposure and risk of multiple primary melanomas. Cancer Causes Control 2007; 18(3):295–304.
2. Wang SQ, Setlow R, Berwick M, et al. Ultraviolet A and melanoma: a review. J Am Acad Dermatol 2001; 44:837–846.
3. Pfeifer GP, You YH, Besaratinia A. Mutations induced by ultraviolet light. Mutat Res 2005; 571:19–31.
4. Thomas NE, Berwick M, Cordeiro-Stone M. Could BRAF mutations in melanocytic lesions arise from DNA damage induced by ultraviolet radiation? J Invest Dermatol 2006; 126:1693–1696.
5. Nelemans PJ, Rampen FH, Ruiter DJ, et al. An addition to the controversy on sunlight exposure and melanoma risk: a meta-analytical approach. J Clin Epidemiol 1995; 48:1331–1342.

6. Elwood JM, Jopson J. Melanoma and sun exposure: an overview of published studies. Int J Cancer 1997; 73:198–203.
7. Gandini S, Sera F, Cattaruzza MS, et al. Meta-analysis of risk factors for cutaneous melanoma: II. Sun exposure. Eur J Cancer 2005; 41(1):45–60.
8. Gallagher RP, Elwood JM, Yang CP. Is chronic sunlight exposure important in accounting for increases in melanoma incidence? Int J Cancer 1989; 44(5):813–815.
9. Boscoe FP, Schymura MJ. Solar ultraviolet-B exposure and cancer incidence and mortality in the United States, 1993–2002. BMC Cancer 2006; 6:264.
10. International Agency for Research on Cancer Working Group on artificial ultraviolet (UV) light and skin cancer. The association of use of sunbeds with cutaneous malignant melanoma and other skin cancers: a systematic review. Int J Cancer 2007; 120(5):1116–1122.
11. Veierød MB, Weiderpass E, Thörn M, et al. A prospective study of pigmentation, sun exposure, and risk of cutaneous malignant melanoma in women. J Natl Cancer Inst 2003; 94:1530–1538.
12. Liu W, Dowling JP, Murray WK, et al. Rate of growth in melanomas. Arch Dermatol 2006; 142(12):1551–1558.
13. Lemish WM, Heenan PJ, Holman CD, et al. Survival from pre-invasive and invasive malignant melanoma in Western Australia. Cancer 1983; 52:580–585.
14. Burton RC, Armstrong BK. Current melanoma epidemic: a non-metastasizing form of melanoma? World J Surg 1995; 19:330–333.
15. Dennis L. Analysis of the melanoma epidemic, both apparent and real. Arch Dermatol 1999; 135:275–280.
16. Welch HG, Woloshin S, Schwartz LM. Skin biopsy rates and incidence of melanoma: population-based ecological study. BMJ 2005; 331:481–485.
17. Berwick M, Armstrong BK, Ben-Porat L, et al. Sun Exposure and mortality from Melanoma. J Natl Cancer Inst 2005; 97:195–198.
18. Barnhill RL, Fine JA, Roush GC, et al. Predicting five-year outcome for patients with cutaneous melanoma in a population-based study. Cancer 1996; 78:427–432.
19. Heenan PJ, English DR, Holman CD, et al. Survival among patients with clinical stage I cutaneous malignant melanoma diagnosed in Western Australia in 1975/76 and 1980/81. Cancer 1991; 65:2079–2087.
20. Diffey B. A contemporary strategy for sun exposure. Expert Rev Dermatol 2007; 2: 139–142.
21. Bataille V, Bykov VJ, Sasieni P, et al. Photoadaptation to ultraviolet (UV) radiation in vivo: photoproducts in epidermal cells following UVB therapy for psoriasis. Br J Dermatol 2000; 143:77–83.
22. Eller M, Maeda T, Magnini C, et al. Enhancement of DNA repair in human skin cells by thymidine dinucleotides: evidence for a p53-mediated mammalian SOS response. Expert Rev Dermatol 1997; 94:12627–12632.
23. Gilchrest BA, Eller MS, Geller AC, et al. The pathogenesis of melanoma induced by ultraviolet radiation. N Engl J Med 1999; 340(17):1341–1348.
24. Kadekaro AL, Wakamatsu K, Ito S, et al. Cutaneous photoprotection and melanoma susceptibility: reaching beyond melanin content to the frontiers of DNA repair. Front Biosci 2006; 11:2157–2173 (review).
25. Yang S, Misner B, Chiu R, et al. Redox Effector Factor-1, combined with reactive oxygen species, plays an important role in the transformation of JB6 cells. Carcinogenesis 2007; 28:2382–2390.

2

Overview of Molecular Pathways in Melanoma

Leslie A. Fecher

*Abramson Cancer Center of the University of Pennsylvania,
Philadelphia, Pennsylvania, U.S.A.*

INTRODUCTION

In the majority of cases, the accumulation of multiple defects rather than a single aberration leads to carcinogenesis. Thus, the discussion of multiple genetic and molecular entities is germane to understanding and treating melanoma. Evidenced by the data reviewed in this book, melanoma is a heterogeneous disease. Our knowledge of molecular and genetic events relevant to melanoma biology has exploded over the past decade, and as our understanding of basic and subtle differences expands, so does our ability to subclassify melanomas. As has been accomplished in other malignancies, we expect tumor profiles will prognosticate as well as predict response to various treatments. In the long run, it is expected that we will utilize individual molecular and genetic tumor features to choose and combine therapies in a rational fashion. The goal of this chapter is to review current clinicopathologic classification of melanoma as well as to provide a brief overview of pathways deemed relevant or potentially relevant to melanoma biology and their status as therapeutic targets (Fig. 1).

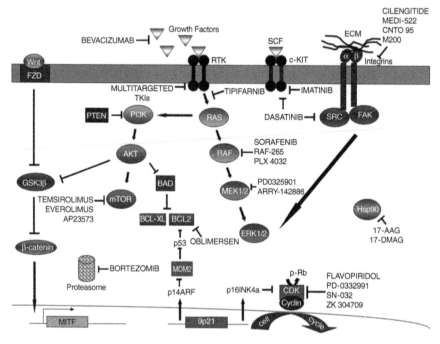

Figure 1 Current pathways relevant to melanoma and associated therapeutic agents. *Source*: Data taken from Ref. 112.

MELANOMA: CLINICOPATHOLOGIC TYPES

Melanocytes are pigment-producing cells of neural crest origin that migrate during embryogenesis and reside predominantly in the basal layer of the epidermis. Melanocytes may proliferate, resulting in a nevus if the melanocytes are benign or in a melanoma if these are malignantly transformed. Histologic assessment of tumor cell morphology is the cornerstone of cancer diagnosis, staging, and therapy. Melanomas are classified according to type and growth pattern of tumor cells in the primary lesion. Melanoma in situ consists of malignant melanocytes that demonstrate a radial growth phase (RGP) without penetrating through the basement membrane, thus confined to the epidermis. Microinvasive RGP melanomas demonstrate malignant cells that penetrate the basement membrane to focally invade the dermis. Dermal involvement with large nests or nodules of malignant melanocytes is characterized as a vertical growth phase (VGP) melanoma. The Clark progression model of melanoma emphasized a stepwise progression from normal melanocyte, to benign nevus, to dysplastic nevus, to RGP melanoma, to VGP melanoma, and to metastatic melanoma (1). The caveat to this model is that not all melanomas develop along the same path.

Most melanomas fall into one of four growth patterns or clinicopathologic subtypes: superficial spreading, lentigo maligna, nodular, or acral lentiginous (2,3). Rarer variants include desmoplastic neurotropic melanomas, nevoid melanomas, and malignant blue nevi. Superficial spreading melanoma is the most common type of melanoma which often occurs in intermittently sun exposed areas (4,5). Second most common are lentigo maligna melanomas, which often occur in chronically sun damaged (CSD) skin in the elderly. Nodular melanomas do not possess a precursor RGP. Acral lentiginous melanomas, localized to the palmar, plantar, and subungual regions, are more common in darker-pigmented individuals. In addition to varied pathologic features and clinical presentation, melanomas in each of these subtypes may display distinct clinical behavior. For example, most lentigo maligna melanomas are thinner and less lethal, while desmoplastic melanomas typically present as thicker lesions and may carry a high incidence of local recurrence (4,5). Melanomas are also categorized according to primary site. Ninety percent of melanomas are cutaneous in origin. Less frequent primary sites include mucosal, uveal, leptomeningeal, and melanoma of soft parts (also known as clear cell sarcoma) characterized by t(12;22) *EWS-ATF-1* translocation (6). Primary site may also portend distinct clinical behavior.

This array of growth patterns, primary sites, and clinical behavior highlights the diversity of this group of cancers. A subclassification system for melanoma that will incorporate distinct types and groups of molecular and genetic changes is gaining momentum in the melanoma community. We are discovering and clarifying varied genetic profiles of melanomas of different primary sites as well as for melanomas stratified according to degree and type of UV exposure (7–11). Several current and future clinical trials are being designed to target certain pathways according to these phenotypic subgroups and incorporate detailed correlative studies. If successful, traditional clinicopathologic subtypes may serve as phenotypic correlates of specific genotypes. Evaluating for correlation between tumor features and clinical endpoints to gauge susceptibility and response to specific therapeutic agents and strategies is difficult but imperative. The scientific community must strive to determine and understand not only the 'target' but also the 'off-target' effects of therapies. In this era of targeting tumor cell signaling and intracellular processes, we must also continue to reevaluate and revise our criteria for tumor responses to include molecular and genetic effects that may be delayed or manifest as stable disease.

PATHWAYS RELEVANT TO MELANOMA

Fearon and Vogelstein clearly demonstrated the relationship between genetic events and neoplastic progression with their colon cancer model (12). In this model, not only the genetic event but the timing of the event is relevant to outcome. In melanoma, several genes and pathways have been identified as aberrant (Fig. 1). Many of these pathways intersect and have overlapping functions, such as proliferation, survival, and angiogenesis. Utilizing the Clark progression model of melanoma (1), the timing of some of the known genetic/molecular events in melanomagenesis has been proposed (13).

Signal Transduction: RAS-RAF-MEK-ERK, PI3K-Akt-mTOR, and c-KIT

A pivotal discovery in the field of melanoma was the documentation of the V600E-activating mutation in the BRAF kinase in a majority of melanomas (14). Subsequently, this same mutation was demonstrated in a majority of benign nevi as well (15). While not sufficient for melanoma initiation, it appears to provide an early and necessary signal for aberrant proliferation. The RAF-MEK-ERK signal transduction pathway, composed of a series of serine-threonine kinases, is activated by RAS. After multiple phosphorylation events, phospho-ERK exerts myriad effects through phosphorylation of factors in the cytoplasm and nucleus of the cell. In addition to *BRAF* mutations, *NRAS* mutations also can lead to constitutive activation of the mitogen-activated protein kinase (MAPK) pathway in melanoma.

The phosphatidylinositol-3-kinase (PI3K)-Akt-mammalian target of rapamycin (mTOR) signaling pathway is involved in proliferation, motility, apoptosis, chemoresistance, and angiogenesis (16,17). Receptor tyrosine kinases (RTKs) or RAS activate PI3K, which converts phosphatidylinositol-4,5-biphosphate (PIP2) to phosphatidylinositol-3,4,5-triphosphate (PIP3) through a phosphorylation event and in turn activates Akt. Akt exerts primarily prosurvival effects through phosphorylation of mTOR, MDM2, human telomerase reverse transcriptase (hTERT), and other factors (16). Through dephosphorylation of PIP3, PTEN (phosphatase and tensin homolog deleted on chromosome 10) negatively regulates the PI3K pathway (16). As both a lipid and protein phosphatase, PTEN exerts a tumor-suppressive effect on other molecular pathways, affecting proliferation, migration, and apoptosis (18). Mutations of *PI3K* are rare in melanoma (19,20). However, loss of chromosome 10 (including *PTEN*) or mutation/deletion/silencing of *PTEN* is seen (18,21–23), as is Akt overexpression (24).

As opposed to the Clark progression model, Curtin and colleagues have proposed a subclassification system for melanoma on the basis of body site and type of UV exposure, consisting of four distinct groups: CSD (with solar elastosis histologically), non-CSD, mucosal, and acral melanomas (10). Utilizing comparative genomic hybridization and sequencing, Curtin et al. evaluated the incidence of copy number changes and mutations in *BRAF, NRAS, PTEN, CDK4,* and *cyclin D1,* as well as *c-KIT* in a subsequent publication, in these subsets (11). They detected isolated genetic changes, as well as groups of changes, and subsequently were able to predict melanoma subset according to specific abnormalities with high accuracy. Several overlying themes were demonstrated, most corroborated by other scientists. *BRAF* mutations are most prominent in melanomas from intermittently sun-exposed sites (non-CSD) and least common in CSD and noncutaneous melanomas (8,9,25–27). *NRAS* mutations are found across subtypes, but at a fairly constant rate (9). *PTEN* loss often accompanies *BRAF* mutations, but not *NRAS* mutations (28,29). Amplification of *CDK4* or *cyclin D1* is found in melanomas that do not demonstrate MAPK mutations (*BRAF* or *NRAS*). Alterations of the Rb pathway, namely *p16* deletions and *CDK4* amplifications, were more common in mucosal and acral melanomas, which rarely demonstrated MAPK alterations. *c-KIT* aberrations (including amplifications and mutations), while not seen in non-CSD melanomas, were found in 28% of CSD, 36% of acral, and 39% of mucosal melanomas (20). This research highlights the interplay of these pathways and probable success of combinatorial therapeutic strategies to avoid targeting nondominant or irrelevant pathways and prevent compensatory changes that may result in tumor escape.

Therapeutic Relevance

The RAS-RAF-MEK-ERK pathway and its therapeutic targeting are explored in depth in another chapter. Briefly, impairment of MAPK signaling is one of many focal points in melanoma research where most attention has been focused on RAS and BRAF. Sorafenib (BAY 43-9006, Nexavar; Bayer, West Haven, Connecticut and Onyx, Richmond, California, U.S.), a multityrosine kinase inhibitor, has shown single-agent efficacy in renal cell and hepatocellular carcinomas, but not in melanoma (30–32). Currently, it is being assessed in combination with other cytotoxic and molecular agents in melanoma. Additionally, more specific and potent BRAF kinase inhibitors as well as MEK inhibitors are under evaluation in clinical trials (33–35) (Fig. 1). These agents may prove more successful in inhibiting the MAPK pathway. However, isolated inhibition of MAPK signaling in melanoma may be insufficient to translate into a clinical benefit.

mTOR inhibitors, such as temsirolimus (CCI-779; Wyeth-Ayerst, Madison, New Jersey, U.S.), everolimus (RAD-001, Novartis Pharmaceuticals, Basel, Switzerland), and AP-23573 (Ariad, Cambridge, Massachusetts, U.S.), are under evaluation in melanoma given the evidence of PI3K pathway activation as well as possible synergistic activity with other therapeutic agents (36,37). In a phase II study in metastatic melanoma, 33 patients were treated with weekly temsirolimus, which resulted in a median time-to-disease progression of 10 weeks and an overall survival of five months (38). The only objective response was one partial response lasting for two months, with stomatitis, rash, and hyperlipidemia as the predominant toxicities. Current ongoing phase II studies in unresectable advanced melanoma combine temsirolimus with sorafenib, bevacizumab (Avastin, Genentech, South San Francisco, California, U.S.) or with bortezomib (Velcade, Millenium Pharmaceuticals Inc., Cambridge, Massachusetts, U.S.). Another phase II study in advanced unresectable melanoma randomizes patients to sorafenib in combination with either temosirolimus or tipifarnib (R115777, Zarnestra, Johnson & Johnson, New Brunswick, New Jersey, U.S.), a farnesyltransferase inhibitor. A two-stage phase II trial of the oral mTOR inhibitor, everolimus, in unresectable stage IV melanoma showed an improvement in progression free survival on interim analysis and good tolerability. However, accrual to the second stage was suspended when the

PFS target was not met and increased toxicity was seen at the higher dose level (39). Other methods of inhibiting signaling pathways include targeting RTKs and growth factors. Anti-angiogenesis agents such as bevacizumab and multitargeted kinase inhibitors are of interest and relevance, but beyond the scope of this chapter.

Previously postulated to be lost with transformation to melanoma because of widely variable expression (40), *c-KIT* encodes an RTK essential for normal melanocyte development and survival (41). The identification of *c-KIT* aberrations in certain melanomas was reinvigorating to the melanoma community for many reasons (11). One, this provided a clear and plausible role for c-KIT in melanoma biology, which has long been an area of uncertainty. Next, it highlighted an abnormality that already possessed a means of successful therapeutic targeting, imatinib (Gleevec, Novartis). Finally, it supported the concept of phenotypic and genotypic correlations in melanoma that may guide future therapeutic choices. Previously, imatinib had been explored in melanoma with disappointing results (42–44). However, in light of recent research, the one near-complete response in a patient with metastatic acral melanoma becomes more significant (42). There are several ongoing studies of imatinib in melanoma as a single agent as well as in combination with bevacizumab or temozolomide (Temodar, Schering-Plough, Kenilworth, New Jersey, U.S.) (45) that select for these melanoma subsets and involve various correlative studies. While all of the melanomas with increased copy number or mutation showed increased c-KIT protein expression (11), it remains to be seen if c-KIT overexpression or mutational status will be predictive factors in melanoma and if attention should be given to uveal melanomas as well (46,47).

Agents interesting for their potential impact on multiple pathways include histone deacetylase (HDAC) and DNA methyltransferase inhibitors, heat shock protein-90 (Hsp90) inhibitors, and bortezomib, as well as others. Epigenetic events are increasingly evident in cancer biology and progression. These modifications, which include methylation and acetylation, impact gene transcription. Both forms of epigenetic silencing of a variety of genes have been documented in melanoma (48). DNA methyltransferase inhibitors, such as 5-azacitadine (Vidaza, Pharmion Corp., Boulder, Colorado, U.S.) and 5-aza-2′-deoxycytidine (decitabine, Dacogen, MGI Pharma, Bloomington, Minnesota, U.S.), have shown benefit in myelodysplastic syndromes (49,50). In metastatic melanoma and renal cell carcinoma, decitabine was evaluated in combination with standard high-dose bolus interleukin-2 (HD IL-2) in a dose-escalation phase I trial that treated 21 patients (51). The dose was escalated from 0.1 to 0.25 mg/kg, with prolonged grade 4 neutropenia as the only dose-limiting toxicity. Thirty-one percent of melanoma patients showed an objective response, and addition of decitabine did not impact HD IL-2 tolerability. The number of HDAC inhibitors, and trials investigating them, is greater than for methyltransferase inhibitors. Within melanoma, SAHA (vorinostat, Zolinza, Merck & Co. Inc., Whitehouse Station, New Jersey, U.S.) and MS-275 have progressed furthest in clinical investigation. There is an ongoing phase II study of SAHA in advanced unresectable melanoma evaluating response to treatment, time to progression, as well as gene expression profiles posttreatment as potential predictive factors. An industry-sponsored phase II study in Europe to evaluate efficacy and toxicity of 3-mg biweekly versus 7-mg weekly dosage of MS-275 in advanced unresectable melanoma recently completed accrual (52). In 28 treated patients, there were no objective responses, but stable disease was seen in 29% and 21% of patients on the two respective dosage arms, lasting from 8 to 48 weeks. Common toxicities included diarrhea, nausea, and hypophosphatemia.

Inhibition of Hsp90 via 17-allylamino-17-demethoxygeldanamycin (17-AAG) or 17-dimethylaminoethylamino-17-demethoxy-geldanamycin (17-DMAG) occurs through degradation of Hsp90-chaperoned proteins. Chaperoned proteins include but are not limited to RAF, Akt, VEGF, HIF-1, CDK4, survivin, hTERT, Met, and MMP2 (53). Hsp90 inhibition is interesting for melanoma, not only for the potential impact on multiple pathways but also for the possible selectivity for V600E BRAF. Serial tumor biopsies of melanoma patients pre- and posttreatment with 17-AAG showed downregulation of the MAPK pathway as evidenced by decreased phospho-ERK expression that was not accompanied by decreased wild-type BRAF expression (54), corroborating preclinical findings (55). Several phase I trials of 17-AAG in combination with other therapies are open, and a phase II trial of single agent 17-AAG recently completed accrual.

Bortezomib directly binds the proteasome, inhibiting ubiquitin-mediated proteolysis. One of the effects of bortezomib treatment is NF-κB inhibition, a possible factor in melanoma invasion (56). Among other roles, bortezomib is believed to enhance susceptibility to chemotherapy- and radiotherapy-induced apoptosis. It is under evaluation in unresectable advanced melanoma in combination with temozolomide or with carboplatin and paclitaxel. The lack of activity of single agent bortezomib in metastatic melanoma (57) may be explained by compensatory accumulation of antiapoptotic factors such as Bcl-x(L) and Mcl-1 (58). Gossypol, a BH3 mimetic, inhibits these antiapoptotic proteins, as well as others, and showed antimelanoma activity in vivo and in vitro in combination with bortezomib. Interestingly, this combinatorial therapy did not increase normal melanocyte death in vitro.

Cell Adhesion: Src/Integrins/Focal Adhesion Kinase and Wnt/β-catenin

Src, the first known proto-oncogene, encodes a nonreceptor membrane tyrosine kinase involved in cellular proliferation, adhesion, migration, and invasion (59). It impacts cellular adhesion and motility through interaction with RTKs, such as epidermal growth factor receptor (EGFR), or with transmembrane integrin receptors and focal adhesion kinase (FAK) (Fig. 1). In cancers, upregulation of *Src* is often seen (59), as is increased FAK expression/activity (60), and altered expression of integrins (61). Src affects multiple downstream targets including cadherins, vascular endothelial growth factor (VEGF), matrix metalloproteinases (MMPs), signal transducer and activator of transcription 3 (STAT3) and STAT5, PTEN, and KIT (62). In melanoma, phospho-Src expression was seen in 61% of cutaneous primaries, 31% of mucosal primaries, and 55% of metastases (63). In vitro, Src inhibitors (dasatinib, SKI-606, and PD180970) inhibited proliferation of melanoma cell lines and were synergistic with cisplatin and topoisomerase I inhibitors, but not with temozolomide (63).

Integrins link the extracellular matrix and the intracellular environment. Involved in adhesion, cytoskeletal structure, and signaling, each integrin consists of α and β subunits that span the cell membrane (64). Different α and β combinations connote distinct ligand binding and functions. In melanoma, $\alpha_v\beta_3$ integrin expression is associated with melanoma progression from RGP to VGP and invasion (65,66), while $\alpha_5\beta_1$ integrin has been associated with angiogenesis and invasion (64). These integrin pathways also regulate cell survival through modulation of bcl-2 expression (67,68).

The Wnt/β-catenin canonical signal transduction pathway regulates gene transcription impacting many cellular processes during development including differentiation, proliferation, and motility (69,70). Extracellular Wnt proteins bind the Frizzled (Fzd) family of G-protein-coupled receptors, inactivating glycogen synthase kinase 3β (GSK-3β) and allowing free β-catenin to accumulate. Accumulated β-catenin then is able to translocate to the nucleus where it interacts with various proteins, including Tcf/Lef-1, to activate transcription. Target genes include *cyclin D1*, *c-myc*, and *MITF*. β-catenin also influences cell-cell adhesion through association with E-cadherin, linking it to the cytoskeleton (70). When Wnt is unbound, any free (non-cadherin bound) β-catenin forms a multiprotein complex, which includes adenomatous polyposis coli (APC), GSK-3β, and axin, marking it for ubiquitinated proteasomal degradation. Aberrant activation of the Wnt/β-catenin pathway is present in approximately 30% of human melanomas, evidenced by elevated β-catenin levels (71). The etiology of this is still under investigation, but epigenetic silencing of *APC* appears to play a role as mutations in *β-catenin* or *APC* are rare (71,72). A recent publication linked the Wnt/β-catenin and MAPK pathways in melanoma initiation by demonstrating spontaneous melanomas in transgenic mice carrying both activated β-catenin and *NRAS* mutation (73). Also of interest in melanoma is Wnt-5a, which not only signals via the Wnt/Ca^{2+} pathway but also can affect β-catenin degradation (74). Wnt5a expression correlates with melanoma invasion and metastasis in vitro and in vivo (75,76).

Therapeutic Relevance

Recently, the Food and Drug Administration (FDA) granted approval for dasatinib (BMS-354825 or Sprycel, Bristol-Myers Squibb Co., Princeton, New Jersey, U.S.A.), a small-molecule multi-targeted kinase inhibitor that inhibits c-KIT, PDGFR, and Src in addition to Bcr-Abl and others, treatment-resistant or treatment-intolerant chronic myelogenous leukemia (CML) (77). Currently, a phase II study of dasatinib in unresectable advanced melanoma is open and another phase II study in unresectable advanced melanoma with mucosal, acral, or CSD primaries is planned and will be conducted under the auspices of the Eastern Cooperative Oncology Group.

Monoclonal antibodies and peptide inhibitors against various integrins are in clinical trials for melanoma and other malignancies. Eight-week progression free survival (PFS) in advanced unresectable melanoma was evaluated in a randomized phase II study of 500-mg versus 2000-mg intravenous dosing of cilengitide (EMD121974, Merck &Co. Inc., Whitehouse Station, New Jersey, U.S.), a peptide selective inhibitor of α_v integrins (78). Of the 26 patients treated, three were progression free at eight weeks. Mainly grade 1 and 2 toxicities were seen including fatigue, lymphopenia, and peripheral neuropathy. Of interest, all patients had pretreatment tumor biopsies to assess $\alpha_v\beta_3$ expression; assessments of $\alpha_v\beta_3$ expression in optional day 8 posttreatment tumor biopsies are pending. A randomized phase II trial of Medi-522 (Vitaxin, MedImmune, Gaithersburg, Maryland, U.S.), a human monoclonal antibody against $\alpha_v\beta_3$, alone or in combination with dacarbazine (DTIC) in advanced unresectable melanoma enrolled and treated 112 patients, 57 with Medi-522 alone and 55 with Medi-522 and DTIC (79). Trial results showed an overall response rate of 0% and median PFS of 1.4 months for Medi-522 alone and an overall response rate of 13% and median PFS of 2.6 months for the combination arm. While most adverse events were grade 1/2, there was one treatment-related death (myocardial infarction and pulmonary embolus) in each arm. A phase I study of Medi-522 in advanced unresectable melanoma requiring tumor biopsies to evaluate tumor tissue saturation is active. CNTO95 (Centocor, Horsham, Pennsylvania, U.S.), a fully human monoclonal antibody against the α_v integrins, is under investigation alone and in combination with DTIC in a randomized phase I/II study in advanced unresectable melanoma given antitumor activity in melanoma xenografts (80). Lastly, a pilot phase II study of M200 (volociximab, PDL BioPharma, Redwood City, California, U.S.), a chimeric monoclonal antibody directed against $\alpha_5\beta_1$, in combination with DTIC in advanced unresectable melanoma has been completed. Nausea, constipation, and vomiting were common adverse events for M200; however, two serious adverse events of hypertension and deep vein thrombosis were possibly related to M200 (81). Of the 30 patients evaluable for response, 16 demonstrated stable disease and 14 had progressive disease.

At this time, specific inhibitors of the Wnt-signaling pathways are still in preclinical development. The only available means of targeting the Wnt/β-catenin pathway is via nonsteroidal anti-inflammatory drugs that can influence β-catenin expression, localization, interactions, and degradation (82).

Miscellaneous Pathways

Microphthalmia-Associated Transcription Factor

Microphthalmia-associated transcription factor (MITF) is essential for melanocyte development and melanin production (83). Various signaling pathways and transcription factors exert control over MITF gene and protein expression, including c-KIT-MAPK, Wnt/β-catenin, α-MSH-MC1R, PAX3, and SOX10 (83). On the basis of evidence of amplification in primary and metastatic melanomas as well as the ability to transform melanocytes in conjunction with V600E *BRAF*, *MITF* is proposed as a melanoma oncogene (84). Additionally, increased *MITF* copy number in cell lines appeared to correlate with resistance to cytotoxic chemotherapy. The data regarding MITF and its role in melanocyte and melanoma biology will be examined in a subsequent chapter. At this time, therapeutic interference with the MITF pathway is not possible.

Telomerase

Over the life span of a normal cell, the tandem repeat sequences that cap and protect the ends of chromosomes, known as telomeres, shorten and ultimately result in replicative senescence and apoptosis (85). Telomerase, an enzyme comprised of hTERT and hTR components, maintains telomere length, thereby preventing cell senescence and death. Its expression is rare in normal somatic cells, but has been documented in germ cells, hematopoetic stem cells, as well as in many malignancies, including melanoma (86,87). Germline mutations of *hTERT* and *hTR* are associated with dyskeratosis congenita, idiopathic pulmonary fibrosis, and aplastic anemia (88–90). The original telomerase hypothesis stated that it was present in germ/stem cells, inactivated in somatic cells, and reactivated late in carcinogenesis (91). Given the stem cell theory of cancer, an alternate hypothesis that telomerase is present from the beginning of carcinogenesis within tumor stem cells and its expression increases with tumor progression has been proposed (92). Because of widespread expression in malignancies, telomerase and its components are of interest as therapeutic targets. Thus far, utilization of hTERT as a tumor antigen in a variety of cancer vaccines and tumor models has been shown to safely induce hTERT-specific immunity (93).

The Cell Cycle: p16^{INK4a}-Retinoblastoma and p53

Thus far, we have concentrated on somatic mutations associated with melanoma. However, the best-characterized genetic abnormality in human melanoma is germline mutation of *p16^{INK4a}* (also known as *CDKN2A* and located on chromosome 9p21). Mutations are rare in sporadic melanoma but are present in 20% to 40% of familial melanoma with a variable penetrance (94,95). p16^{INK4a} and p14^{ARF}, two distinct tumor suppressor proteins, are both encoded on the 9p21 locus and produced by alternative splicing (Fig. 1). Both proteins independently regulate cell cycle progression via the retinoblastoma (Rb) and p53 pathways, respectively. Germline mutations of *p14^{ARF}* and *CDK4* have also been documented in familial melanomas, but are quite rare (96,97).

The Rb and p53 pathways regulate cell cycle progression, but through very different means. Rb controls entrance into S phase, where p16^{INK4a} functions as a cyclin-dependent kinase (CDK) inhibitor; p53 is a transcription factor that can induce expression of genes that prevent cell cycling under conditions of cellular stress (98). Mutations and deletions of $p16^{INK4a}$ have been described in various cancers, in particular melanoma (99), while mutations of *p53* are rare in melanoma (100) but present in most other human cancers. To effect cell cycle progression from G1 to S phase, Rb is inactivated through CDK phosphorylation, resulting in E2F release and activation, followed by DNA replication (98). Under normal circumstances, p16^{INK4a} inhibits cyclin D/CDK4 phosphylation of Rb, causing G1 arrest. In melanomas with mutation or deletion of $p16^{INK4a}$, this negative regulatory control is lost and cell cycle progression is allowed (98,99). Inactivation of the Rb pathway through alternative mechanisms including epigenetic silencing or decreased expression of $p16^{INK4a}$ or *Rb,* or through overexpression or amplification of *CDK4* and/or *CDK6* or *cyclin D1,* may be more relevant to a broader group of melanomas (10,101).

p53 is a transcription factor activated in response to DNA damage. As the "guardian of the genome," it halts cell cycle progression in order to accelerate DNA repair if possible, or to facilitate apoptosis if the damage is irreparable (98). MDM2 negatively regulates p53 by binding and marking it for ubiquitin-mediated proteasomal degradation, while p14^{ARF} is a positive regulator of p53 that binds MDM2 and prevents its interaction with p53. Aside from *p53* mutations, altered expression of *p53* and *MDM2* overexpression has been documented in melanoma (101,102).

Therapeutic Relevance

While unable to therapeutically replace deleted tumor-suppressor proteins, there are other ways of mechanistically repairing and/or restoring cell cycle regulation. Varied drugs that function as CDK inhibitors are being investigated and include older agents, such as flavopiridol (alvocidib, Aventis Pharmaceuticals, Inc., Bridgewater, New Jersey, U.S.), as well as newer selective inhibitors that target one or several CDKs (103,104). The therapeutic goal of CDK inhibitors is to effect cell cycle arrest in lieu of aberrant regulatory controls, facilitating apoptotic tumor cell death (103). In metastatic melanoma, flavopiridol, a pan-CDK inhibitor, demonstrated stable disease in 7 of 16 patients treated but no objective responses (105). Novel small-molecule inhibitors, all under phase I investigation, include: PD-0332991 (Pfizer) which inhibits CDK 4/6 (106), SNS-032 (BMS-387032, Sunesis, South San Francisco, California, U.S.) which inhibits CDK 2/7/9, and ZK 304709 (Schering AG, Berlin, Germany) which inhibits CDK 1/2/4/7/9 as well as VEGFR 1/2/3 and PDGFR-β (107,108). Therapeutic agents aimed at epigenetic alterations as well as at the proteasome may be relevant in tumors with aberrant cell cycle controls.

APAF-1, a proapoptotic factor downstream of p53, interacts with cytochrome c and procaspase-9 to induce apoptosis via the effector caspase pathway. Inactivation of *APAF-1* through mutation and methylation has been shown in melanoma (109). Further, the proapoptotic activity of APAF-1, as well as chemo-sensitivity, was restored in melanoma cells by treatment with the DNA methyl-transferase inhibitor, 5-aza-2′-deoxycitadine.

Bcl-2, an inhibitor of apoptosis protein, can modulate cytochrome c release and APAF-1/procaspase-9 interaction and is overexpressed in melanoma (110). Oblimersen sodium (Genasense, Genta Inc., Berkeley Heights, New Jersey, U.S.) is an antisense oligonucleotide designed to block such inhibition, enhancing cytotoxic antitumor effects. Unfortunately, only small improvements in response rate, complete response, and PFS were seen when DTIC in combination with oblimersen was compared with single agent DTIC in a randomized phase III study in advanced unresectable melanoma (111). On subset analysis, there was a survival benefit in patients with normal serum lactate dehydrogenase (LDH). Thus, a phase 3 randomized double-blind, placebo controlled trial of oblimersen plus dacarbazine versus dacarbazine alone in advanced melanoma (AGENDA) was designed for patients with normal LDH.

CONCLUSIONS

This is an exciting time in the field of melanoma. As illustrated above, carcinogenesis is a multistep process that requires multiple therapeutic steps. Clearly, there are several relevant and therapeutically interesting pathways that interact in melanoma initiation and progression. Ultimately, therapeutic success will likely involve defining and targeting such pathways with combinatorial strategies on an individual level. Continued collaboration between scientists and physician scientists is imperative to rationally design in vitro and in vivo investigation that informs and guides clinical investigation and therapeutic studies. As we continue to gather information to better understand and classify melanoma, our therapeutic options and strategies will evolve.

REFERENCES

1. Clark WH Jr., Elder DE, Guerry D IV, et al. A study of tumor progression: the precursor lesions of superficial spreading and nodular melanoma. Hum Pathol 1984; 15:1147–1165.
2. Clark WH Jr., From L, Bernardino EA, et al. The histogenesis and biologic behavior of primary human malignant melanomas of the skin. Cancer Res 1969; 29:705–727.
3. Arrington JH III, Reed RJ, Ichinose H, et al. Plantar lentiginous melanoma: a distinctive variant of human cutaneous malignant melanoma. Am J Surg Pathol 1977; 1:131–143.
4. Gershenwald JE, Balch CM, Soong SJ, et al. Prognostic factors and natural history. In: Balch CM, Houghton A, Sober A, et al., eds. Cutaneous Melanoma, 4th ed. St. Louis: Quality Medical Publishing, Inc., 2003:25–54.
5. Crowson AN, Magro CM, Barnhill RL, et al. Pathology. In: Balch CM, Houghton A, Sober A, et al., eds. Cutaneous Melanoma, 4th ed. St. Louis: Quality Medical Publishing, Inc., 2003:171–208.

6. Reeves BR, Fletcher CD, Gusterson BA. Translocation t(12;22)(q13;q13) is a nonrandom rearrangement in clear cell sarcoma. Cancer Genet Cytogenet 1992; 64:101–103.
7. Parrella P, Sidransky D, Merbs SL. Allelotype of posterior uveal melanoma: implications for a bifurcated tumor progression pathway. Cancer Res 1999; 59: 3032–3037.
8. Cohen Y, Rosenbaum E, Begum S, et al. Exon 15 BRAF mutations are uncommon in melanomas arising in nonsun-exposed sites. Clin Cancer Res 2004; 10: 3444–3447.
9. Wong CW, Fan YS, Chan TL, et al. BRAF and NRAS mutations are uncommon in melanomas arising in diverse internal organs. J Clin Pathol 2005; 58:640–644.
10. Curtin JA, Fridlyand J, Kageshita T, et al. Distinct sets of genetic alterations in melanoma. N Engl J Med 2005; 353:2135–2147.
11. Curtin JA, Busam K, Pinkel D, et al. Somatic activation of KIT in distinct subtypes of melanoma. J Clin Oncol 2006; 24:4340–4346.
12. Fearon ER, Vogelstein B. A genetic model for colorectal tumorigenesis. Cell 1990; 61:759–767.
13. Miller AJ, Mihm MC Jr. Melanoma. N Engl J Med 2006; 355:51–65.
14. Davies H, Bignell GR, Cox C, et al. Mutations of the BRAF gene in human cancer. Nature 2002; 417:949–954.
15. Pollock PM, Harper UL, Hansen KS, et al. High frequency of BRAF mutations in nevi. Nat Genet 2003; 33:19–20.
16. Cully M, You H, Levine AJ, et al. Beyond PTEN mutations: the PI3K pathway as an integrator of multiple inputs during tumorigenesis. Nat Rev Cancer 2006; 6:184–192.
17. Jiang BH, Liu LZ. PI3K/PTEN signaling in tumorigenesis and angiogenesis. Biochim Biophys Acta 2008; 1784(1):150–158.
18. Wu H, Goel V, Haluska FG. PTEN signaling pathways in melanoma. Oncogene 2003; 22:3113–3122.
19. Omholt K, Krockel D, Ringborg U, et al. Mutations of PIK3CA are rare in cutaneous melanoma. Melanoma Res 2006; 16:197–200.
20. Curtin JA, Stark MS, Pinkel D, et al. PI3-kinase subunits are infrequent somatic targets in melanoma. J Invest Dermatol 2006; 126:1660–1663.
21. Tsao H, Zhang X, Benoit E, et al. Identification of PTEN/MMAC1 alterations in uncultured melanomas and melanoma cell lines. Oncogene 1998; 16:3397–3402.
22. Zhou XP, Gimm O, Hampel H, et al. Epigenetic PTEN silencing in malignant melanomas without PTEN mutation. Am J Pathol 2000; 157:1123–1128.
23. Mirmohammadsadegh A, Marini A, Nambiar S, et al. Epigenetic silencing of the PTEN gene in melanoma. Cancer Res 2006; 66:6546–6552.
24. Stahl JM, Sharma A, Cheung M, et al. Deregulated Akt3 activity promotes development of malignant melanoma. Cancer Res 2004; 64:7002–7010.
25. Maldonado JL, Fridlyand J, Patel H, et al. Determinants of BRAF mutations in primary melanomas. J Natl Cancer Inst 2003; 95:1878–1890.
26. Edwards RH, Ward MR, Wu H, et al. Absence of BRAF mutations in UV-protected mucosal melanomas. J Med Genet 2004; 41:270–2.
27. Deichmann M, Krahl D, Thome M, et al. The oncogenic B-raf V599E mutation occurs more frequently in melanomas at sun-protected body sites. Int J Oncol 2006; 29:139–145.
28. Tsao H, Goel V, Wu H, et al. Genetic interaction between NRAS and BRAF mutations and PTEN/MMAC1 inactivation in melanoma. J Invest Dermatol 2004; 122:337–341.

29. Goel VK, Lazar AJ, Warneke CL, et al. Examination of mutations in BRAF, NRAS, and PTEN in primary cutaneous melanoma. J Invest Dermatol 2006; 126:154–160.
30. Escudier B, Eisen T, Stadler WM, et al. Sorafenib in advanced clear-cell renal-cell carcinoma. N Engl J Med 2007; 356:125–134.
31. Llovet J, Ricci S, Mazzaferro V, et al. Sorafenib improves survival in advanced hepatocellular carcinoma (HCC): results of a phase III randomized placebo-controlled trial (SHARP trial). J Clin Oncol 2007; 25 (supplement 18S):1s (abstr LBA1).
32. Eisen T, Ahmad T, Flaherty KT, et al. Sorafenib in advanced melanoma: a phase II randomised discontinuation trial analysis. Br J Cancer 2006; 95:581–586.
33. Amiri P, Aikawa ME, Dove J, et al. CHIR-265 is a potent selective inhibitor of c-Raf/ B-Raf/$_{mut}$B-Raf that effectively inhibits proliferation and survival of cancer cell lines with Ras/Raf pathway mutations. Proc Amer Assoc Cancer Res 2006; 47 (abstr 4855).
34. Tsai J, Zhang J, Bremer R, et al. Development of a novel inhibitor of oncogenic b-raf. Proc Amer Assoc Cancer Res 2006; 47 (abstr 2412).
35. Yeh TC, Marsh V, Bernat BA, et al. Biological characterization of ARRY-142886 (AZD6244), a potent, highly selective mitogen-activated protein kinase kinase 1/2 inhibitor. Clin Cancer Res 2007; 13:1576–1583.
36. Molhoek KR, Brautigan DL, Slingluff CL Jr. Synergistic inhibition of human melanoma proliferation by combination treatment with B-Raf inhibitor BAY43-9006 and mTOR inhibitor Rapamycin. J Transl Med 2005; 3:39.
37. Meier F, Busch S, Lasithiotakis K, et al. Combined targeting of MAPK and AKT signaling pathways is a promising strategy for melanoma treatment. Br J Dermatol 2007; 156:1204–1213.
38. Margolin K, Longmate J, Baratta T, et al. CCI-779 in metastatic melanoma: a phase II trial of the California Cancer Consortium. Cancer 2005; 104:1045–1048.
39. Rao RD, Allred JB, Windschitl HE, et al. N0377: Results of NCCTG phase II trial of the mTOR inhibitor RAD-001 in metastatic melanoma. J Clin Oncol 2007; 25 (supplement 18S):479s (abstr 8530).
40. Montone KT, van Belle P, Elenitsas R, et al. Proto-oncogene c-kit expression in malignant melanoma: protein loss with tumor progression. Mod Pathol 1997; 10:939–944.
41. Grichnik JM. Kit and melanocyte migration. J Invest Dermatol 2006; 126:945–947.
42. Eton O, Billings L, Kim K, et al. Phase II trial of imatinib mesylate (STI-571) in metastatic melanoma (MM). J Clin Oncol 2004; 22 (supplement 14S):717s (abstr 7528).
43. Wyman K, Atkins MB, Prieto V, et al. Multicenter phase II trial of high-dose imatinib mesylate in metastatic melanoma: significant toxicity with no clinical efficacy. Cancer 2006; 106:2005–2011.
44. Ugurel S, Hildenbrand R, Zimpfer A, et al. Lack of clinical efficacy of imatinib in metastatic melanoma. Br J Cancer 2005; 92:1398–1405.
45. Schuchter LM, Flaherty KT, Davidson R, et al. Phase I trial of imatinib and temozolomide in patients with metastatic melanoma. J Clin Oncol 2004; 22 (supplement 14S):728s (abstr 7572).
46. Pache M, Glatz K, Bosch D, et al. Sequence analysis and high-throughput immunohistochemical profiling of KIT (CD 117) expression in uveal melanoma using tissue microarrays. Virchows Arch 2003; 443:741–744.
47. Lefevre G, Glotin AL, Calipel A, et al. Roles of stem cell factor/c-Kit and effects of Glivec/STI571 in human uveal melanoma cell tumorigenesis. J Biol Chem 2004; 279:31769–31779.

48. Rothhammer T, Bosserhoff AK. Epigenetic events in malignant melanoma. Pigment Cell Res 2007; 20:92–111.
49. Silverman LR, Demakos EP, Peterson BL, et al. Randomized controlled trial of azacitidine in patients with the myelodysplastic syndrome: a study of the Cancer and Leukemia Group B. J Clin Oncol 2002; 20:2429–2440.
50. Kantarjian H, Issa JP, Rosenfeld CS, et al. Decitabine improves patient outcomes in myelodysplastic syndromes: results of a phase III randomized study. Cancer 2006; 106:1794–1803.
51. Gollob JA, Sciambi CJ, Peterson BL, et al. Phase I trial of sequential low-dose 5-aza-2'-deoxycytidine plus high-dose intravenous bolus interleukin-2 in patients with melanoma or renal cell carcinoma. Clin Cancer Res 2006; 12:4619–4627.
52. Hauschild A, Trefzer U, Garbe C, et al. A phase II multicenter study on the histone deacetylase (HDAC) inhibitor MS-275, comparing two dosage schedules in metastatic melanoma. J Clin Oncol 2006; 24 (supplement 18S):463s (abstr 8044).
53. Powers MV, Workman P. Targeting of multiple signaling pathways by heat shock protein 90 molecular chaperone inhibitors. Endocr Relat Cancer 2006; 13(suppl 1): S125–S135.
54. Friedlander P, Solit D, Osman I, et al. Treatment of melanoma patients with 17AAG results in downregulation of the MAPK pathway in melanoma tumors. Proc Amer Assoc Cancer Res 2005; 46 (abstr 1503).
55. Grbovic OM, Basso AD, Sawai A, et al. V600E B-Raf requires the Hsp90 chaperone for stability and is degraded in response to Hsp90 inhibitors. Proc Natl Acad Sci U S A 2006; 103:57–62.
56. Ryu B, Kim DS, Deluca AM, et al. Comprehensive expression profiling of tumor cell lines identifies molecular signatures of melanoma progression. PLoS ONE 2007; 2:E594.
57. Markovic SN, Geyer SM, Dawkins F, et al. A phase II study of bortezomib in the treatment of metastatic malignant melanoma. Cancer 2005; 103:2584–2589.
58. Wolter KG, Verhaegen M, Fernandez Y, et al. Therapeutic window for melanoma treatment provided by selective effects of the proteasome on Bcl-2 proteins. Cell Death Differ 2007; 14:1605–1616.
59. Irby RB, Yeatman TJ. Role of Src expression and activation in human cancer. Oncogene 2000; 19:5636–5642.
60. Gabarra-Niecko V, Schaller MD, Dunty JM. FAK regulates biological processes important for the pathogenesis of cancer. Cancer Metastasis Rev 2003; 22:359–374.
61. Mizejewski GJ. Role of integrins in cancer: survey of expression patterns. Proc Soc Exp Biol Med 1999; 222:124–138.
62. Homsi J, Cubitt C, Daud A. The Src signaling pathway: a potential target in melanoma and other malignancies. Expert Opin Ther Targets 2007; 11:91–100.
63. Homsi J, Messina J, Cubutt C, et al. Targeting Src/Stat3 pathway in malignant melanoma. J Clin Oncol 2006; 24 (supplement 18S):459s (abstr 8025).
64. Kuphal S, Bauer R, Bosserhoff AK. Integrin signaling in malignant melanoma. Cancer Metastasis Rev 2005; 24:195–222.
65. Danen EH, Ten Berge PJ, Van Muijen GN, et al. Emergence of alpha 5 beta 1 fibronectin- and alpha v beta 3 vitronectin-receptor expression in melanocytic tumour progression. Histopathology 1994; 24:249–256.

66. Hsu MY, Shih DT, Meier FE, et al. Adenoviral gene transfer of beta3 integrin subunit induces conversion from radial to vertical growth phase in primary human melanoma. Am J Pathol 1998; 153:1435–1442.
67. Petitclerc E, Stromblad S, von Schalscha TL, et al. Integrin alpha(v)beta3 promotes M21 melanoma growth in human skin by regulating tumor cell survival. Cancer Res 1999; 59:2724–2730.
68. Lee BH, Ruoslahti E. alpha5beta1 integrin stimulates Bcl-2 expression and cell survival through Akt, focal adhesion kinase, and Ca2+/calmodulin-dependent protein kinase IV. J Cell Biochem 2005; 95:1214–1223.
69. Weeraratna AT. A Wnt-er wonderland–the complexity of Wnt signaling in melanoma. Cancer Metastasis Rev 2005; 24:237–250.
70. Larue L, Delmas V. The WNT/Beta-catenin pathway in melanoma. Front Biosci 2006; 11:733–742 (review).
71. Rimm DL, Caca K, Hu G, et al. Frequent nuclear/cytoplasmic localization of beta-catenin without exon 3 mutations in malignant melanoma. Am J Pathol 1999; 154:325–329.
72. Worm J, Christensen C, Gronbaek K, et al. Genetic and epigenetic alterations of the APC gene in malignant melanoma. Oncogene 2004; 23:5215–5226.
73. Delmas V, Beermann F, Martinozzi S, et al. Beta-catenin induces immortalization of melanocytes by suppressing p16INK4a expression and cooperates with N-Ras in melanoma development. Genes Dev 2007; 21:2923–2935.
74. Topol L, Jiang X, Choi H, et al. Wnt-5a inhibits the canonical Wnt pathway by promoting GSK-3-independent beta-catenin degradation. J Cell Biol 2003; 162:899–908.
75. Bittner M, Meltzer P, Chen Y, et al. Molecular classification of cutaneous malignant melanoma by gene expression profiling. Nature 2000; 406:536–540.
76. Weeraratna AT, Jiang Y, Hostetter G, et al. Wnt5a signaling directly affects cell motility and invasion of metastatic melanoma. Cancer Cell 2002; 1:279–288.
77. Lombardo LJ, Lee FY, Chen P, et al. Discovery of N-(2-chloro-6-methyl-phenyl)-2-(6-(4-(2-hydroxyethyl)-piperazin-1-yl)-2-methylpyrimidin-4-ylamino)thiazole-5-carboxamide (BMS-354825), a dual Src/Abl kinase inhibitor with potent antitumor activity in preclinical assays. J Med Chem 2004; 47:6658–6661.
78. Kim KB, Diwan AH, Papadopoulos NE, et al. A randomized phase II study of EMD 121974 in patients (pts) with metastatic melanoma (MM). J Clin Oncol 2007; 25 (supplement 18S):484s (abstr 8548).
79. Hersey P, Sosman J, O'Day S, et al. A phase II, randomized, open-label study evaluating the antitumor activity of MEDI-522, a humanized monoclonal antibody directed against the human alpha v beta 3 (avb3) integrin, +/− dacarbazine (DTIC) in patients with metastatic melanoma (MM). J Clin Oncol 2005; 23 (supplement 16S):711s (abstr 7507).
80. Trikha M, Zhou Z, Nemeth JA, et al. CNTO 95, a fully human monoclonal antibody that inhibits αv integrins, has antitumor and antiangiogenic activity in vivo. Int J Cancer 2004; 110:326–335.
81. Cranmer LD, Bedikian AY, Ribas A, et al. Phase II study of volociximab (M200), an alpha5beta1 anti-integrin antibody in metastatic melanoma. J Clin Oncol 2006; 24 (supplement 18S):455s (abstr 8011).
82. Dihlmann S, von Knebel Doeberitz M. Wnt/beta-catenin-pathway as a molecular target for future anti-cancer therapeutics. Int J Cancer 2005; 113:515–524.

83. Widlund HR, Fisher DE. Microphthalamia-associated transcription factor: a critical regulator of pigment cell development and survival. Oncogene 2003; 22:3035–3041.
84. Garraway LA, Widlund HR, Rubin MA, et al. Integrative genomic analyses identify MITF as a lineage survival oncogene amplified in malignant melanoma. Nature 2005; 436:117–122.
85. Holt SE, Shay JW, Wright WE. Refining the telomere-telomerase hypothesis of aging and cancer. Nat Biotechnol 1996; 14:836–839.
86. Kim NW, Piatyszek MA, Prowse KR, et al. Specific association of human telomerase activity with immortal cells and cancer. Science 1994; 266:2011–2015.
87. Miracco C, Pacenti L, Santopietro R, et al. Evaluation of telomerase activity in cutaneous melanocytic proliferations. Hum Pathol 2000; 31:1018–1021.
88. Mitchell JR, Wood E, Collins K. A telomerase component is defective in the human disease dyskeratosis congenita. Nature 1999; 402:551–555.
89. Yamaguchi H, Calado RT, Ly H, et al. Mutations in TERT, the gene for telomerase reverse transcriptase, in aplastic anemia. N Engl J Med 2005; 352:1413–1424.
90. Armanios MY, Chen JJ, Cogan JD, et al. Telomerase mutations in families with idiopathic pulmonary fibrosis. N Engl J Med 2007; 356:1317–1326.
91. Feldser DM, Hackett JA, Greider CW. Telomere dysfunction and the initiation of genome instability. Nat Rev Cancer 2003; 3:623–627.
92. Armanios M, Greider CW. Telomerase and cancer stem cells. Cold Spring Harb Symp Quant Biol 2005; 70:205–208.
93. Vonderheide RH. Prospects and challenges of building a cancer vaccine targeting telomerase. Biochimie 2008; 90:173–180.
94. Bataille V. Genetics of familial and sporadic melanoma. Clin Exp Dermatol 2000; 25:464–470.
95. Pho L, Grossman D, Leachman SA. Melanoma genetics: a review of genetic factors and clinical phenotypes in familial melanoma. Curr Opin Oncol 2006; 18:173–179.
96. Zuo L, Weger J, Yang Q, et al. Germline mutations in the p16INK4a binding domain of CDK4 in familial melanoma. Nat Genet 1996; 12:97–99.
97. Harland M, Taylor CF, Chambers PA, et al. A mutation hotspot at the p14ARF splice site. Oncogene 2005; 24:4604–4608.
98. Sherr CJ, McCormick F. The RB and p53 pathways in cancer. Cancer Cell 2002; 2:103–112.
99. Liggett WH Jr., Sidransky D. Role of the p16 tumor suppressor gene in cancer. J Clin Oncol 1998; 16:1197–1206.
100. Lubbe J, Reichel M, Burg G, et al. Absence of p53 gene mutations in cutaneous melanoma. J Invest Dermatol 1994; 102:819–821.
101. Li W, Sanki A, Karim RZ, et al. The role of cell cycle regulatory proteins in the pathogenesis of melanoma. Pathology 2006; 38:287–301.
102. Polsky D, Bastian BC, Hazan C, et al. HDM2 protein overexpression, but not gene amplification, is related to tumorigenesis of cutaneous melanoma. Cancer Res 2001; 61:7642–7646.
103. Schwartz GK, Shah MA. Targeting the cell cycle: a new approach to cancer therapy. J Clin Oncol 2005; 23:9408–9421.
104. Shapiro GI. Cyclin-dependent kinase pathways as targets for cancer treatment. J Clin Oncol 2006; 24:1770–1083.

105. Burdette-Radoux S, Tozer RG, Lohmann RC, et al. Phase II trial of flavopiridol, a cyclin dependent kinase inhibitor, in untreated metastatic malignant melanoma. Invest New Drugs 2004; 22:315–322.
106. O'Dwyer PJ, LoRusso P, DeMichele A, et al. A phase I dose escalation trial of daily oral CDK 4/6 inhibitor PD-0332991. J Clin Oncol 2007; 25 (supplement 18S):150s (abstr 3550).
107. Ahmed S, Molife R, Shaw H, et al. Phase I dose-escalation study of ZK 304709, an oral multitarget tumor growth inhibitor (MTGI), administered for 14 days of a 28-day cycle. J Clin Oncol 2006; 24 (supplement 18S):98s (abstr 2076).
108. Graham J, Wagner K, Plummer R, et al. Phase I dose-escalation study of novel oral multitarget tumor growth inhibitor (MTGI) ZK 304709 administered daily for 7 days of a 21-day cycle to patients with advanced solid tumors. J Clin Oncol 2006; 24 (supplement 18S):97s (abstr 2073).
109. Soengas MS, Capodieci P, Polsky D, et al. Inactivation of the apoptosis effector Apaf-1 in malignant melanoma. Nature 2001; 409:207–211.
110. Soengas MS, Lowe SW. Apoptosis and melanoma chemoresistance. Oncogene 2003; 22:3138–3151.
111. Bedikian AY, Millward M, Pehamberger H, et al. Bcl-2 antisense (oblimersen sodium) plus dacarbazine in patients with advanced melanoma: the Oblimersen Melanoma Study Group. J Clin Oncol 2006; 24:4738–4745.
112. Fecher LA, Cummings SD, Keefe MJ, et al. Towards a molecular classification of melanoma. J Clin Oncol 2007; 25:1606–1620.

3

Challenging Melanocytic Neoplasms: Spitzoid Melanoma Vs. Spitz Nevus

Julide T. Celebi

Department of Dermatology, Columbia University, New York, New York, U.S.A.

Jane L. Messina

H. Lee Moffitt Cancer Center and the Department of Pathology and Cell Biology, University of South Florida College of Medicine, Tampa, Florida, U.S.A.

INTRODUCTION

Melanoma in the pediatric patient remains a relatively rare event, comprising 1% to 3% of all childhood cancers (1). Early diagnosis remains a challenge, with the median tumor thickness of 3.5 mm at diagnosis significantly thicker than that of adult melanomas (2). The emphasis on early diagnosis and increasing public awareness of melanoma in children has renewed interest as well as debate concerning the melanocytic neoplasms of childhood, especially Spitz nevus and the melanoma that resembles it, so-called Spitzoid melanoma.

In 1948, Sophie Spitz described a series of 13 cases of "melanomas in childhood" with distinct histopathologic features and benign clinical courses. It was recognized subsequently that these lesions represented an entity distinct from melanoma due to their indolent behavior, and thus the lesion was renamed "Spitz nevus" or "spindle and epithelioid cell nevus" (3,4). In her landmark paper, Spitz reported 1 of the 13 cases to result in a fatal outcome from metastatic melanoma. Even after an exhaustive detailing of the histopathologic features of the case series, only the presence of multinucleated giant cells distinguished the case eventuating in death of a patient from those with a benign course. Indeed, since this original description, distinguishing Spitz nevus from melanoma—and thereby predicting biologic behavior of a tumor with Spitzoid features—has been one of the most challenging issues facing dermatopathologists and melanoma researchers.

While "classic" Spitz nevus is considered a benign melanocytic neoplasm, at the opposite end of the biologic spectrum is a subset of melanoma that can mimic Spitz nevus both clinically and histopathologically. These are referred to as "Spitzoid melanoma" or "melanoma with Spitz nevus-like features" (5). Although the diagnosis of most Spitz nevi and Spitzoid melanomas can be achieved by clinicopathologic correlation and application of standard histopathologic criteria, there is a subset of cases for which the biologic potential cannot be discerned by these means alone. These lesions simultaneously exhibit histopathologic features of both Spitz nevus and Spitzoid melanoma, making the diagnosis difficult and controversial. These melanocytic lesions that do not fall into either of the two categories have been designated as "atypical Spitz tumors" or "atypical Spitz nevi" (6). As a result of these diagnostic difficulties, there are well-documented cases of Spitzoid melanomas that were originally diagnosed as Spitz nevi or atypical Spitz tumors, that resulted in fatal outcomes (6).

Spitz nevi typically occur in children and adolescents, although they can occur in adults. By contrast, melanomas of all types, including Spitzoid melanoma, are rare in children and occur typically in adults. The Centers for Disease Control and Prevention estimated 475 new cases of melanoma in the United States in 2002 for persons aged 19 years or below and only 47 new cases in children aged below 10 years (7). Therefore, the diagnosis of Spitzoid melanoma in children is especially difficult, and accurate diagnosis is most challenging in this age group.

CLINICAL FEATURES

Clinically, Spitz nevi present as pink or brown-black papules, typically less than 1 cm in size, often resembling hemangiomas. In rare cases, they occur as multiple grouped papules, named "agminated Spitz nevus." The clinical features of Spitzoid melanoma are less well characterized; they can have similar features as in Spitz nevi, and present as solitary papules or nodules that may or may not exhibit pigmentation (Fig. 1) (8). Of note, the ABCD rule (asymmetry, border irregularity, color variation, diameter >6mm) for diagnosis of most types of melanoma does not apply well to Spitzoid melanomas, making them difficult to recognize as melanoma on clinical examination.

HISTOPATHOLOGY

The classic Spitz nevus (4) is dome shaped, symmetrical in silhouette, laterally well marginated, and consists of large melanocytes with both spindle and epithelioid morphology, uniformly arrayed as vertically oriented nests along the junction of hyperplastic epidermis. Artifactual clefts may be seen around

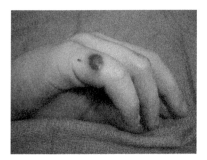

Figure 1 Symmetrical, dome-shaped brown papule on the finger of a five-year-old male. Clinically consistent with either a Spitz nevus or a Spitzoid melanoma, this lesion proved to be a benign Spitz nevus (Fig. 2) (*See Color Insert*).

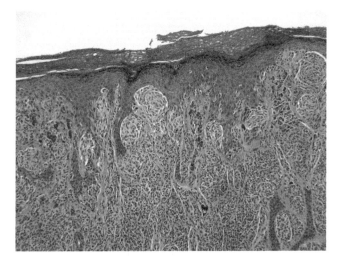

Figure 2 Histopathologic examination of lesion shown in Figure 1. Nests of spindle and epithelioid melanocytes, many vertically oriented, extend from the epidermis into the dermis, where they show evidence of maturation. A lack of atypia and no mitotic activity are seen in this compound Spitz nevus (H&E, 200X).

junctional nests. Eosinophilic hyaline globules (Kamino bodies) are commonly noted along the dermoepidermal interface. Dermal melanocytes show maturation with descent into the dermis and lack significant pleomorphism or deep mitotic activity (Fig. 2).

In Spitzoid melanoma, the spindle and epithelioid melanocytic proliferation shows some histologic attributes of Spitz nevus, but the predominant features are those of conventional melanoma. Thus, these lesions tend to be broad,

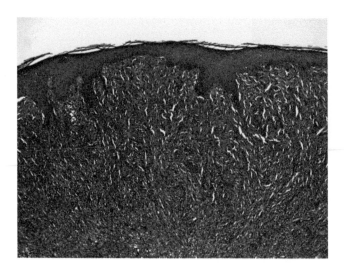

Figure 3 Histopathologic examination of a lesion from the thigh of a 14-year-old female. This Spitzoid melanoma shows sheet-like growth of large, pleomorphic spindled melanocytes beneath an effaced epidermis. The lesion measured 3 mm in thickness. Metastases were found in 3 of 19 inguinal lymph nodes (H&E, 200X).

poorly circumscribed, and asymmetrical. If a spindle and epithelioid tumor demonstrates many or most of the following features, it is categorized as Spitzoid melanoma: abundant pagetoid spread, high-grade nuclear atypia, high mitotic rate with deep dermal mitoses or atypical mitoses, no or only focal maturation at the base, deep penetration into lower dermis or subcutis, ulceration, and large lesional size (Fig. 3) (9,10).

There are a number of spindle and epithelioid melanocytic neoplasms that share some histologic features of both Spitz nevus and Spitzoid melanoma and do not fit neatly into either category. This borderline group of tumors has been variously termed atypical Spitz nevus, atypical Spitz tumor (5), diagnostically controversial Spitzoid melanocytic tumors (11), and Spitz-like lesion in the borderline category of indeterminate malignant potential (12). If a Spitz nevus-like lesion demonstrates involvement of subcutaneous fat, ulceration, poor circumscription, pagetoid melanocytosis, confluence of melanocytes, high cellularity, lack of maturation, asymmetry, significant mitotic rate ($>2–6/mm^2$), deep mitoses, or atypical nuclear features (loss of delicate chromatin, hyperchromasia, large nucleoli, high nucleus to cytoplasm ratio), it should be classified in this borderline category (13).

Despite detailed characterization of the histologic features of these tumors over the past few decades, there still remains a void in delineation of definitive, objective criteria for differentiating Spitz nevus from Spitzoid melanoma. An elegant study by Barnhill et al. illustrated the lack of consensus among pathologists in diagnosing Spitz tumors and the difficulties in predicting clinical outcome on the basis of histologic examination (6). In this study, 13 of the 19 Spitzoid melanomas, which were confirmed as melanoma by regional or systemic metastases, were designated as Spitz nevus or atypical Spitz tumor by some of the pathologists. Furthermore, there are well-documented cases of Spitzoid melanomas in the literature that were initially misdiagnosed as Spitz nevus leading to fatal outcomes. Taken together, these data justify the need to identify molecular markers to classify Spitzoid tumors and predict patient outcome.

PROGNOSIS

The prognosis for Spitz nevus, a benign neoplasm, is excellent. Since recurrence of incompletely excised lesions is well documented, most advocate complete but conservative excision of these lesions. Controversy remains concerning the prognosis of the lesion called "malignant Spitz nevus" by Smith et al. (14). In their group of 33 patients with lesions demonstrating most features of Spitz nevus, regional nodal disease developed in six, but all remained disease free after six years. This prompted speculation that a subset of Spitz nevi harbor the potential for limited metastatic spread. The long-term follow-up of these patients has not been presented, and the existence of a Spitzoid lesion of intermediate malignancy remains extremely controversial.

The prognosis of pediatric melanoma is also controversial, mainly due to small numbers and limited follow-up. It is unclear whether the outcome of childhood melanoma differs significantly from adults in outcome, or whether its behavior in older children differs substantially from younger children. Because of rarity of these tumors in this age group, childhood melanoma remains understudied. The treatment strategies employed for adults, both surgical and medical, are typically applied to this age group. Thus, wide local excision remains the primary treatment, with sentinel node biopsies for lesions thicker than 1 mm. Adjuvant interferon is used in the setting of regional disease. Although a few limited studies suggest that the prognosis of childhood melanomas is similar to those in adults, and is dependent on the initial stage of the tumor, there is controversy with respect to the biologic behavior of childhood melanomas (2,7,15). A recent study of 20 children aged below 20 years undergoing sentinel node biopsy demonstrated a higher rate of nodal involvement compared with adults (40% vs. 18%) but no recurrences after limited (35 month) follow-up (16). Some studies suggest certain histologic subtypes, such as Spitzoid melanoma subtype, confer a survival advantage. Spitzoid melanomas with regional lymph node metastasis but no further progression have been reported (14). By contrast, cases leading to widespread metastasis and fatal outcomes are also well documented (17). Other studies suggest younger age (<10 years) as a favorable prognostic factor, regardless of the histologic subtype (2,18). However, in the absence of large studies with long-term follow-up, survival characteristics of childhood melanoma and thus Spitzoid melanoma remain unclear.

GENETIC STUDIES

DNA Copy Number Changes in Spitzoid Tumors

DNA copy number changes, gains or losses, in melanocytic tumors using comparative genomic hybridization have been studied extensively in recent years. In one study, it has been shown that most nevi do not show any chromosomal aberrations, whereas most "conventional" melanomas (96%) show some form of DNA copy number change (19). The most frequent alteration is loss of 9p (64.4%) due to deletion or inactivation of the *CDKN2A* locus encoding for p16 and ARF. Of interest, in this study, 13% of benign nevi showed gains of 11p, all of which were Spitz nevi. All other types of benign acquired nevi, congenital nevi, and blue nevi showed no aberrations in this series. Analysis of a larger series of 102 Spitz nevi using fluorescence in situ hybridization found at least threefold gains of 11p in 12 cases (11.8%) (20). 11p gains in Spitz nevi were confirmed by another group (21). Recurrent gains of 11p implicated *HRAS* as a candidate oncogene located on 11p, and activating mutations in *HRAS* have been identified in majority of Spitz nevi with increased copy numbers of 11p (20). As in other benign melanocytic nevi, Spitz nevi also have strong expression of the p16 protein, supporting the notion that intact p16 in the presence of a gain-of-function mutation is protective against transformation to melanoma.

In summary, gains of 11p are found in a subset of Spitz nevi ($\sim$ 10%) and are associated with activating mutations in *HRAS*. However, the majority of Spitz nevi do not show DNA copy number changes. Since majority of "conventional" melanomas have chromosomal aberrations, it has been suggested that this information can be used to distinguish Spitz nevi from Spitzoid melanomas. Therefore, if a Spitzoid tumor harbors DNA copy number changes common to "conventional" melanomas, such as loss of 9p, then this information can be helpful in the clinical decision-making process. However, to date, studies specifically examining Spitzoid melanomas and atypical Spitz tumors for chromosomal aberrations are lacking. Therefore, until these studies are conducted, the utility of DNA copy number changes by comparative genomic hybridization as an ancillary diagnostic test for classifying Spitzoid tumors and distinguishing Spitz nevi from Spitzoid melanoma remains unclear, and therefore this test should be used and interpreted with caution.

NRAS, *HRAS*, and *BRAF* Mutations in Spitzoid Tumors

The Ras-Erk pathway is hyperactivated in 90% of melanomas. In melanoma, it can be activated by autocrine growth factors or in rare cases by mutational activation of growth factor receptor such as c-Kit. A more common mechanism is through gain-of-function mutations in *NRAS* or *BRAF* (22). *NRAS* is mutated in 10% to 15% of melanomas, and *BRAF* is mutated in 50% to 70% of melanomas (23). Interestingly, melanocytic nevi also harbor high rates of *BRAF* or *NRAS* mutations. *BRAF* mutations are often observed among common acquired

Table 1 Gain-of-Function Mutations in *BRAF*, *NRAS*, and *HRAS* among Spitzoid Tumors

Tumor type	Number	BRAF	NRAS	HRAS	Refs.
Spitz nevus	30	0/30 (0%)			26
	21	0/21 (0%)			27
	14	0/14 (0%)	0/14 (0%)	4/14 (29%)	28
	48[a]	10/48 (21%)[a]	0/48 (0%)		31
	12	0/12 (0%)	0/12 (0%)	0/12 (0%)	29
	22	1/22 (4.5%)	0/22 (0%)	1/22 (4.5%)	30
Atypical Spitz tumor	16	0/16 (0%)	0/16 (0%)	2/16 (13%)	28
	7	0/7 (0%)	1/7 (14%)		31
	16	1/16 (6%)	0/16 (0%)	0/16 (0%)	29
Spitzoid melanoma	33	1/33 (3%)	0/33 (0%)		32,33
	6	2/6 (33%)			27
	36	23/36 (64%)	7/36 (19%)	0/36 (0%)	28
	13	2/13 (15%)	0/13 (0%)		31

[a]Some Spitz nevi mentioned in this study were reported to have atypical features.

melanocytic nevi (70–80%) (24), whereas *NRAS* is frequently mutated in congenital melanocytic nevi ($\sim 80\%$)(25).

Several groups have examined Spitzoid tumors for mutations in *NRAS*, *HRAS*, and *BRAF*, which harbor gain-of-function mutations among melanocytic nevi and melanomas. These studies are summarized in Table 1. The majority of classic Spitz nevi show no or very low frequency of mutations in *BRAF* (0–4.5%) (26–30), and no mutations in *NRAS* have been identified (28–30). However, one study showed 21% *BRAF* mutation frequency among Spitz nevi (31). Of note, the authors indicated that some of the Spitz nevi in this study had atypical features. Therefore, it is possible that the discrepancy of this report with others may be due to selection of heterogeneous group of Spitz nevi rather than classic Spitz nevi. In one study, 4 of the 14 Spitz nevus cases were found to have *HRAS* mutations (28). Taken together, the mutation frequency of *NRAS*, *HRAS*, and *BRAF* among Spitz nevi is very low in contrast to other melanocytic nevi, suggesting other gene/s or mechanisms for their development.

Several studies, most with limited number of cases, have examined atypical Spitz tumors and Spitzoid melanoma for gain-of-function mutations of the molecules that signal through the Ras-Erk pathway. On the basis of three studies, *BRAF* mutation frequency appears to be low among atypical Spitz tumors (0–6%). However, mutation frequency of *BRAF* in Spitzoid melanomas is quite variable ranging from 3% to 64%. It is possible that this discrepancy is due to histopathologic classification; as previously stated, it may be difficult at times to differentiate Spitzoid melanoma from other nodular spindle cell melanomas. Two groups studied metastatic Spitzoid melanomas. In one study, no mutations in *BRAF* or *NRAS* were identified in 14 metastatic cases (32), of which the majority were tumors from children. By contrast, another study showed *BRAF* mutations in four of the seven metastatic melanomas from adult patients (28).

On the basis of studies that classify Spitz tumors by histopathology, *BRAF* and *NRAS* mutation status does not reliably distinguish Spitz nevi from Spitzoid melanomas and cannot be relied upon as a specific ancillary diagnostic tool by itself.

CONCLUSION

Sixty years after its original description, Spitzoid tumors continue to be one of the most challenging melanocytic tumors with respect to diagnosis, classification, and management. Currently, there is no molecular marker that has been proven to unequivocally differentiate Spitz nevus and Spitzoid melanoma. Moreover, the molecular basis of Spitzoid tumors remains uncharacterized. Future studies will focus on identifying molecular signatures that predict patient outcome as well as establishing a molecular-based understanding of these tumors.

REFERENCES

1. Pappo AS. Melanoma in children and adolescents. Eur J Cancer 2003; 39(18): 2651–2661.
2. Ferrari A, Bono A, Baldi M, et al. Does melanoma behave differently in younger children than in adults? A retrospective study of 33 cases of childhood melanoma from a single institution. Pediatrics 2005; 115(3):649–654.
3. Weedon D, Little JH. Spindle and epithelioid cell nevi in children and adults. A review of 211 cases of the Spitz nevus. Cancer 1977; 40(1):217–225.
4. Paniago-Pereira C, Maize JC, Ackerman AB. Nevus of large spindle and/or epithelioid cells (Spitz's nevus). Arch Dermatol 1978; 114(12):1811–1823.
5. Barnhill RL, Flotte TJ, Fleischli M, et al. Cutaneous melanoma and atypical Spitz tumors in childhood. Cancer 1995; 76(10):1833–1845.
6. Barnhill RL, Argenyi ZB, From L, et al. Atypical Spitz nevi/tumors: lack of consensus for diagnosis, discrimination from melanoma, and prediction of outcome. Hum Pathol 1999; 30(5):513–520.
7. Lange JR, Palis BE, Chang DC, et al. Melanoma in children and teenagers: an analysis of patients from the National Cancer Data Base. J Clin Oncol 2007; 25(11): 1363–1368.
8. Mehregan AH, Mehregan DA. Malignant melanoma in childhood. Cancer 1993; 71(12):4096–4103.
9. Piepkorn M. On the nature of histologic observations: the case of the Spitz nevus. J Am Acad Dermatol 1995; 32(2 pt 1):248–254.
10. Peters MS, Goellner JR. Spitz naevi and malignant melanomas of childhood and adolescence. Histopathology 1986; 10(12):1289–1302.

11. Lohmann CM, Coit DG, Brady MS, et al. Sentinel lymph node biopsy in patients with diagnostically controversial spitzoid melanocytic tumors. Am J Surg Pathol 2002; 26(1):47–55.

12. Reed RJ. Atypical spitz nevus/tumor. Hum Pathol 1999; 30(12):1523–1526.

13. Barnhill RL. The Spitzoid lesion: rethinking Spitz tumors, atypical variants, 'Spitzoid melanoma' and risk assessment. Mod Pathol 2006; 19(suppl 2):S21–S33.

14. Smith KJ, Barrett TL, Skelton HG III. Spindle cell and epithelioid cell nevi with atypia and metastasis (malignant Spitz nevus). Am J Surg Pathol 1989; 13(11): 931–939.

15. Fabrizi G, Massi G. Spitzoid malignant melanoma in teenagers: an entity with no better prognosis than that of other forms of melanoma. Histopathology 2001; 38(5): 448–453.

16. Roaten JB, Partrick DA, Bensard D, et al. Survival in sentinel lymph node-positive pediatric melanoma. J Pediatr Surg 2005; 40(6):988–992 (discussion 92).

17. Melnik MK, Urdaneta LF, Al-Jurf AS, et al. Malignant melanoma in childhood and adolescence. Am Surg 1986; 52(3):142–147.

18. Gibbs P, Moore A, Robinson W, et al. Pediatric melanoma: are recent advances in the management of adult melanoma relevant to the pediatric population? J Pediatr Hematol Oncol 2000; 22(5):428–432.

19. Bastian BC, Olshen AB, LeBoit PE, et al. Classifying melanocytic tumors based on DNA copy number changes. Am J Pathol 2003; 163(5):1765–1770.

20. Bastian BC, LeBoit PE, Pinkel D. Mutations and copy number increase of HRAS in Spitz nevi with distinctive histopathological features. Am J Pathol 2000; 157(3): 967–972.

21. Harvell JD, Kohler S, Zhu S, et al. High-resolution array-based comparative genomic hybridization for distinguishing paraffin-embedded Spitz nevi and melanomas. Diagn Mol Pathol 2004; 13(1):22–25.

22. Gray-Schopfer V, Wellbrock C, Marais R. Melanoma biology and new targeted therapy. Nature 2007; 445(7130):851–857.

23. Davies H, Bignell GR, Cox C, et al. Mutations of the BRAF gene in human cancer. Nature 2002; 417(6892):949–954.

24. Pollock PM, Harper UL, Hansen KS, et al. High frequency of BRAF mutations in nevi. Nat Genet 2003; 33(1):19–20.

25. Bauer J, Curtin JA, Pinkel D, et al. Congenital melanocytic nevi frequently harbor NRAS mutations but no BRAF mutations. J Invest Dermatol 2007; 127(1):179–182.

26. Gill M, Renwick N, Silvers DN, et al. Lack of BRAF mutations in Spitz nevi. J Invest Dermatol 2004; 122(5):1325–1326.

27. Palmedo G, Hantschke M, Rutten A, et al. The T1796A mutation of the BRAF gene is absent in Spitz nevi. J Cutan Pathol 2004; 31(3):266–270.

28. van Dijk MC, Bernsen MR, Ruiter DJ. Analysis of mutations in B-RAF, N-RAS, and H-RAS genes in the differential diagnosis of Spitz nevus and spitzoid melanoma. Am J Surg Pathol 2005; 29(9):1145–1151.

29. Takata M, Lin J, Takayanagi S, et al. Genetic and epigenetic alterations in the differential diagnosis of malignant melanoma and spitzoid lesion. Br J Dermatol 2007; 156(6):1287–1294.

30. Indsto JO, Kumar S, Wang L, et al. Low prevalence of RAS-RAF-activating mutations in Spitz melanocytic nevi compared with other melanocytic lesions. J Cutan Pathol 2007; 34(6):448–455.

31. Fullen DR, Poynter JN, Lowe L, et al. BRAF and NRAS mutations in spitzoid melanocytic lesions. Mod Pathol 2006; 19(10):1324–1332.
32. Lee DA, Cohen JA, Twaddell WS, et al. Are all melanomas the same? Spitzoid melanoma is a distinct subtype of melanoma. Cancer 2006; 106(4):907–913.
33. Gill M, Cohen J, Renwick N, et al. Genetic similarities between Spitz nevus and Spitzoid melanoma in children. Cancer 2004; 101(11):2636–2640.

4

Melanoma Genomics—Techniques and Implications for Therapy

Adil I. Daud

*Department of Medicine, University of California San Francisco,
San Francisco, California, U.S.A.*

Vernon K. Sondak

*H. Lee Moffitt Cancer Center and the Departments of Oncologic
Sciences and Surgery, University of South Florida College of Medicine,
Tampa, Florida, U.S.A.*

Ashani Weeraratna

*Laboratory of Immunology, National Institute on Aging, National Institutes of
Health, Baltimore, Maryland, U.S.A.*

INTRODUCTION

In the last decade, the advent of high-throughput gene expression profiling technology opened up a myriad of possibilities for the targeted therapy of many diseases. High-throughput gene expression profiling techniques such as microarray technology and serial analysis of gene expression (SAGE) have now been in use for several years, but it was not until the complete sequencing of the human genome that these techniques truly burgeoned. SAGE technologies expanded to include longer tags, and more tags could be sequenced per library. Microarrays went from containing 8000 to 10,000 sequences to encompassing 44,000 to 60,000 clones, encompassing the entire human genome. Sequences corresponding to single nucleotide polymorphisms (SNPs) allow for the arraying of SNPs onto high-density

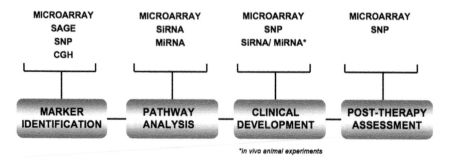

*In vivo animal experiments

Figure 1 A schematic of melanoma progression and of the stages along the progression continuum at which genomic therapies are being used.

chips, and techniques such as comparative genomic hybridization (CGH) could be translated to an array-based platform to allow for a comprehensive study of genomic changes. In this chapter, we will provide an overview of these commonly used technologies and discuss the latest applications of these technologies to melanoma research and the utility of these current findings in the clinic (Fig. 1).

SERIAL ANALYSIS OF GENE EXPRESSION AND LARGE-SCALE SEQUENCING PROJECTS

The development of sequencing machines capable of handling large volumes of sequence information in a short amount of time has led to the large-scale sequencing of transcripts, or expressed sequence tags (ESTs), generated from random-primed complementary DNA (cDNA) libraries. Such effort has been pioneered by the Merck/Washington University (1) and is being extended by the Cancer Genome Anatomy Project (CGAP) (2). On their Web site (http://cgap.nci.nih.gov/), CGAP currently lists over one million ESTs from normal, premalignant, and malignant cells in its Tumor Gene Index (2). In an attempt to make the process of sequencing ESTs more efficient, massively parallel signature sequencing (MPSS) (3) and SAGE were developed (4). MPSS is a gene expression profiling method that sequences 16 to 20 base pair (bp) transcripts using a novel nongel-based signature-sequencing technique. MPSS can reliably generate an impressive two million tags from approximately 500 ng of messenger RNA (mRNA) (3). However, MPSS is a complex technique and is currently only available from Lynx Therapeutics Inc (Hayward, California, U.S.) (http://www.lynxgen.com).

SAGE is a technique based on the principle that a 10- to14-bp piece of mRNA can uniquely identify a transcript, provided that it is derived from a unique region within that transcript (4). These unique identifiers are referred to as SAGE tags and are generated by cleavage of the transcript with a specific four-base-recognizing restriction endonuclease (*Nla*III, referred to as the anchoring enzyme), at a fixed distance from the poly(A) tail. The human genome is estimated to contain 33,000 to 35,000 genes (5); therefore, in theory, the variety provided by the possible combinations of the four bases of DNA into 10 bp sequences (4^{10}) is sufficient to identify all expected transcripts from the human genome. These 10 bp sequences can be joined together (concatemerized), so that a single sequencing reaction can identify several transcripts at once, making the sequencing of SAGE libraries an order of magnitude more efficient than the sequencing of EST libraries. Like other EST-sequencing projects, it does not necessitate a prior knowledge of genes, and instead identifies and tallies mRNA transcripts, thereby providing a comprehensive profile of gene expression of a cell. Modifications of this technique include small amplified RNA-SAGE (SAR-SAGE) (6), polymerase chain reaction-SAGE (PCR-SAGE) (7), SAGE-lite (8), and micro-SAGE (9), and involve PCR amplification of template cDNA to generate larger quantities of double-strand (ds) cDNA, which is used as the template for subsequent SAGE analysis. These techniques allow for the use of minute quantities of RNA, thus expanding the range of studies that can be performed using this technique.

A method that is increasingly used over the original SAGE protocol is that of LongSAGE. LongSAGE was developed to experimentally assess whether many of the hypothetical genes generated by computational gene predictions of sequences derived from the human genome map exist in vivo (10). The technical aspect of this procedure is almost identical to the original approach but uses a different type of (II)S restriction endonuclease, *Mme* I, to generate longer transcript tags. The use of *Mme* I as a tagging enzyme results in tags that are 21 bps in length, consisting of a constant 4-bp sequence attached to a unique 17-bp tag. LongSAGE allows for unique assignment of tags to genomic sequences and, unlike conventional SAGE, is not restricted to only ESTs and previously characterized transcripts. This technique allows us to merge experimental and computational biology and allows for a high-throughput validation of gene predictions. For example, using a DLD-1 colon cancer line, LongSAGE methodology provided in vivo evidence for the expression of 245 predicted genes, half of which had no previous experimental proof of their existence (10). The Robust Long (RL) SAGE protocol developed by Gowda et al. (11) was developed to overcome the low efficiency of cloning often found with LongSAGE and promises high cloning efficiency, large concatemer inserts, and deep transcriptome analyses that are not possible with conventional SAGE or LongSAGE protocols. In fact, this protocol promises libraries of up to 4.5 million tags in a much shorter time than either conventional or LongSAGE.

SAGE AND OTHER LARGE-SCALE SEQUENCING PROJECTS IN MELANOMA

Because of the tedious and costly nature of large-scale sequencing projects, many laboratories tend to conduct high-throughput gene expression studies using techniques such as microarray analysis. However, of the sequencing studies that have been conducted, some fundamental observations that have literally refocused the field of melanoma research have emerged. Perhaps, the most critical gene identified by one of these techniques, a genome-wide scan conducted by researchers at the Sanger Institute, is the gene *BRAF* (12), which is discussed in greater detail elsewhere in this volume. Data from this study showed that *BRAF* was mutated in 66% of melanomas, and data from a follow-up study confirmed this and also discovered that *BRAF* was mutated in roughly the same proportion of nevi as well (13). As BRAF signaling involves a cascade of events, including farnesylation, BRAF kinase activity, and the activation of downstream kinases such as ERK and MAPK, there are many potential targets for therapy (14). Indeed, inhibitors to all the above-mentioned steps in the cascade are in preclinical and clinical development (15). Other sequencing projects in combination techniques, such as single-strand conformation polymorphism (SSCP), have identified other key melanoma genes such as *CDKN2A*, *CDK4*, and *MC1R* (16–18).

Another advance in the characterization of the molecular progression of melanoma is the use of SAGE or variants of this technique. Currently available to the public, on the CGAP Web site, are three SAGE libraries, made from two melanomas in vertical growth phase, and one visceral metastasis. The analysis of these libraries, when subjected to methods more commonly reserved for microarray analysis suggested the involvement of a variety of genes such as *calpain*, *CD74*, *ATM*, *HEI10*, *PKD1*, *KAI1*, *IL-10R*, and various members of the Wnt pathway (19,20). Another gene identified in these SAGE libraries was the gene *Claudin-1*, a tight junction protein, and in a follow-up study it was shown that *Claudin-1* is aberrantly expressed in melanoma and regulated by protein kinase C (PKC) and its expression correlates to increases in MMP-2 and invasion. These effects can be reversed by either *Claudin-1* knockdown or PKC inhibition (21). In a recent SAGE study, LongSAGE was used to determine if a melanoma derived from a positive lymph node bore a resemblance to the primary tumor, and indeed the profiles were quite similar. These data were also assayed using antibody arrays and they identified Ubc9 as a molecule involved in the chemosensitivity of melanoma (22). Another study involving a modification of the SAGE technique known as digital karyotyping allowed for the analysis of over 800,000 tags and identified a deletion of the Duchenne Muscular Dystrophy (*DMD*) gene in melanoma (23). Follow-up analysis suggested that the loss of *DMD* may contribute to the migration of melanoma cells. SAGE has also allowed for the identification of novel vaccine targets, such as P. polypeptide (24). What sort of impact these SAGE-based discoveries will have on melanoma biology and therapy remains to be seen.

MICROARRAY ANALYSIS

With the sequencing of the human genome came the ability to design oligomers corresponding to all known genes and ESTs. The majority of arrays used today are oligomer based and are either manufactured by in situ synthesis on glass using photolithography, or manufactured in vitro and then robotically spotted onto glass, or synthesized onto microbeads, which is a cheaper technique. Oligomers range from about 25 to 70 bp and encompass anywhere from 44,000 to 60,000 genes and ESTs. cDNA can then be made by reverse transcribing RNA, during which process fluorescent dyes can be incorporated into the cDNA. Two different fluorochromes are often used to differentiate between and compare samples on the basis of the relative abilities of each sample to hybridize to the same elements on the microarray chip (25). Microarray-based platforms have been used to examine not only gene expression but also copy number changes and gene polymorphisms (both described below) as well as epigenetic phenomena such as methylation (26). Microarray technology is by far the most commonly used high-throughput genomic analysis tool.

Unlike SAGE, microarray analysis is a ratio-based comparison, which often accounts for the large variability among studies from multiple laboratories, as changes in gene expression are dependent on the reference sample used. However, microarrays are a much cheaper, less laborious technique than SAGE, and with the newer chips that encompass sequences from the whole genome, they give comparable data. As with any high-throughput technique, it is not just the experiment and generation of data that is the challenge for both array and SAGE analysis but the analysis of the generated data. The tools that are currently available to analyze microarray data and, to a lesser extent, SAGE data are too abundant to discuss in this chapter, but the reader is referred to some comprehensive reviews and book chapters on this topic (27–29).

MICROARRAY ANALYSIS IN MELANOMA— PAST, PRESENT, AND FUTURE

Unlike the other three genomic techniques described in this chapter, microarray analysis has evolved beyond a discovery tool that identifies potential markers or targets for melanoma, simply on the basis of tumor grade or subtype. In addition, more follow-up studies have been performed on microarray data than any of the other techniques discussed here. For example, some of the seminal initial studies identified genes and pathways important to melanoma biology, including genes such as *Wnt5A* (30) and *RhoC* (31). Follow-up studies on both *RhoC* and *Wnt5A* have confirmed the initial observations and highlighted two important pathways in melanoma biology. These early studies also demonstrated the power of the technique itself, as well as highlighted how complex mathematical analyses could translate into real biology and tumor classification. Today microarray technology is being used in a more focused manner, often combining other genomic approaches to address specific experimental conditions. For example, as a further follow-up to the above-mentioned study on *Wnt5A*, we have recently used a combination of small interfering RNA (siRNA) technology (described below) and microarray analysis to comprehensively examine the effects of Wnt5A on melanoma cells. This study implicated Wnt5A in the suppression of metastasis suppressors such as Kiss-1 and in the initiation of the epithelial to mesenchymal transition, characterized by the loss of E-cadherin, and the upregulation of the transcriptional repressor, Snail (32). Other focused applications of microarray technology include the use of a more specific tissue or cell type for analysis using techniques such as laser capture microdissection, allowing for specific profiling of melanoma cells in relation to their microenvironment (33). Other specific interactions have also been examined, such as those of the interplay between melanoma cells and the immune system by arraying peripheral blood lymphocytes from melanoma patients with metastatic disease (34), which showed that T cells from melanoma patients have defects in interferon signaling. In another study, profiling of $CD8^+$ T cells from melanoma patients post-immunotherapy (35) supported this observation, as patients who were able to secrete interferon gamma and tumor necrosis factor alpha in response to vaccination had a better outcome.

Other studies have used microarrays to focus on very specific subsets of genes, rather than the initial large "fishing expeditions" of first-generation array studies, which were important for identifying the types of gene expression signatures we now use to study melanoma and other diseases. For example, a recent study found that the inhibition of apoptosis is an early event in melanoma, with the greatest downregulation of apoptosis-related genes occurring in the transition from thin to thick melanomas (36). This is informative, not just biologically but also clinically, as these data suggest that these tumors may be less susceptible to agents that would otherwise cause them to apoptose. Another study used a focused cytokine array to distinguish sentinel lymph nodes with melanoma micrometastases from tumor-negative sentinel nodes and compared both with nonsentinel nodes (37). This revealed a small signature of genes including *leptin* and *IL10* that correlated to tumor-positive nodes. Other chips focused on highly specific genes such as mitochondrial genes (38) and calcium channels (39) have also identified pathway or organelle-specific changes in melanoma. Finally, microarray studies to analyze how specimen collection affects data production are also being carried out. In a recent trial, microarray analysis was performed prospectively on metastatic liver tumors in patients with colorectal adenocarcinoma undergoing chemotherapy with either capecitabine/oxaliplatin/bevacizumab or capecitabine/irinotecan/bevacizumab. Analysis of RNA quality showed that core biopsies were preferable to fine-needle aspirates and that biopsies collected in RNAlater reagent were preferable to those flash-frozen in liquid nitrogen. Technical aspects of biopsy collection were also important, including biopsy of peripheral rather than central regions of the tumor and touch preparations to verify the presence of viable tumor (40). This "fine-tuning" approach to generating reliable, high-quality microarray data is promising for targeted therapy and can eventually be correlated to outcome data.

Microarray analysis has also recently been used to classify tumors according to gene expression in the context of genomic alterations such as *BRAF* mutations. This has resulted in some conflicting data. Some studies have stated that there is indeed a *BRAF*-specific gene expression signature (41,42). Another study, however, determined that there is no *BRAF*-specific gene expression signature, and instead tumors are better subclassified by their transforming growth factor (TGF)-β susceptibility and Wnt status (43). This type of discrepancy highlights the need for better uniformity of data analysis tools, experimental techniques (e.g., standard reference samples across studies), and array platforms. In fact, there are currently studies that compare gene expression data from various studies and find very little correlation among them. One study created a web-based data "warehouse" of gene expression in melanoma and demonstrated that there was a huge disparity among data from the existing studies (44). A second study recently compared all the major studies of microarray analysis of melanoma and determined that only three genes were consistently found and validated across multiple genomic studies. These genes were *Wnt5A, β-3 integrin*, and *syndecan-4* (45).

Despite these discrepancies, microarray technology is still a vitally important technique not just in the study of melanoma biology but also for its therapy and diagnosis. Perhaps the most exciting application of this technique is its use in individualized therapy. This type of therapy involves profiling the mRNA in a patient's tumor and reveals various targets that can be treated by conventional or targeted therapy. This would obviate the need for these patients to enter a clinical trial, or at least increase the likelihood that clinical trials would be positive, since these patients would be far more likely to be responsive to the therapeutic agent. As a very simple example, if a patient's tumor expresses elevated levels of Her-2/Neu, the tumor might be treatable with trastuzumab (Herceptin). Currently, such information can only be provided to inform an oncologist of possible choices they may wish to consider when dealing with a patient with advanced refractory cancer for which the standard lines of treatment have failed. This type of effort is already underway in a collaborative clinical trial being carried out between the Molecular Profiling Institute and the Translational Genomics Research Institute (Phoenix, Arizona, U.S.). Future directions in which this type of research could go, although currently pure speculation, would be to "re-array" the patient posttreatment and ask if the treatment is working (based on downregulation of the target gene), and finally, if the tumor recurs, to array the patient once more to find other potential targets that may now be expressed in the tumor.

COMPARATIVE GENOMIC HYBRIDIZATION

Microarray-based techniques can be expanded to identify changes such as chromosomal amplification via a technique known as CGH. This technique is based on the fact that cancer cells are inherently genetically unstable, and their DNA often undergoes copy number changes. Test and reference DNAs are labeled with different fluorochromes, and their differential binding to genomic DNA is examined (46). Conventional CGH compares the mixtures of test and reference DNAs directly on metaphase chromosomes, whereas array CGH involves hybridization to genomic DNA that has been spotted onto an array (47).

As with cDNA microarray, the ratio of test to reference DNA can be assessed by the relative intensity of fluorescence in each sample. In CGH, this corresponds to increases or decreases in copy number of the specific gene locus represented by the array elements. Array CGH is logarithmically more sensitive than conventional CGH and can reliably detect single-copy changes (47).

CGH in Melanoma

CGH was used quite early on in melanoma research and identified key changes in melanoma cells, including the loss of 9p, 3p, and 6q; monosomy of chromosome 3; and increases in 6p and 8q (48). In a recent study, DNA was recovered from over 100 formalin-fixed paraffin-embedded (FFPE) uveal melanomas and subjected to CGH analysis (49). The power of this particular study was that the large number of samples examined could be correlated to outcome data. The authors found that there were gains in the following genomic regions: 18q11.2, 6q16, 21q11.2, 9q12, and 3q12 and a loss at 1p33, with the 18q11.2 gain having the most significant correlation to survival. Interestingly, in male patients with poor outcome there was a gain at Xq21, a change not seen in females or males who survived more than nine years post diagnosis (49). In primary cutaneous melanomas, CGH on FFPE tissues has revealed a large number of changes, including most commonly the loss of 9p and others, e.g., 10, 6q, and 8p, and gains at 7, 8, 6p, 1q, 20, 17, and 2 (50).

In addition, CGH is particularly useful as a diagnostic tool for distinguishing between melanocytic lesions such as nevi, which rarely exhibit chromosomal changes, Spitz nevi, which exhibit specific chromosomal changes (predominantly gains in 11p) not seen in other tumors, and melanoma, over 95% of which have chromosomal alterations (50). In a recent comprehensive study, 186 melanocytic lesions were examined using CGH. Of the 54 nevi in this subset, only seven exhibited any form of chromosomal aberration, and all of these were Spitz nevi. Of the 132 melanoma samples, 127 exhibited some form of chromosomal alteration. What makes this study particularly elegant is that the researchers then expanded their analysis to include the correlation between chromosomal alterations and parameters such as anatomical site, sun exposure, and Clark's level (51). These studies have been expanded to identify various oncogenes such as c-KIT, which is altered in a large proportion of melanomas arising in chronically or heavily sun-damaged skin (52). Because drugs such as imatinib are used to target c-KIT in other cancers, this observation raises the possibility that the same drugs may be used to target a subset of melanoma. Since other molecules such as BRAF are not commonly mutated in tumors from heavily sun-exposed skin (53), the available inhibitors to this pathway are less useful in these tumors, so this type of discovery has great value. Taken together, all of these results demonstrate that not only can CGH be used as a tool to differentiate nevi from melanoma but may also identify key differences among different subtypes of melanoma that can be used to tailor therapy.

SINGLE NUCLEOTIDE POLYMORPHISMS

Studies have shown that patients' immune and drug responses may have a genetic basis and that identifying these hereditary genetic variations between patients could help to optimize therapy as well as identify molecular targets for therapy (54). These variations take the form of single nucleotide changes or SNPs within the genome and are quite abundant, occurring once every 1000 bps in the human genome (which has a total of 3 billion bps), resulting in an estimated total of over 10 million SNPs (55). The mapping of the human genome has also allowed for genome-wide association studies, giving researchers the ability to link genetic traits to drug response, without the necessity of an a priori knowledge of the SNPs that need to be included. Public databases such as http://www.ncbi.nlm.nih.gov/SNP, HapMap (56), jSNp (57) exist, and over six million SNP sequences have been deposited into these types of databases (58). *In silico* mapping of SNPs is also being performed by private groups such as The SNP Consortium (TSC) (a private, not-for-profit alliance of 13 major multinational companies and the Wellcome Trust; http://snp.cshl.org) (59). The National Institutes of Health have established a Pharmacogenetics Research Network group (60), and this group has developed a research tool known as PharmGKB that allows for the researching and comparison of existing SNP databases. Other tools such as PolyMAPr also exist (61). Such cataloguing and identification of SNPs allow for their production and synthesis, and currently, the most commonly used technique is to analyze SNPs using a microarray-based platform (62). Unlike microarray analysis, SNP analysis yields a binary answer; so data analysis is much simpler, which allows for the analysis of a greater number of sequences. Recent studies have demonstrated that the higher the density of SNPs used (over half a million SNPs on 1 chip), the more precisely a locus can be identified (63). In addition, SNP analysis appears to be even more sensitive than array CGH (64). These types of studies may herald the advent of individualized therapy and improved diagnostics for patients suffering from various diseases, including melanoma.

SNPs in Melanoma

SNP analysis in melanoma has identified polymorphisms in several genes, ranging from matrix metalloproteinases to cytokines (65,66). The use of high-density SNP arrays has allowed for the identification of both tumor suppressor genes and oncogenes. In a recent study, whole-genome SNP array analysis on 76 melanoma cell lines confirmed many of the CGH-identified allelic changes mentioned above (67). Additionally, tumor suppressor genes were detected via homozygous deletions, and these corresponded to the loss of genes such as *CDKN2A, PTEN, PTPRD*, and *HDAC4*. Amplifications were detected that correspond to *NRAS, BRAF, CCND1*, and *MITF* (67). *MITF*, which encodes a key transcription factor in melanocyte biology, was initially identified as an oncogene in melanoma in an elegant study that combined SNP analysis with gene expression signatures derived from the NCI60 microarray database (68). In this study, the authors also determined that *MITF* was predominantly amplified in more aggressive tumors, along with *BRAF* and *p16* alterations. *MITF* and *BRAF* alterations in primary human melanocytes resulted in their transformation, and the knockdown of *MITF* sensitized melanomas to chemotherapy. Because MITF represents a melanocyte lineage-restricted alteration, it holds a lot of promise as a target for specific therapy against melanoma. Other SNP studies have identified changes in cytokines (65), matrix metalloproteinases (66), *BRAF* (69), epidermal growth factor (70,71), and vascular endothelial growth factor (*VEGF*) (72).

RNA—HARNESSING CELLULAR MECHANISMS OF MESSAGE REGULATION

A relatively recent advent in molecular biology has been the discovery of cellular mechanisms of gene regulation in response to the introduction of double-stranded RNA into eukaryotic organisms such as nematodes. On introduction of double-stranded RNA into a cell, an adenosine triphosphate (ATP)-dependent cleavage of the dsRNA into smaller 21 to 25 nucleotide fragments occurs. This is mediated by the dsRNA-specific endonuclease, Dicer, producing siRNAs with a phosphate group on their 5' end, and a hydroxyl group on their 3' end. These fragments are then incorporated into a protein complex where they are unwound into single-stranded RNAs that then target their corresponding mRNAs for degradation by recruiting them to a protein complex known as the RNA-induced silencing complex (RISC) (73). Because of the transient nature of siRNA transfection, researchers have attempted to make more stable transfectants, known as short hairpin RNA (shRNA). This again harnesses the endogenous machinery of the cell, as shRNAs are designed so that they are transcribed off a sequence that contains a stem or hairpin loop using an RNA polymerase promoter (74). However, the mechanisms of shRNA processing are not yet clear, and the efficiency of this technique is not yet on a par with the transient technique of siRNA delivery. For both techniques, validation of protein downregulation following message reduction is key.

Another small RNA species that is receiving considerable attention is microRNA (miRNA). Although the same size as siRNA, miRNAs are endogenously generated and are transcribed either from introns, 5' untranslated RNA or intergenic regions (75). Often, miRNAs derived from intronic sequences are coexpressed with their mRNA, indicating a common origin, and many miRNAs are coexpressed with proximal miRNAs within 50 kilobases (kb) (76). Currently, over 600 miRNAs have been discovered that are responsible for regulating 30% of the genome, and these are listed in a publicly available registry (77). Recently it has been shown that miRNAs use two methods to inhibit mRNA translation. One method involves the binding of miRNAs to a protein complex that closely resembles a ribosome. This complex then binds the corresponding mRNA and makes it inaccessible to actual ribosomes, thereby inhibiting translation (78). The

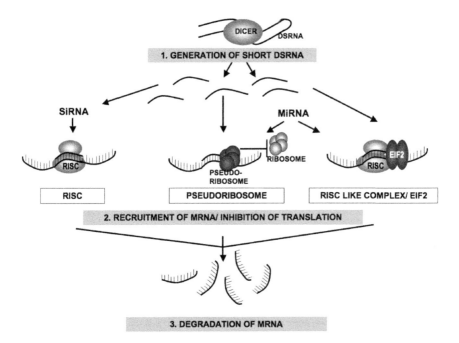

Figure 2 Mechanisms of RNA regulation. Small RNAs are generated by cleavage of ds RNA by the enzyme Dicer. Small RNAs can either be siRNA or microRNAs. SiRNAs regulate message by binding to target mRNAs in the RISC complex, by allowing for their silencing, and ultimately by degradation. MicroRNAs can bind to a protein complex that closely resembles a ribosome. This complex then binds the corresponding mRNA and makes it inaccessible to actual ribosomes, thereby inhibiting translation. The second mechanism involves the RISC complex, but unlike in siRNA-mediated gene silencing, this complex binds to a second multiprotein complex that contains elongation initiation factor 6 (eIF6), a protein known to inhibit ribosome assembly. The ultimate result is the regulation RNA translation. *Abbreviations*: ds, double-strand; siRNA, small interfering RNA; mRNA, messenger RNA; RISC, RNA-induced silencing complex.

second mechanism involves the RISC complex, but unlike in siRNA-mediated gene silencing, this complex binds to a second multiprotein complex that contains elongation initiation factor 6 (eIF6), a protein known to inhibit ribosome assembly (79). This effectively inhibits translation of the mRNA (Fig. 2). The efficiency of both siRNA and miRNA at silencing gene expression makes them valuable research tools and promising therapeutic agents because of their highly specific nature.

Applications of RNAi in Melanoma Research

One of the first uses of siRNA as a tool in melanoma involved the targeting of *BRAF* is to determine if the suppression of *BRAF* could affect melanoma tumorigenesis. Knockdown of *BRAF* indeed resulted in an ablation of the transforming ability of *BRAF*, but knockdown of *CRAF* did not alter the melanoma phenotype (80). Since then, over a hundred studies have used siRNA as a tool to ascertain the effects of various genes on melanoma biology. Large-scale analyses of the effects of various siRNAs are also being developed using siRNA arrays (81). Further, the successful use of siRNAs in vivo also holds great promise for targeted therapy. Perhaps the most promising study for the treatment of cancer using siRNA involved the treatment of subcutaneously injected breast cancer cells with siRNA against *CXCR4* (82). This study examined the most efficacious way of in vivo treatment of cells with siRNA: cells were either transfected prior to tail vein injection, followed by intermittent injections of siRNA (twice weekly) or untransfected cells were injected into the tail vein, followed by twice weekly injections. Other control groups were also included, but, in short, this experiment showed that even simple injection of siRNA posttail vein injection of untransfected cells could inhibit metastasis by over 50% (the pretransfected cells had a decrease in metastasis of over 70%). Given the abundance of data regarding *CXCR4* in melanoma (83,84), these results have specific implications for melanoma therapy as well as hold promise for the general use of siRNA molecules in an in vivo setting.

MicroRNAs are a very new field, and currently only a handful of studies exist in the melanoma literature. One study used a highly sensitive PCR technique to assess the expression of 241 miRNAs across the NCI-60 human tumor cell line database. These analyses showed that the large majority of miRNAs are downregulated in human tumors (85). Specific miRNA signatures could be assigned to specific tumor types, including melanoma. Another impressive study used array-based CGH to assess abnormalities in genomic loci harboring miRNA genes in a panel of tumors (86). Of the tumors analyzed, melanoma had the largest number of abnormal miRNAs, with over 85% of the loci showing alterations in greater than 15% of the tumors. These copy number changes correlated to the expression of the mature miRNA and were largely representative of genes involved in oncogenesis. Because of the endogenous nature of these molecules and their significant level of alteration in melanoma, miRNA species represent valuable targets for both diagnosis and therapy.

MOVING FROM RESEARCH AND DISCOVERY INTO THE CLINIC: THE NEXT GENERATION OF GENOMIC RESEARCH

The vast potential of genomic technology to transform the diagnosis of melanocytic neoplasms and the therapy of advanced melanoma is beginning to be felt. CGH has been useful to differentiate melanocytic lesions for melanoma and potentially could be useful in subcategorizing melanoma for therapeutic and prognostic purposes. RNA microarray, SAGE, and CGH analyses have yielded fundamental insights into melanoma biology that will be translated into novel therapeutic targets and novel molecules that may improve the treatment of this resistant cancer. SNPs appear to be useful to determine the clearance and metabolism of drugs and potentially could improve the therapeutic index and confidence with which these drugs can be administered. Given current in vivo experiments being conducted using siRNAs, it is not inconceivable that small molecule inhibitors designed along these lines may soon be viable for use in the clinic. In short, the repertoire of genomic therapies currently available provides us with a formidable array of tools with which to tackle the problem of recurrent melanoma.

REFERENCES

1. Williamson AR. The Merck Gene Index project. Drug Discov Today 1999; 4(3): 115–122.
2. Strausberg RL, Buetow KH, Emmert-Buck MR, et al. The cancer genome anatomy project: building an annotated gene index. Trends Genet 2000; 16(3):103–106.
3. Brenner S, Johnson M, Bridgham J, et al. Gene expression analysis by massively parallel signature sequencing (MPSS) on microbead arrays. Nat Biotechnol 2000; 18(6):630–634.
4. Velculescu VE, Zhang L, Vogelstein B, et al. Serial analysis of gene expression. Science 1995; 270(5235):484–487.
5. Lander ES, Linton LM, Birren B, et al. Initial sequencing and analysis of the human genome. Nature 2001; 409(6822):860–921.
6. Vilain C, Vassart G. Small amplified RNA-SAGE. Methods Mol Biol 2004; 258: 135–152.
7. Neilson L, Andalibi A, Kang D, et al. Molecular phenotype of the human oocyte by PCR-SAGE. Genomics 2000; 63(1):13–24.
8. Peters DG, Kassam AB, Yonas H, et al. Comprehensive transcript analysis in small quantities of mRNA by SAGE-lite. Nucleic Acids Res 1999; 27(24):e39.
9. Datson NA, van der Perk-de Jong J, van den Berg MP, et al. MicroSAGE: a modified procedure for serial analysis of gene expression in limited amounts of tissue. Nucleic Acids Res 1999; 27(5):1300–1307.
10. Saha S, Sparks AB, Rago C, et al. Using the transcriptome to annotate the genome. Nat Biotechnol 2002; 20(5):508–512.
11. Gowda M, Jantasuriyarat C, Dean RA, et al. Robust-LongSAGE (RL-SAGE): a substantially improved LongSAGE method for gene discovery and transcriptome analysis. Plant Physiol 2004; 134(3):890–897.
12. Davies H, Bignell GR, Cox C, et al. Mutations of the BRAF gene in human cancer. Nature 2002; 417(6892):949–954.
13. Pollock PM, Meltzer PS. A genome-based strategy uncovers frequent BRAF mutations in melanoma. Cancer Cell 2002; 2(1):5–7.
14. Smalley KS, Herlyn M. Targeting intracellular signaling pathways as a novel strategy in melanoma therapeutics. Ann N Y Acad Sci 2005; 1059:16–25.
15. Kalinsky K, Haluska FG. Novel inhibitors in the treatment of metastatic melanoma. Expert Rev Anticancer Ther 2007; 7(5):715–24.
16. Monzon J, Liu L, Brill H, et al. CDKN2A mutations in multiple primary melanomas. N Engl J Med 1998; 338(13):879–87.

17. Holland EA, Schmid H, Kefford RF, et al. CDKN2A (P16(INK4a)) and CDK4 mutation analysis in 131 Australian melanoma probands: effect of family history and multiple primary melanomas. Genes Chromosomes Cancer 1999; 25(4):339–348.
18. Papp T, Pemsel H, Zimmermann R, et al. Mutational analysis of the N-ras, p53, p16INK4a, CDK4, and MC1R genes in human congenital melanocytic naevi. J Med Genet 1999; 36(8):610–614.
19. Smith AP, Weeraratna AT, Spears JR, et al. SAGE identification and fluorescence imaging analysis of genes and transcripts in melanomas and precursor lesions. Cancer Biol Ther 2004; 3(1):104–109.
20. Weeraratna AT, Becker D, Carr KM, et al. Generation and analysis of melanoma SAGE libraries: SAGE advice on the melanoma transcriptome. Oncogene 2004; 23(12):2264–2274.
21. Leotlela PD, Wade MS, Duray PH, et al. Claudin-1 overexpression in melanoma is regulated by PKC and contributes to melanoma cell motility. Oncogene 2007; 26(26):3846–3856.
22. Moschos SJ, Smith AP, Mandic M, et al. SAGE and antibody array analysis of melanoma-infiltrated lymph nodes: identification of Ubc9 as an important molecule in advanced-stage melanomas. Oncogene 2007; 26(29):4216–4225.
23. Korner H, Epanchintsev A, Berking C, et al. Digital karyotyping reveals frequent inactivation of the dystrophin/DMD gene in malignant melanoma. Cell Cycle 2007; 6(2):189–198.
24. Touloukian CE, Leitner WW, Robbins PF, et al. Mining the melanosome for tumor vaccine targets: P.polypeptide is a novel tumor-associated antigen. Cancer Res 2001; 61(22):8100–8104.
25. Weeraratna AT, Nagel JE, de Mello-Coelho V, et al. Gene expression profiling: from microarrays to medicine. J Clin Immunol 2004; 24(3):213–224.
26. Kim B, Kim H, Song BJ, et al. Oligonucleotide DNA chips are useful adjuncts in epigenetic studies of glioblastomas. Neuropathology 2006; 26(5):409–416.
27. Greer BT, Khan J. Diagnostic classification of cancer using DNA microarrays and artificial intelligence. Ann N Y Acad Sci 2004; 1020:49–66.
28. Kim S, Dougherty ER, Bittner ML, et al. General nonlinear framework for the analysis of gene interaction via multivariate expression arrays. J Biomed Opt 2000; 5(4):411–424.
29. Mocellin S, Rossi CR. Principles of gene microarray data analysis. Adv Exp Med Biol 2007; 593:19–30.
30. Bittner M, Meltzer P, Chen Y, et al. Molecular classification of cutaneous malignant melanoma by gene expression profiling. Nature 2000; 406(6795):536–540.
31. Clark EA, Golub TR, Lander ES, et al. Genomic analysis of metastasis reveals an essential role for RhoC. Nature 2000; 406(6795):532–535.
32. Dissanayake SK, Wade M, Johnson CE, et al. The Wnt5A/protein kinase C pathway mediates motility in melanoma cells via the inhibition of metastasis suppressors and initiation of an epithelial to mesenchymal transition. J Biol Chem 2007; 282(23): 17259–17271.
33. Jaeger J, Koczan D, Thiesen HJ, et al. Gene expression signatures for tumor progression, tumor subtype, and tumor thickness in laser-microdissected melanoma tissues. Clin Cancer Res 2007; 13(3):806–815.
34. Critchley-Thorne RJ, Yan N, Nacu S, et al. Down-regulation of the interferon signaling pathway in T lymphocytes from patients with metastatic melanoma. PLoS Med 2007; 4(5):e176.

35. Chen DS, Soen Y, Stuge TB, et al. Marked differences in human melanoma antigen-specific T cell responsiveness after vaccination using a functional microarray. PLoS Med 2005; 2(10):e265.
36. Jensen EH, Lewis JM, McLoughlin JM, et al. Down-regulation of pro-apoptotic genes is an early event in the progression of malignant melanoma. Ann Surg Oncol 2007; 14(4):1416–1423.
37. Torisu-Itakura H, Lee JH, Scheri RP, et al. Molecular characterization of inflammatory genes in sentinel and nonsentinel nodes in melanoma. Clin Cancer Res 2007; 13(11):3125–3132.
38. Bai X, Wu J, Zhang Q, et al. Third-generation human mitochondria-focused cDNA microarray and its bioinformatic tools for analysis of gene expression. Biotechniques 2007; 42(3):365–375.
39. Deli T, Varga N, Adam A, et al. Functional genomics of calcium channels in human melanoma cells. Int J Cancer 2007; 121(1):55–65.
40. Aea D, Chodkiewicz C, Garrett C, et al. Microarray analysis of colon cancer outcome: Preliminary results of a randomized phase II study. Presented at: Gastrointestinal Cancers Symposium, ASCO GI 2006, Orlando, FL.
41. Pavey S, Johansson P, Packer L, et al. Microarray expression profiling in melanoma reveals a BRAF mutation signature. Oncogene 2004; 23(23):4060–4067.
42. Johansson P, Pavey S, Hayward N. Confirmation of a BRAF mutation-associated gene expression signature in melanoma. Pigment Cell Res 2007; 20(3):216–221.
43. Hoek KS, Schlegel NC, Brafford P, et al. Metastatic potential of melanomas defined by specific gene expression profiles with no BRAF signature. Pigment Cell Res 2006; 19(4):290–302.
44. Gyorffy B, Lage H. A Web-based data warehouse on gene expression in human malignant melanoma. J Invest Dermatol 2007; 127(2):394–399.
45. Timar J, Meszaros L, Ladanyi A, et al. Melanoma genomics reveals signatures of sensitivity to bio- and targeted therapies. Cell Immunol 2006; 244(2):154–157.
46. Kallioniemi OP, Kallioniemi A, Sudar D, et al. Comparative genomic hybridization: a rapid new method for detecting and mapping DNA amplification in tumors. Semin Cancer Biol 1993; 4(1):41–46.
47. Oostlander AE, Meijer GA, Ylstra B. Microarray-based comparative genomic hybridization and its applications in human genetics. Clin Genet 2004; 66(6):488–495.
48. Speicher MR, Prescher G, du Manoir S, et al. Chromosomal gains and losses in uveal melanomas detected by comparative genomic hybridization. Cancer Res 1994; 54(14): 3817–3823.
49. White JS, McLean IW, Becker RL, et al. Correlation of comparative genomic hybridization results of 100 archival uveal melanomas with patient survival. Cancer Genet Cytogenet 2006; 170(1):29–39.
50. Bastian BC, Wesselmann U, Pinkel D, et al. Molecular cytogenetic analysis of Spitz nevi shows clear differences to melanoma. J Invest Dermatol 1999; 113(6): 1065–1069.
51. Bastian BC, Olshen AB, LeBoit PE, et al. Classifying melanocytic tumors based on DNA copy number changes. Am J Pathol 2003; 163(5):1765–1770.
52. Curtin JA, Busam K, Pinkel D, et al. Somatic activation of KIT in distinct subtypes of melanoma. J Clin Oncol 2006; 24(26):4340–4346.
53. Maldonado JL, Fridlyand J, Patel H, et al. Determinants of BRAF mutations in primary melanomas. J Natl Cancer Inst 2003; 95(24):1878–1890.

54. McLeod HL, Yu J. Cancer pharmacogenomics: SNPs, chips, and the individual patient. Cancer Invest 2003; 21(4):630–640.

55. Velasquez JL, Lipkin SM. What are SNPs and haplotypes and how will they help us manage the prevention of adult cancer? Curr Oncol Rep 2005; 7(6):475–479.

56. Schmidt CW. HapMap: building a database with blocks. EHP Toxicogenomics 2003; 111(1T):A16.

57. Hirakawa M, Tanaka T, Hashimoto Y, et al. JSNP: a database of common gene variations in the Japanese population. Nucleic Acids Res 2002; 30(1):158–162.

58. Jiang R, Duan J, Windemuth A, et al. Genome-wide evaluation of the public SNP databases. Pharmacogenomics 2003; 4(6):779–789.

59. Thorisson GA, Stein LD. The SNP Consortium website: past, present and future. Nucleic Acids Res 2003; 31(1):124–127.

60. Giacomini KM, Brett CM, Altman RB, et al. The pharmacogenetics research network: from SNP discovery to clinical drug response. Clin Pharmacol Ther 2007; 81(3): 328–345.

61. Freimuth RR, Stormo GD, McLeod HL. PolyMAPr: programs for polymorphism database mining, annotation, and functional analysis. Hum Mutat 2005; 25(2): 110–117.

62. Sapolsky RJ, Hsie L, Berno A, et al. High-throughput polymorphism screening and genotyping with high-density oligonucleotide arrays. Genet Anal 1999; 14(5–6): 187–192.

63. Komura D, Shen F, Ishikawa S, et al. Genome-wide detection of human copy number variations using high-density DNA oligonucleotide arrays. Genome Res 2006; 16(12): 1575–1584.

64. Onken MD, Worley LA, Person E, et al. Loss of heterozygosity of chromosome 3 detected with single nucleotide polymorphisms is superior to monosomy 3 for predicting metastasis in uveal melanoma. Clin Cancer Res 2007; 13(10):2923–2927.

65. Howell WM, Turner SJ, Theaker JM, et al. Cytokine gene single nucleotide polymorphisms and susceptibility to and prognosis in cutaneous malignant melanoma. Eur J Immunogenet 2003; 30(6):409–414.

66. Benbow U, Tower GB, Wyatt CA, et al. High levels of MMP-1 expression in the absence of the 2G single nucleotide polymorphism is mediated by p38 and ERK1/2 mitogen-activated protein kinases in VMM5 melanoma cells. J Cell Biochem 2002; 86(2):307–319.

67. Stark M, Hayward N. Genome-wide loss of heterozygosity and copy number analysis in melanoma using high-density single-nucleotide polymorphism arrays. Cancer Res 2007; 67(6):2632–2642.

68. Garraway LA, Widlund HR, Rubin MA, et al. Integrative genomic analyses identify MITF as a lineage survival oncogene amplified in malignant melanoma. Nature 2005; 436(7047):117–122.

69. James MR, Roth RB, Shi MM, et al. BRAF polymorphisms and risk of melanocytic neoplasia. J Invest Dermatol 2005; 125(6):1252–1258.

70. James MR, Hayward NK, Dumenil T, et al. Epidermal growth factor gene (EGF) polymorphism and risk of melanocytic neoplasia. J Invest Dermatol 2004; 123(4): 760–762.

71. Packer LM, Pavey SJ, Boyle GM, et al. Gene expression profiling in melanoma identifies novel downstream effectors of p14ARF. Int J Cancer 2007; 121(4):784–790.

72. Howell WM, Bateman AC, Turner SJ, et al. Influence of vascular endothelial growth factor single nucleotide polymorphisms on tumour development in cutaneous malignant melanoma. Genes Immun 2002; 3(4):229–232.
73. Caplen NJ, Mousses S. Short interfering RNA (siRNA)-mediated RNA interference (RNAi) in human cells. Ann N Y Acad Sci 2003; 1002:56–62.
74. Fewell GD, Schmitt K. Vector-based RNAi approaches for stable, inducible and genome-wide screens. Drug Discov Today 2006; 11(21–22):975–982.
75. Bartel DP. MicroRNAs: genomics, biogenesis, mechanism, and function. Cell 2004; 116(2):281–297.
76. Sen CK, Roy S. miRNA: licensed to kill the messenger. DNA Cell Biol 2007; 26(4): 193–194.
77. Griffiths-Jones S. The microRNA Registry. Nucleic Acids Res 2004; 32(database issue):D109–D111.
78. Thermann R, Hentze MW. Drosophila miR2 induces pseudo-polysomes and inhibits translation initiation. Nature 2007; 447(7146):875–878.
79. Chendrimada TP, Finn KJ, Ji X, et al. MicroRNA silencing through RISC recruitment of eIF6. Nature 2007; 447(7146):823–828.
80. Hingorani SR, Jacobetz MA, Robertson GP, et al. Suppression of BRAF(V599E) in human melanoma abrogates transformation. Cancer Res 2003; 63(17):5198–5202.
81. Mousses S, Caplen NJ, Cornelison R, et al. RNAi microarray analysis in cultured mammalian cells. Genome Res 2003; 13(10):2341–2347.
82. Liang Z, Yoon Y, Votaw J, et al. Silencing of CXCR4 blocks breast cancer metastasis. Cancer Res 2005; 65(3):967–971.
83. Payne AS, Cornelius LA. The role of chemokines in melanoma tumor growth and metastasis. J Invest Dermatol 2002; 118(6):915–922.
84. Scala S, Giuliano P, Ascierto PA, et al. Human melanoma metastases express functional CXCR4. Clin Cancer Res 2006; 12(8):2427–2433.
85. Gaur A, Jewell DA, Liang Y, et al. Characterization of microRNA expression levels and their biological correlates in human cancer cell lines. Cancer Res 2007; 67(6): 2456–2468.
86. Zhang L, Huang J, Yang N, et al. microRNAs exhibit high frequency genomic alterations in human cancer. Proc Natl Acad Sci U S A 2006; 103(24):9136–9141.

5

RAS Signaling in Melanoma Development and Prevention

Marie-France Demierre

Boston University School of Medicine, Boston University Medical Center, Boston, Massachusetts, U.S.A.

INTRODUCTION

Cutaneous melanoma has continued to increase at a skyrocketing pace. In the United States alone, 62,480 newly diagnosed invasive melanomas have been estimated in 2008 along with an additional 54,020 cases of in situ melanomas (1,2). At this rate, currently, one in 59 Americans will develop invasive melanoma during their lifetime, a significant increase from 1 in 1500 in 1930. Of significant concern has been the lack of impact, in the last two decades, of prevention strategies on the incidence of thick melanomas (3). The extremely poor survival of patients with advanced or metastatic melanoma and inherent aggressive nature of the disease has underlined the ineffectiveness of current treatment strategies (4). Chemoprevention has remained an underexplored prevention approach that could target this fatal cancer by preventing, delaying, or reversing the malignant transformation of a melanocyte and its subsequent invasion (5). Chemoprevention should ideally complement ongoing prevention approaches.

Examples of successful chemoprevention approaches include tamoxifen for the reduction of breast cancer, the first Food and Drug Administration (FDA)-approved chemopreventive agent celecoxib for familial adenomatous polyposis, and both topical diclophenac and imiquimod for actinic keratoses.

Table 1 Prerequisites for a Valid Melanoma Chemoprevention Strategy

Elements of a strong scientific rationale
- Determination of the underlying molecular mechanisms of carcinogenesis
- Discovery of genetic markers that identify the early events in the carcinogenic process
- Availability of drugs that can target the molecular mechanism of carcinogenesis

Long-term safety of potential candidate agents
- Availability of long-term human safety data
- Availability of animal tumor models that permit preclinical trials of evaluation of drug toxicity

Critical elements of a rigorous chemoprevention clinical trial design
- Availability of animal tumor models that permit preclinical trials evaluation of drug efficacy
- Compilation of data from epidemiologic, basic science, and cancer research literature that can yield candidate prevention agents for in vitro or in vivo testing
- Availability of molecular or histologic markers of the carcinogenic process to be used as endpoints and to obviate the need for prolonged and costly trials
- Access to defined groups at very high risk for the disease

Despite these successes, in other settings, large randomized trials based on epidemiologic observations yielded disappointing results in cervical cancer (6), colorectal cancers (7), lung cancer (8), and an increased incidence of second primary head and neck cancers with oral α-tocopherol supplementation (9). These failures have highlighted the critical need for a strong scientific rationale, long-term safety of potential agents, and rigorous chemoprevention trial design (10,11). A scientific rationale is of particular relevance to melanoma (12,13). Recently, several lines of data have indicated that RAS signaling, an important early event in melanoma carcinogenesis, could represent a potential target for melanoma chemoprevention (12). In the context of known prerequisites needed for a valid melanoma chemoprevention strategy (Table 1) (13,14), the scientific rationale of targeting RAS signaling in melanoma chemoprevention is discussed.

RAS SIGNALING AND MELANOMA

Cutaneous melanoma is a cancer resulting from detrimental gene-environment interactions, with the environmental agent widely accepted as ultraviolet (UV) radiation (15). The understanding that UV-induced melanoma is a multistep process (16) provides opportunities to intervene and possibly reverse the process. The effects of UV radiation on the skin are complex and include UV signature mutations, DNA oxidative damage, and immunosuppression. It is likely that several pathways can lead to cutaneous melanoma. Recent epidemiologic data as well as molecular data provide early support for at least two divergent pathways, one associated with melanocytic proliferation and the other one with chronic sun exposure (17–20). In developing agents for the chemoprevention of melanoma, scientific rationale must be consistent with known pathways implicated in the pathogenesis of cutaneous melanoma. Data have suggested that alterations of RAS pathway genes (21) are critically important in the pathogenesis of sporadic cutaneous melanoma, with *NRAS* and *BRAF* mutations rarely overlapping (22–25). Activating *BRAF* mutations are present in up to 66% of melanomas (22). *BRAF* mutations are found in melanomas that occur in intermittently sun-exposed body sites but are rare or absent in melanomas developing in completely sun-protected areas, e.g., mucosal melanomas (18). *NRAS* mutations have been reported in 5% to 33% of melanomas (26,27). *RAS* genes are clearly a target of UV light with identifiable UV signature mutations, although the role of UV is not as evident in *BRAF* mutations (28). To date, in one study, epidemiologic data indicated that high UV exposure in early age was associated with melanoma with *BRAF* mutation while later-life UV exposure was associated with melanoma with *NRAS* mutations (29). The constellation of findings suggests that *BRAF* mutations in cutaneous melanoma do not occur in the absence of sun exposure.

The role of RAS signaling in melanoma is likely multifaceted. Transgenic murine models have suggested an essential role of RAS in tumor maintenance and angiogenesis (30,31). In in vitro and in vivo models, *NRAS* mutations have been associated with chemoresistance to cisplatin (32). *NRAS* and *BRAF* mutations represent alternative genetic changes resulting in the activation of the same signaling pathway, the RAS/ERK/MAPK cascade, driving tumorigenesis. Activated BRAF kinase phosphorylates downstream targets via MEK such as ERK, ultimately influencing aberrant growth. With regard to oncogenic relevance, it is known that processes involved in tumor growth, progression, and metastasis are mediated by signaling pathways initiated by activated receptor tyrosinase kinases (Fig. 1) (33). Since RAS functions downstream of several receptor tyrosine kinases, RAS activation represents an important oncogenic mechanism.

RAS SIGNALING AND NEVI

NRAS mutations have been found not only in cutaneous melanoma but also in adjacent congenital nevi, as well as in adjacent dysplastic nevi in some cases, reinforcing the notion that nevi and cutaneous melanoma have a shared cellular response to some mutagenic agents (e.g., UV) (26,34). Overall, there appears to be a low frequency of *NRAS* mutations in dysplastic nevi (35–38) as compared with congenital melanocytic nevi, whereby reported rates varying from 28% to 56% (37,39,40). In one study, congenital nevi known to be present at birth harbored no *BRAF* mutations, while nevi with histologic features described as "congenital pattern," but not present at birth, had *BRAF* mutations, further supporting the finding that *BRAF* mutations were uncommon in the absence of sun exposure (40).

There exists a scientific rationale for targeting RAS signaling in melanoma chemoprevention, as exemplified by early clinical data on sorafenib (BAY

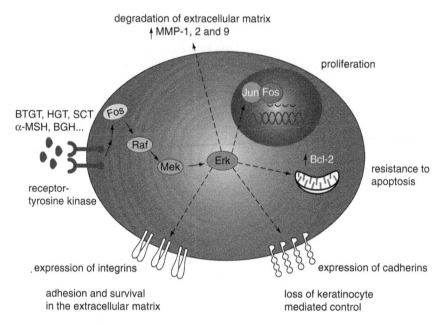

Figure 1 The RAS-MAPK signal transduction pathway. RAF kinases are serine/threonine protein kinases that initiate the mitogenic kinase cascade that ultimately modulates gene expression by way of the phosphorylation of transcription factors such as Jun, Elk1, c-Ets1/2, STAT 1/3, or Myc. *Source*: From Ref. 33 (*See Color Insert*).

43-9006, a C-RAF/BRAF inhibitor) (33) in metastatic melanoma. Sorafenib in combination with chemotherapeutic drugs initially showed long-lasting clinical responses in a subset of melanoma patients. However, sorafenib's important side effects of hypertension and skin eruptions have precluded its use in the prevention setting. While RAS signaling might not be relevant to all forms of cutaneous melanoma—for example, the desmoplastic variant frequently does not harbor an activating mutation of *BRAF* (41)—this signaling pathway appears to represent a reasonable target for chemoprevention given its mutation rate in approximately 50% of cutaneous melanomas. The current strategy of evaluating drugs targeting RAS signaling in breast cancers harboring *RAS* mutations (42) provides further support for focusing on RAS signaling in melanoma chemoprevention.

PREREQUISITES TO DEVELOPING MELANOMA CHEMOPREVENTION

Proof of Effectiveness: Data on Agents Targeting RAS Signaling

A potential chemoprevention intervention should have a broad spectrum of activity that addresses aspects of the "hallmarks of cancer," namely, (*i*) self sufficiency in growth signals, (*ii*) insensitivity to antigrowth signals, (*iii*) apoptosis evasion, (*iv*) unlimited replicative potential, (*v*) sustained angiogenesis, and (*vi*) tissue invasion and metastasis (43,44). Among the three agents that target RAS signaling—statins, apomine, and perillyl alcohol—all fulfill the prerequisite of scientific rationale of chemoprevention; however, statins have the most data and a broad spectrum of activity (12). Mounting evidence indicates that statins have a role in cancer prevention, with preclinical data on anti-proliferative, proapoptotic, angiostatic, anti-invasive, and immunomodulatory effects (45). The rate-limiting step of the mevalonate pathway is the conversion of 3-hydroxy-3-methylglutaryl coenzyme A (HMG-CoA) to mevalonate, cata-lyzed by HMG-CoA reductase. Blockade of the rate-limiting step results in decreased levels of mevalonate and its downstream products, including the isoprenoids geranylgeranyl pyrophosphate (GGPP) and farnesyl pyrophosphate (FPP), needed for the posttranslational modification of RAS proteins and small GTP-binding proteins of the Rab, Rac, and Rho family, belonging to the RAS superfamily (Fig. 2). Statins' inhibition of protein prenylation results in the absence of posttranslational modification, thus impacting RAS proteins' function and their oncogenicity. In one in vitro cancer model, statins reduced proliferation and survival signals in susceptible phenotypes (42). There may be differences between hydrophilic and lipophylic statins. The lipophilicity of statins like lovastatin, fluvastatin, and simvastatin allow them to directly cross cell mem-branes and exert pleiotropic effects in many extrahepatic tissues (46).

There is a strong rationale for statin use as a melanoma chemoprevention agent (12). Data indicate that statin effects on melanoma development appear to be principally via inhibiting geranylgeranylation of Rho and other small G-proteins and less by inhibiting farnesylation of RAS. RhoA and RhoC are known to be widely expressed in human melanoma and have been implicated in causing melanoma metastases. Overexpressed RhoA and RhoC must be ger-anylgeranylated before melanoma reaches its full invasive potential. In pre-clinical models, lovastatin induced caspase-dependent apoptosis in multiple human melanoma cell lines via a geranylation-specific mechanism (47). The statin atorvastatin, at doses used in treating hypercholesterolemia, could revert the metastatic phenotype in human melanoma cells expressing RhoC (48).

Although compelling preclinical data have supported the development of statins in melanoma chemoprevention, to date, epidemiologic data have not confirmed these preclinical results. One meta-analysis of randomized control trials of statins in cardiovascular disease, with patients receiving therapy for at least four years, revealed no significant difference between statin and observa-tion groups with regard to the secondary outcome of melanoma incidence (49). Similarly, in other cancers, the epidemiologic data has also failed to demonstrate consistent findings across studies (50). This is due in part to the recognized difficulties with publication bias, incomplete acquisition of unpublished data, and the fact that most studies have been designed around cardiac and vascular endpoints (49,50). Data indicating that lipophilic statins could exert direct

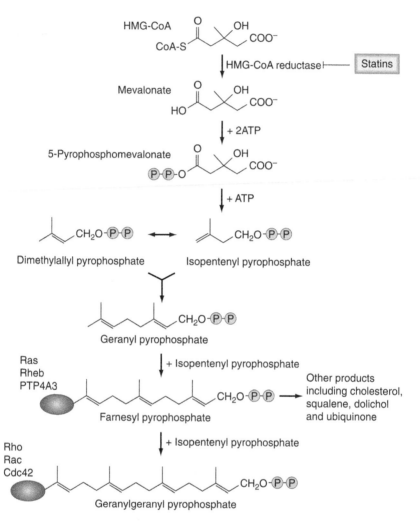

Figure 2 Mevalonate pathway. Statins inhibit the conversion of HMG-CoA to mevalonate. Molecules of ATP are then used to phosphorylate mevalonate to pyrophosphomevalonate, which is then converted to IPP. IPP can be reversibly converted to DMAPP. IPP and DMAPP can then be combined to form the 10-carbon isoprenoid GPP. Additional IPPs can be added to produce FPP, the 15-carbon isoprenoid, and GGPP, the 20-carbon isoprenoid. Inhibition of this pathway by statins prevents the formation of both mevalonate and its downstream product IPP. This inhibition can be reversed completely with mevalonate. Supplementation with FPP will restore farnesylation but not geranylgeranylation, as IPP is not available to convert FPP into GGPP. Supplementation with GGPP will only restore geranylgeranylation. Several other branches of this pathway can convert FPP into various other products, including cholesterol. In general, FPP helps prenylate proteins in the RAS, Rheb, and PTP4A3 families, whereas GGPP helps prenylate proteins in the Rho, Rac, and Cdc42 families. A few G-proteins (including RHOB and *NRAS*) can be either farnesylated or geranylgeranylated. *Abbreviations*: HMG-CoA, 3-hydroxy-3-methylglutaryl coenzyme A; ATP, adenosine triphosphate; IPP, isopentenyl pyrophosphate; DMAPP, dimethylallyl pyrophosphate; GPP, geranyl pyrophosphate; FPP, farnesyl pyrophosphate; GGPP, geranylgeranyl pyrophosphate. *Source*: From Ref. 45 (*See Color Insert*).

anticancer activity on in vitro and in vivo tumor growth inhibition of breast cancer, while hydrophilic statins did not (42) suggest that statins' inherent properties may impact cancer prevention activity.

Apomine, a novel biphosphonate ester with nonmyelosuppressive properties, has been noted to activate the farnesoid X receptor, increase the rate of degradation of HMG-CoA reductase, inhibit cell proliferation, and induce tumor-cell apoptosis (51). It also appears to have a membrane-mediated cytolytic mechanism, independent of *NRAS* farnesylation and caspase-3 activation (52). This agent was evaluated in a murine chemoprevention model. Powell et al. used a transgenic mouse model, the TPRAS model, that expressed a human-activated Ha-RAS gene driven by a mouse tyrosinase promoter, in which cutaneous melanomas could be induced with topical application of 7,12-dimethylbenz[a] anthracene (DMBA) (53). In this model, topical application of apomine to TPRAS mice resulted in a 55% reduction in melanoma incidence (54). The TPRAS model was used to screen another agent targeting RAS signaling, perillyl alcohol, a monoterpene isolated from essential oils (54,55). In vitro data had suggested that perillyl alcohol inhibited detectable RAS protein expression and the activation of downstream targets, including mitogen-activated protein kinases and Akt (55). Topical application of perillyl alcohol to TPRAS mice resulted in delay of melanoma and a 25% to 35% reduction in melanoma incidence (55). Early phase studies with topical perillyl alcohol have been initiated at the University of Arizona.

Topical Vs. Oral Administration

A relevant consideration for melanoma chemoprevention is the administration of the agent itself (43). While most prevention interventions are given orally, to adequately deliver the drug to the organ or tissue of interest, a topical approach could be considered in melanoma. However, early studies of topical retinoids as chemoprevention agents for melanoma illustrated the challenges of providing sufficient drug delivery to all areas of the body. Possibly, daily application might not be necessary to achieve a biological effect, especially if the agent could repair DNA or existing photodamage or induce cell death of a DNA-damaged melanocyte. Furthermore, for some individuals, daily oral administration may not be acceptable, with even minimal side effects affecting compliance. In contrast, oral administration could potentially deliver an agent to all tissues, affecting the risk of developing melanoma anywhere in the body, although drug delivery would be quite variable depending on the tissue of interest. Ultimately, both approaches deserve further study.

Long-Term Safety of Candidate Agents

The cardiovascular toxicities and enhanced cardiovascular events with use of COX-2 inhibitors have highlighted the critical need for long-term safety data for agents used in chemoprevention. Chemoprevention studies differ significantly from therapeutic trials where toxic therapies would be accepted in exchange for prolonged survival, disease-free interval, or quality of life. In chemoprevention trials, however, the "at risk" individuals are "healthy." The potential benefit (prevention or delay in cancer occurrence) must be large and the risk small; in other words, the "therapeutic index" for a chemoprevention intervention must be acceptable (14). Using transgenic murine models to evaluate toxicity and dose limitations of new drugs is therefore appropriate. Among the potential chemoprevention agents for melanoma that satisfy the scientific rationale, statins have known and acceptable toxicities. Is this sufficient to move forward with large-scale phase III studies? No. While statins can be given for a long period (13), subtle minor toxicities that could affect drug compliance should be evaluated in placebo-controlled randomized phase II studies.

Indeed, in other cancers, failures to carefully evaluate parameters that can modulate relevant endpoints (10) have led to overestimation of the potential chemoprevention benefit and underestimation of the risks (11). How can melanoma chemoprevention move forward? As a first step, validating biomarkers that will help predict the likelihood of developing cancer or melanoma (prognostic marker) (56) is necessary. Studies are underway at the University of California, Irvine, evaluating possible biomarkers of melanoma. While in melanoma the best type of intermediate marker, one that will have prognostic value as to the likelihood of developing melanoma, has not yet been identified, tumor angiogenesis represents an appropriate target of cancer prevention, as RAS signaling appears to be involved in tumor angiogenesis in melanoma (57). Studies of vascular endothelial growth factor (VEGF) in dysplatic nevi may provide further clues to the relevance of angiogenesis in melanoma (58). Taking advantage of genetically engineered murine models to validate biomarkers will also be helpful. Once prognostic markers are identified, prospective clinical studies and trials determining the cancer preventive role, for example, of statins in high-risk groups and in patients with a history of melanoma and multiple nevi or dysplastic nevi, will allow for a better assessment of the true effect of statins on melanoma incidence.

Chemoprevention Agent Development

In moving a potential chemoprevention agent forward, the level of evidence must be critically assessed (10) (Table 2). All of the evidence should be weighted, experimental, epidemiologic, and clinical data, and should be that obtained in early phase studies prior to moving a candidate agent forward. While epidemiologic data allows hypotheses to be generated, supporting preclinical (in vitro, in vivo) and clinical data, as well as results from well-designed phase I and II chemoprevention studies are necessary prior to moving to full-scale phase III trials (10–12). Statins appear to satisfy the majority of the prerequisites for a valid melanoma chemoprevention strategy (12,13). The rationale is clear and the pleiotropic effects of statins would target the "hallmarks of cancer." Long-term safety

Table 2 Criteria of Evidence to Move Chemopreventive Agents to Large Randomized Trials

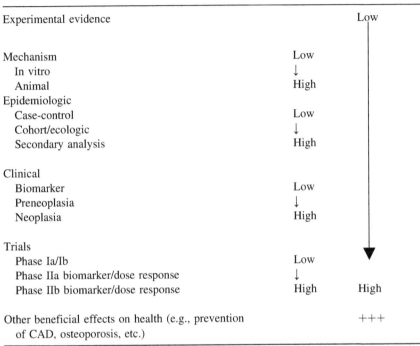

Experimental evidence		Low
Mechanism	Low	
In vitro	↓	
Animal	High	
Epidemiologic		
Case-control	Low	
Cohort/ecologic	↓	
Secondary analysis	High	
Clinical		
Biomarker	Low	
Preneoplasia	↓	
Neoplasia	High	
Trials		
Phase Ia/Ib	Low	
Phase IIa biomarker/dose response	↓	
Phase IIb biomarker/dose response	High	High
Other beneficial effects on health (e.g., prevention of CAD, osteoporosis, etc.)		+++

⁺⁺⁺Very High.
Abbreviation: CAD, coronary artery disease.
Source: From Ref. 10.

data on statins have been established in cardiovascular disease. Since the evaluation of dose-response relationships and phase II (biomarker) efficacy studies are integral components of a chemoprevention agent development strategy (10), initiating a phase IIB chemoprevention (biomarker) trial of statins (two different doses) in early stage melanoma patients with at least two clinical atypical nevi is a reasonable first step toward this goal. At least one such trial is currently underway.

CONCLUSION

A chemoprevention strategy that would target early molecular events in melanoma could potentially result in profound improvements in the incidence and morbidity and mortality from melanoma. This chemoprevention strategy should ultimately complement ongoing melanoma-prevention/sun-protection approaches. RAS signaling is an appropriate chemoprevention target for UV-induced cutaneous melanoma. While apomine, perillyl alcohol, and statins all target RAS signaling, currently, the strongest cancer prevention data appear to be with the latter, which not only target RAS signaling but also affect the hallmarks of cancer (45). Carefully establishing valid biomarkers in melanoma chemoprevention and determining dose-response relationships will be necessary before one can prospectively evaluate the role of statins in melanoma prevention.

REFERENCES

1. Jemal A, Siegel R, Ward E, et al. Cancer statistics, 2008. CA Cancer J Clin 2008; 58:71–96.
2. ACS. Facts and Figures. American Cancer Society. 2007.
3. Demierre MF, Chung C, Miller DR, et al. Early detection of thick melanomas in the US? "Beware" of the nodular subtype. Arch Dermatol 2005; 141:745–750.
4. Tsao H, Atkins MB, Sober AJ. Management of cutaneous melanoma. N Engl J Med 2004; 351(10):998–1012.
5. Demierre MF, Nathanson L. Chemoprevention of melanoma: an unexplored strategy. J Clin Oncol 2003; 21(1):158–165.
6. Follen M, Vlastos AT, Meyskens FL Jr., et al. Why phase II trials in cervical chemoprevention are negative: what have we learned? Cancer Causes Control 2002; 13(9):855–873.
7. Viner JL, Umar A, Hawk ET. Chemoprevention of colorectal cancer: problems, progress, and prospects. Gastroenterol Clin North Am 2002; 31(4):971–999.
8. Omenn GS, Goodman GE, Thornquist MD, et al. Effects of a combination of beta carotene and vitamin A on lung cancer and cardiovascular disease. N Engl J Med 1996; 334(18):1150–1155.
9. Bairati I, Meyer F, Gelinas M, et al. A randomized trial of antioxidant vitamins to prevent second primary cancers in head and neck cancer patients. J Natl Cancer Inst 2005; 97(7):481–488.
10. Meyskens FL, Szabo E. How should we move the field of chemopreventive agent development forward in a productive manner? Recent Results Cancer Res 2005; 166:113–124.
11. Brenner DE, Gescher AJ. Cancer chemoprevention: lessons learned and future directions. Br J Cancer 2005; 93(7):735–739.
12. Demierre MF, Sondak VK. Cutaneous melanoma: pathogenesis and rationale for chemo-prevetion. Crit Rev Oncol Hematol 2005; 53:225–239.
13. Demierre MF, Sondak VK. Chemoprevention of melanoma: theoretical and practical considerations. Cancer Control 2005; 12(4):219–222.
14. Demierre MF. What about chemoprevention for melanoma? Curr Opin Oncol 2006; 18(2):180–184.
15. Merlino G, Noonan FP. Modeling gene-environment interactions in malignant melanoma. Trends Mol Med 2003; 9(3):102–108.
16. Dlugosz A, Merlino G, Yuspa SH. Progress in cutaneous cancer research. J Investig Dermatol Symp Proc 2002; 7(1):17–26.
17. Whiteman DC, Watt P, Purdie DM, et al. Melanocytic nevi, solar keratoses, and divergent pathways to cutaneous melanoma. J Natl Cancer Inst 2003; 95(11): 806–812.
18. Maldonado JL, Fridlyand J, Patel H, et al. Determinants of BRAF mutations in primary melanomas. J Natl Cancer Inst 2003; 95(24):1878–1890.

19. Whiteman DC, Stickley M, Watt P, et al. Anatomic site, sun exposure, and risk of cutaneous melanoma. J Clin Oncol 2006; 24(19):3172–3177.

20. Lee EY, Williamson R, Watt P, et al. Sun exposure and host phenotype as predictors of cutaneous melanoma associated with neval remnants or dermal elastosis. Int J Cancer 2006; 119(3):636–642.

21. Gray-Schopfer VC, da Rocha Dias S, Marais R. The role of B-RAF in melanoma. Cancer Metastasis Rev 2005; 24(1):165–183.

22. Davies H, Bignell GR, Cox C, et al. Mutations of the BRAF gene in human cancer. Nature 2002; 417(6892):949–954.

23. Brose MS, Volpe P, Feldman M, et al. BRAF and RAS mutations in human lung cancer and melanoma. Cancer Res 2002; 62(23):6997–7000.

24. Pollock PM, Harper UL, Hansen KS, et al. High frequency of BRAF mutations in nevi. Nat Genet 2003; 33(1):19–20.

25. Reifenberger J, Knobbe CB, Sterzinger AA, et al. Frequent alterations of Ras signaling pathway genes in sporadic malignant melanomas. Int J Cancer 2004; 109:377–384.

26. Demunter A, Stas M, Degreef H, et al. Analysis of N- and K-ras mutations in the distinctive tumor progression phases of melanoma. J Invest Dermatol 2001; 117(6): 1483–1489.

27. Omholt K, Karsberg S, Platz A, et al. Screening of N-ras Codon 61 mutations in paired primary and metastatic cutaneous melanomas: mutations occur early and persist throughout tumor progression. Clin Cancer Res 2002; 8(11):3468–3474.

28. Thomas NE, Berwick M, Cordeiro-Stone M. Could BRAF mutations in melanocytic lesions arise from DNA damage induced by ultraviolet radiation? J Invest Dermatol 2006; 126(8):1693–1696.

29. Thomas NE, Edmiston SN, Alexander A, et al. Number of nevi and early-life ambient UV exposure are associated with BRAF-mutant melanoma. Cancer Epidemiol Biomarkers Prev 2007; 16(5):991–997.

30. Chin L, Tam A, Pomerantz J, et al. Essential role for oncogenic Ras in tumour maintenance. Nature 1999; 400(6743):468–472.

31. Wong AK, Chin L. An inducible melanoma model implicates a role for RAS in tumor maintenance and angiogenesis. Cancer Metastasis Rev 2000; 19(1–2):121–129.

32. Jansen B, Schlagbauer-Wadl H, Eichler HG, et al. Activated N-ras contributes to the chemoresistance of human melanoma in severe combined immunodeficiency (SCID) mice by blocking apoptosis. Cancer Res 1997; 57(3):362–365.

33. Becker JC, Kirkwood JM, Agarwala SS, et al. Molecularly targeted therapy for melanoma: current reality and future options. Cancer 2006; 107(10):2317–2327.

34. Lee JY, Dong SM, Shin MS, et al. Genetic alterations of p16INK4a and p53 genes in sporadic dysplastic nevus. Biochem Biophys Res Commun 1997; 237:667–672.

35. Papp T, Pemsel H, Rollwitz I, et al. Mutational analysis of N-ras, p53, CDKN2A (p16(INK4a)), p14(ARF), CDK4, and MC1R genes in human dysplastic melanocytic naevi. J Med Genet 2003; 40(2):E14.

36. Albino AP, Nanus DM, Mentle IR, et al. Analysis of ras oncogenes in malignant melanoma and precursor lesions: correlation of point mutations with differentiation phenotype. Oncogene 1989; 4:1363–1374.

37. Carr J, Mackie RM. Point mutations in the N-ras oncogene in malignant melanoma and congenital naevi. Br J Dermatol 1994; 131(1):72–77.

38. Jafari M, Papp T, Kirchner S, et al. Analysis of ras mutations in human melanocytic lesions: activation of the ras gene seems to be associated with the nodular type of human malignant melanoma. J Cancer Res Clin Oncol 1995; 121(1):23–30.

39. Papp T, Pemsel H, Zimmermann R, et al. Mutational analysis of the N-ras, p53, p16INK4a, CDK4, and MC1R genes in human congenital melanocytic naevi. J Med Genet 1999; 36(8):610–614.

40. Bauer J, Curtin JA, Pinkel D, et al. Congenital melanocytic nevi frequently harbor *NRAS* mutations but no BRAF mutations. J Invest Dermatol 2007; 127(1):179–182.

41. Davison JM, Rosenbaum E, Barrett TL, et al. Absence of V599E BRAF mutations in desmoplastic melanomas. Cancer 2005; 103(4):788–792.

42. Campbell MJ, Esserman LJ, Zhou Y, et al. Breast cancer growth prevention by statins. Cancer Res 2006; 66(17):8707–8714.

43. Lao CD, Demierre MF, Sondak VK. Targeting events in melanoma carcinogenesis for the prevention of melanoma. Expert Rev Anticancer Ther 2006; 6(11):1559–1568.

44. Hanahan D, Weinberg RA. The hallmarks of cancer. Cell 2000; 100(1):57–70.

45. Demierre MF, Lippman SM, Higgins P, et al. Statins and cancer prevention. Nat Rev Cancer 2005; 5(12):930–942.

46. Ichihara K, Satoh K. Disparity between angiographic regression and clinical event rates with hydrophobic statins. Lancet 2002; 359(9324):2195–2198.

47. Shellman YG, Ribble D, Miller L, et al. Lovastatin-induced apoptosis in human melanoma cell lines. Melanoma Res 2005; 15(2):83–89.

48. Collisson EA, Kleer C, Wei M, et al. Atorvastatin prevents RhoC isoprenylation, invasion and metastasis in human melanoma cells. Molecular Cancer Therapeutics 2003; 2:941–948.

49. Dellavalle RP, Drake A, G Graber M, et al. Statins and fibrates for preventing melanoma: Cochrane Database Syst Rev 2005; (4)CD003697.

50. Bonovas S, Filioussi K, Tsavaris N, et al. Use of statins and breast cancer: a meta-analysis of seven randomized clinical trials and nine observational studies. J Clin Oncol 2005; 23(34):8606–8612.

51. Niesor E, Flach J, Weinberger C, et al. Synthetic farnesoid X receptor (FXR) agonists: a new class of cholesterol synthesis inhibitors and antiproliferative drugs. Drugs Future 1999; 24:431–438.

52. Pourpak A, Dorr RT, Meyers RO, et al. Cytotoxic activity of Apomine is due to a novel membrane-mediated cytolytic mechanism independent of apoptosis in the A375 human melanoma cell line. Invest New Drugs 2007; 25(2):107–114.

53. Powell MB, Gause PR, Hyman P, et al. Induction of melanoma in TPras transgenic mice. Carcinogenesis 1999; 20(9):1747–1753.

54. Powell BM, Alberts DS, Lluria-Prevatt M. Preclinical and clinical activity of Apomine, a novel biophosphonate ester, in the prevention and treatment of melanoma. Proc Am Assoc Cancer Res 2002; 43:1007 (abstr).

55. Lluria-Prevatt M, Morreale J, Gregus J, et al. Effects of perillyl alcohol on melanoma in the TPras mouse model. Cancer Epidemiol Biomarkers Prev 2002; 11(6):573–579.

56. Armstrong WB, Taylor TH, Meyskens FL Jr. Point: Surrogate end point biomarkers are likely to be limited in their usefulness in the development of cancer chemoprevention agents against sporadic cancers. Cancer Epidemiol Biomarkers Prev 2003; 12(7):589–592.

57. Arbiser JL. Molecular regulation of angiogenesis and tumorigenesis by signal transduction pathways: evidence of predictable and reproducible patterns of synergy in diverse neoplasms. Semin Cancer Biol 2004; 14(2):81–91.

58. Einspahr JG, Thomas TL, Saboda K, et al. Expression of VEGF and microvessel density counts in early cutaneous melanocytic lesion progression. Cancer 2007; 110(11):2519–27.

6

Targeting BRAF Activity as a Novel Paradigm for Melanoma Therapy

Keiran S.M. Smalley

H. Lee Moffitt Cancer Center & Research Institute, Tampa, Florida, U.S.A.

Keith T. Flaherty

*Abramson Cancer Center of the University of Pennsylvania,
Philadelphia, Pennsylvania, U.S.A.*

THE MITOGEN-ACTIVATED PROTEIN KINASE PATHWAY AND TRANSLATIONAL RESEARCH IN MELANOMA

It is little exaggeration to say that the discovery of activating BRAF mutations in over 60% of melanomas has revolutionized the expectations for targeted therapy in melanoma. The past 30 years of research effort have yielded very little in the way of progress and median survival for disseminated melanoma remains at 6 to 10 months. Currently, dacarbazine (DTIC) is the only cytotoxic drug approved by the U.S. Food and Drug Administration (FDA) for metastatic melanoma and is associated with response rates between 5% and 10% with little survival advantage. The discovery of *BRAF* as the major melanoma oncogene arrived at an exciting time in the era of targeted therapy development, following in the wake of the success of imatinib (Gleevec) in treating both chronic myeloid leukemia (CML) and gastrointestinal stromal tumors (GIST). The imatinib paradigm offers the tantalizing possibility that inhibiting the key oncogenic mutation responsible for disease progression (*Bcr-Abl* for CML, and *c-Kit* for

GIST) could lead to near-complete remission in the case of CML and arrest of disease progression in GIST.

Maximizing the therapeutic value of mitogen-activated protein kinase (MAPK) pathway inhibition is the central focus of clinical trials with novel RAS, RAF, and MEK inhibitors. To understand the limitations of this approach in humans, it is essential to address the efficacy associated with this approach in the most responsive models such as two-dimensional cell culture. Even in that setting, widespread apoptosis is not induced. A number of downstream consequences of MAPK pathway activity have been elucidated, providing a network of molecular markers that can be prospectively incorporated into the next generation of preclinical and clinical studies of these therapies. Data will be presented regarding the cellular consequences of perturbing the MAPK pathway in melanoma with the purpose of enumerating the potential biomarkers that have emerged in recent years.

THE ROLE OF BRAF IN MELANOMA PROGRESSION

BRAF mutations were first identified in melanoma following a genome-wide screen performed at the Sanger Institute in Cambridge, United Kingdom (1). Since then, over 50 distinct mutations in *BRAF* have been identified (2), of these the *BRAF* V600E mutation is by far the most common, accounting for over 80% of the reported mutations. The *BRAF* V600E mutation results in the substitution of glutamate in place of valine, leading to destabilization of the inactive kinase conformation switching the equilibrium toward the active form (3). Most of the transforming activity of the V600E *BRAF* is thought to result through the activation of the MAPK pathway (1). Under physiological situations, the MAPK pathway is stimulated through the interaction of growth factors with their respective cell surface receptors followed by the transmission of their signals to the interior of the cell through the small GTPase RAS (4). When active in its GTP-bound state, RAS activates a number of downstream effectors, one of which is the Raf family of serine/threonine kinases. There are three isoforms of Raf: A-Raf, BRAF, and C-Raf (also called Raf-1). Once active, Raf activates the MAPK cascade, resulting in the sequential activation of MEK1 and MEK2, which in turn activate ERK1 and ERK2 (5,6). Upon activation, the ERKs can either regulate cytoplasmic targets or can migrate to the nucleus where they phosphorylate a number of transcription factors. The V600E mutation is one of the most active *BRAF* mutations and possesses an in vitro kinase activity 500-fold greater than that of the wild-type BRAF kinase (3).

Regardless of *BRAF* V600E mutational status, virtually all melanomas have high constitutive activity in the MAPK pathway (7). In addition to activating mutations in *BRAF* (1), at least 15% of melanomas have activating mutations in *NRAS* (8–10), and a further 4% of melanomas (mostly acral and mucosal) have activating mutations in *c-Kit* (11). The incidence of *NRAS* and *BRAF* mutations in melanoma appears to be mutually exclusive and the simultaneous coexpression of both NRAS and BRAF in melanoma cells leads to senescence (12). In melanomas that lack *BRAF, NRAS,* and *c-Kit* mutations, MAPK activity arises through autocrine stimulation of growth factor receptors, such as c-met and FGFR1 (13) and cell-cell adhesion interactions, such as N-cadherin and the integrins.

Pathological studies in which melanomas are stained for MAPK pathway activity, using phospho-ERK (pERK) as a surrogate, have shown that signaling through the pathway is correlated with the malignant potential of melanomas, where the levels of pERK staining increase during the progression from dysplastic nevi to melanoma (14). Further support for a role of pERK in the progression of melanoma comes from the finding that higher pERK levels are found at the leading edge of the melanoma where the tumor is invading into the dermis (14).

The acquisition of V600E *BRAF* mutations appears to occur early in the process of oncogenic transformation, and 20% to 80% of otherwise benign melanocytic nevi are known to harbor the mutation (15). Although some nevi do progress to melanoma, this is thought to be relatively rare, and most nevi remain in a growth-arrested state throughout the patient's lifetime. It was recently shown that most nevi display the hallmarks of senescence, staining highly for the tumor suppressor p16 as well as the classical senescence marker β-galactosidase (16,17). In agreement with these findings, overexpression of the V600E BRAF in primary human melanocytes typically leads to a senescence-like phenotype (16). It is worth noting that these studies do show a heterogeneous pattern of p16 staining, and it is suggested that other pathways may also contribute to this oncogene-induced senescence. Taken together, these studies demonstrate that although *BRAF* mutations seem to be acquired at a very early, premalignant stage, there is an initial activation of antioncogenic pathways to stop further progression. It seems possible that the p16/retinoblastoma pathway plays a key role in the suppression of BRAF-mediated transformation of melanocytes.

In Vitro Evidence for BRAF Being the Major Driving Force in Melanoma

The in vitro data supporting a role for *BRAF* as the major melanoma oncogene are compelling. V600E *BRAF* is an oncogene in immortalized mouse melano-cytes (18), and selective downregulation of V600E *BRAF* using RNAi causes cell death and reversal of the melanoma phenotype (19). In vivo studies using an inducible *BRAF* RNAi xenograft model have shown reversible tumor regression, following *BRAF* knockdown (20). Increased *BRAF* activity also suppresses the activity of the melanocyte-specific transcription factor micropthalmia (MITF) diverting the melanoma cells from a differentiation pathway into a highly proliferative state (21).

Most studies of the MAPK pathway in melanoma have focused on its effects on cell proliferation. Under physiological conditions, cell cycle entry is regulated at the G1 checkpoint. Cancer cells acquire the ability to overcome the G1 cell cycle checkpoint, through the loss of key regulatory mechanisms, leading

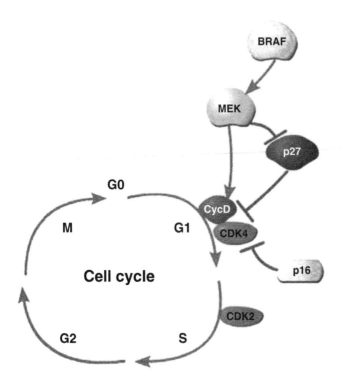

Figure 1 *BRAF* mutations drive melanoma growth by overcoming the G1 phase cell cycle checkpoint. *BRAF* mutations increase MEK activity that downregulates levels of the cell cycle inhibitor p27 and increases expression of cyclin D1 (CycD). Activation of this pathway cooperates with loss of p16 to drive uncontrolled cell growth.

to uncontrolled growth. Progression through the G1 restriction point into S phase is driven by cyclin-dependent kinases (CDK) 4 and 6, which interact with cyclin D1 as well as by CDK2, which interacts with cyclins A/E (22). Constitutive activity in the MAPK pathway resulting from *BRAF* mutation increases cyclin D1 and downregulates p27 expression in melanoma cells (23) and is likely to be one mechanism that melanoma cells use to overcome the G1 checkpoint (Fig. 1).

Activating mutations in *BRAF* also drive other processes important for melanoma progression. One troubling feature of melanoma is their exceptional resistance to apoptosis, and there is some suggestion that BRAF may contribute toward this through MAPK activation. Studies in epithelial cancers have shown that inhibition of ERK increases sensitivity to cisplatin and increases levels of apoptosis following serum withdrawal (24). In a human melanoma cell xenograft model, there is evidence that overexpression of *NRAS* increases chemoresistance (25). A number of groups have demonstrated that *BRAF* knockdown using RNAi induces apoptosis (19,26,27). There is also compelling evidence that constitutive MAPK activity suppresses a number of apoptosis effectors in melanoma. The induction of tumor necrosis factor–related apoptosis-inducing ligand (TRAIL)-induced apoptosis in melanoma proceeds via the release of second mitochondria-derived activator of caspase (SMAC)/direct IAP binding protein with low pl (Diablo) from the mitochondria (28) and can be suppressed by constitutive MAPK activity. Another mechanism by which MAPK activity suppresses apoptosis in melanoma cells is through the RSK-mediated inactivation of the proapoptotic protein BAD (29).

Vascular endothelial growth factor (VEGF) production has been shown to be regulated by MAPK activity in several cancers including melanoma (30–32). Furthermore, downregulation of V600E *BRAF* with siRNA significantly decreases the amount of VEGF produced by melanoma cells (33). This raises the possibility that melanoma-associated angiogenesis is partially mediated by the MAPK pathway and that the successful inhibition of the pathway will impair this process. Other recent work has shown that melanoma cells harboring the *BRAF* V600E mutation express higher levels of hypoxia inducible factor (HIF)-1α, a key mediator of angiogenesis. Knockdown of *BRAF* using specific short hairpin RNA (shRNA) significantly reduces the HIF-1α expression and survival of melanoma cells under hypoxic conditions (34).

One important characteristic of melanoma is its propensity for metastatic spread at an early stage, and there is evidence that BRAF-mediated signaling contributes to this. Initially, nascent melanoma cells remain under the control of the surrounding keratinocytes through homotypic E-cadherin-mediated adhesion (35), and there is evidence that BRAF/MAPK activity downregulates E-cadherin expression (Fig. 2). After escape from keratinocyte control, the melanoma cells must be able to survive in the dermis by resisting anoikis. One mechanism for overcoming anoikis is through the upregulation of the integrin family of heterodimeric adhesion proteins, which generate "outside-in" survival signals. There is strong evidence that $\alpha_v\beta_3$ integrin is critical for the adhesion of melanoma cells to dermal collagen, and the suppression of apoptosis and expression of these integrins correlates well with tumor progression (36–38). Sustained activation of the MAPK pathway increases expression of β_3 integrin, and inhibition of this pathway using the MEK inhibitor U0126 can reduce β_3 integrin expression (39). BRAF/MAPK activity also contributes toward cell invasion through the regulation of the expression of two families of enzymes, the urokinase plasminogen activation (uPA) and matrix metalloproteinases (MMPs). Of these, MMP-1, which is an interstitial collagenase, and MMPs 2-9, which degrade the basement membrane, are thought to be particularly important. In various melanoma cell lines, BRAF/MAPK activity has been shown to induce MMP expression. Conversely, the pharmacological inhibition of BRAF/MEK signaling is known to inhibit invasion of melanoma cells (40–42). Consistent with an antimetastatic role for inhibitors of the MAPK pathway, recent studies have shown that U0126 treatment suppressed lung metastasis in a mouse melanoma model (43).

Escape from the immune system is another important characteristic of melanoma progression, and there is growing evidence that the V600E *BRAF*

Malignantly transformed melanocyte | Early stage melanoma

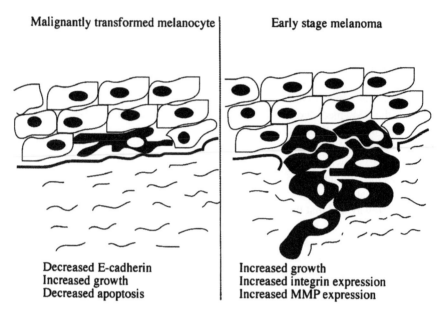

Decreased E-cadherin	Increased growth
Increased growth	Increased integrin expression
Decreased apoptosis	Increased MMP expression

Figure 2 The roles of BRAF/MEK activity in the early progression of melanoma. In the early stages of transformation, high BRAF/MEK activity downregulates the expression of adhesion proteins important for keratinocyte control, such as E-cadherin, as well as increasing melanocyte growth through the stimulation of growth and suppression of apoptosis. As the early melanomas progress, BRAF/MEK activity contributes to dermal invasion through the increased expression of integrins and MMPs. *Abbreviation*: MMPs, matrix metalloproteinases.

mutation contributes to this property. During tumor progression, melanomas tend to lose expression of their highly immunogenic pigmentation antigens, allowing them to evade immune cell attack. High BRAF/MAPK activity seems to play a role in suppressing the release of these antigens, and as inhibition of the pathway using U0126 and RNAi approaches, it increases expression of these antigens (44). It has been further shown that treating melanoma cells with either U0126 or an RNAi to V600E *BRAF* reduces the release of immunosuppressive cytokines from melanoma cells (45), as well as reverses the suppressive effects of melanoma cell culture supernatants upon dendritic cell activation. It is worth noting that the MAPK pathway also plays an important role in normal immune cell function, raising the possibility that small molecule BRAF/MAPK inhibitor treatment may cause unintended immune suppression in patients.

SMALL-MOLECULE INHIBITORS OF BRAF: PRECLINICAL STUDIES

The discovery of the V600E *BRAF* mutation in melanoma has prompted a flurry of activity from both academic labs and pharmaceutical companies to develop small-molecule inhibitors of BRAF and the MAPK pathway. The first inhibitor to be extensively developed as a putative BRAF inhibitor was sorafenib (Nexavar®, BAY 43-9006). A number of studies have shown that sorafenib induces melanoma cell apoptosis in vitro and reduces the growth of human melanoma xenografts in mice (26,43,46). Although it was shown that pMEK was blocked at the concentrations of sorafenib used (26,43), only relatively minor levels of apoptosis were observed in vivo (43), suggesting that there are possible alternative mechanisms of action. It was later shown that sorafenib treatment reduced the vascularization of melanoma xenografts (33) and that the compound was a relatively potent VEGF receptor inhibitor (47). In line with this, sorafenib was recently approved for use in renal cell carcinomas (which do not harbor *BRAF* mutations and where VEGF signaling is critical to tumor progression), where the mechanism of action is thought to be mostly anti-angiogenic. It has been therefore suggested that the effects of sorafenib in melanoma may be largely non-BRAF mediated. Other compounds with a broad spectrum of activity, such as the farnesyl transferase inhibitor SCH66336, also inhibit the MAPK pathway and induce apoptosis in in vitro melanoma cell cultures (48). Again, like sorafenib, the apoptosis induced by FTIs in melanoma are probably non-BRAF/MAPK mediated.

A number of specific BRAF inhibitors have now been developed, some of which have high selectivity for the *BRAF* V600E mutation over wild-type BRAF, such as SB590885 (GlaxoSmithKline) and PLX-4032 (Plexxikon). Meanwhile, inhibitors that are more potent against BRAF than sorafenib but share the general property of cross-reactivty with other kinases are also being developed, such as RAF-265 (Novartis). As selective BRAF-targeted compounds have relatively few off-target effects, it is now possible to assess the effects of specific pharmacological inhibition of BRAF in melanoma. An extensive characterization of SB590885 has shown that the compound is highly selective for cell lines with *BRAF* mutations, accompanied by a profound inhibition of cell growth associated with the induction of G1-phase cell cycle arrest (49). Interestingly, SB590885 activity against human melanoma mouse xenografts is fairly weak, and there is merely a delay in the onset of tumor growth. Here, the low activity levels seen with SB590885 are likely to be a consequence of poor pharmacokinetics. Similar G1-phase growth arrest results have been observed with allosteric MEK inhibitors, such as U0126 and PD0325901, suggesting that inhibition of the MAPK pathway in melanoma is largely cytostatic (50,51). However, there is evidence that PLX-4032, a novel small molecule BRAF inhibitor from Plexxikon, with high selectivity for the V600E mutation over wild-type BRAF, induces some limited apoptosis in melanoma cell lines with the V600E mutation but not those that are *BRAF* wild-type (52).

Given the pivotal role of BRAF in melanoma progression and the obvious ''oncogene addiction'' of melanomas to the *BRAF* mutation, it is somewhat surprising that these pharmacological inhibitors do not induce apoptosis. This is particularly unexpected given that BRAF and MEK act downstream of cytochrome-C and Smac to control caspase activation (53). Recent studies have shown that blocking the MAPK pathway using U0126 did not affect the levels of

Bcl-2, Bcl-XL, or Mcl-1 (53). Knockdown of the BH3-family protein Mcl-1 using shRNA sensitized the melanoma cells to U0126-induced apoptosis, showing that overexpression of these key antiapoptotic proteins in melanoma is a critical barrier to effective BRAF/MEK inhibitor therapy. It also suggests that BRAF/MEK inhibitors may have to be used in combination with other small-molecule inhibitors that modulate apoptosis.

Another unresolved issue in the potential therapeutic use of BRAF inhibitors is the extent of pERK inhibition needed to see a good clinical response. Recent clinical studies of CI-1040 in multiple solid tumor types have shown that although intratumoral pERK levels are inhibited by 80% to 90%, there is little clinical activity (54,55). Similar findings have also come out of the preclinical in vivo studies using sorafenib, where pERK immunoreactivity is still seen even following prolonged drug treatment (26,33). It is highly possible that low levels of pERK may still be able to drive tumor growth. The expression pattern of pERK within a melanoma lesion tends to be very heterogeneous, with the highest levels of staining being seen at the leading edges of the tumor, where most of the growth and invasion is taking place (14). This is an interesting observation as the melanoma itself is assumed to be genetically homogeneous and all of the cells within a given lesion are normally *BRAF*-mutation positive, suggesting that microenvironmental factors regulate pERK activity within a given tumor cell. It further indicates that the bulk of the cells in the tumor may be relatively quiescent and therefore not susceptible to BRAF inhibition. Similar patterns of regional, leading edge–localized, pERK staining are also seen within our three-dimensional organotypic melanoma cultures. Interestingly, growth of the melanoma cell under organotypic culture conditions is associated with much increased MEK inhibitor resistance compared with standard adherent two-dimensional culture conditions (50). It seems that although most melanoma cells within the tumor will have the activating *BRAF* V600E mutation, the signaling activity in the MAPK pathway may be localized to a minority of the cells, possibly limiting therapeutic efficacy. Conversely, the robust activity of RAF and MEK inhibitors in two-dimensional culture may only be realized in the small subpopulation of cells in a three-dimensional tumor that have similar growth properties. Clearly, more work needs to be done to understand the mechanisms of MAPK pathway regulation within V600E *BRAF* melanoma cells in three-dimensional culture and in vivo.

On the basis of the evidence presented above, there is a growing realization that single-agent BRAF inhibitor therapy is not the optimal strategy for treating melanoma. Clinical trials of sorafenib monotherapy yielded little response, and in in vivo human melanoma mouse xenograft studies, sorafenib was associated with cytostasis and limited tumor regression (26,33). An interesting observation from these latter studies was that although sorafenib significantly reduced cell proliferation as measured by 5-bromodeoxyuridine (BrDU)-uptake studies, it did not completely inhibit it, suggesting that melanomas have other, non-BRAF/MAPK-mediated growth pathways. Previous work has shown that melanomas have constitutive activity in a number of other signaling pathways known to regulate growth, including PI3K/Akt, Src/STAT3, NFκB, and Notch (56). To address this issue, we performed a series of studies to determine whether there was a correlation between the inhibition of pERK and the inhibition of cell growth across a panel of melanoma cell lines (57). We found no correlation between the inhibition of growth and the inhibition of pERK levels, suggesting that activity in the MAPK pathway was not a good marker of therapeutic efficacy. Instead, there was a better correlation between the inhibition of Ki67 positivity and inhibition of growth (57). We therefore suggest that any future trials of BRAF/MEK inhibitors in melanoma should use pERK only as a marker of pathway inhibition and that a proliferation marker, such as Ki67, would be a better indicator of therapeutic efficacy. It is expected that any clinical activity would need to be associated with a total inhibition of all proliferative activity within the tumor, which would be admittedly difficult to achieve.

The current expectation is that BRAF inhibitors will be used in combination with either other targeted therapy agents or established chemotherapy regimens. The combination of sorafenib with chemotherapy has generated evidence of activity in phase II trials and has led to phase III trials. The mechanism by which sorafenib appears to enhance the cytotoxicity of chemotherapy remains in question and is complicated by the broad spectrum antikinase activity seen with this drug. While there is evidence that MEK inhibition may sensitize cells to certain chemotherapies, it is not clear whether this mechanism is shared by sorafenib. A number of other studies have shown that inhibitors of VEGF signaling, such as bevacizumab, synergize with chemotherapy drugs, suggesting that the anti-VEGF activity of sorafenib may underlie its interaction with chemotherapy (58). If this proves to be true, we may not expect more highly specific BRAF inhibitors to synergize with chemotherapy. There is, however, a body of literature that suggests that the MAPK pathway regulates DNA repair and can modulate responses to chemotherapy. Two clinical studies have suggested that the presence of *BRAF* mutations confer a lower likelihood of response or disease control with multiagent chemotherapy regimens (59,60). This is clearly an area deserving further investigation.

Another promising strategy is combining BRAF inhibitors with the taxane family of microtubule-stabilizing agents. Sorafenib appears to enhance the effect of paclitaxel in clinical trials of chemotherapy-naïve melanoma, although the mechanism underlying this interaction is not clear. In vitro, MEK inhibitors, such as U0126 are known to have additive growth-inhibitory effects when combined with paclitaxel (61). There is evidence that MEK/ERK signaling is critical for the execution of mitosis, and under these circumstances, pERK inhibition may lead to enhancement in the level of paclitaxel-induced mitotic catastrophe.

Ultimately, combining effective BRAF/MAPK pathway inhibitors with other agents that target other signaling molecules essential for melanoma survival might provide the greatest possibility of durable responses in the metastatic setting or reducing the risk of recurrence in the adjuvant setting. There are many possible suitable drug combinations that need to be considered, and this is very much a work in progress. The PI3K pathway appears to be essential for melanoma progression, and the ability of PI3K and Akt to modulate apoptosis may provide the basis for rational combination with BRAF inhibitors. Preliminary studies from our own laboratory have demonstrated some synergy in three-dimensional organotypic melanoma cultures when MEK and PI3K inhibitors are combined (50). Other groups have also shown that the simultaneous topical application of MEK and PI3K inhibitors leads to melanoma regression in in vivo models of human melanoma (62). Another possible combination target within the PI3K/Akt pathway is the mammalian target of rapamycin (mTOR) and there is evidence of synergy between sorafenib and rapamycin in in vitro melanoma studies (63). Although a recent phase II trial of the clinical mTOR inhibitor temsirolimus showed little single agent activity in melanoma patients, a cooperative group phase II trial will include the combination of temsirolimus with sorafenib.

In the phase I evaluation of one of the second-generation MEK inhibitors, PD0325901, serial tumor biopsies were performed among the majority of patients (64). A disproportionate percentage of study participants had melanoma. Suppression of ERK phosphorylation was investigated with immunohistochemistry. The preliminary assessment of this end point suggested that ERK activity was significantly inhibited in most patients treated at the higher dose levels and that complete inhibition (within the limits of qualitative immunohistochemistry assessments) was rarely seen. The interpatient variability in pERK suppression is not understood and likely depends on drug disposition as well as factors within the tumors. In the ongoing phase I trials of the second-generation RAF inhibitors, PLX4032 and RAF-265, similar methods are being applied to determine the ability of these agents to inhibit ERK activity across dose levels. As discussed previously, it is likely that investigation of additional markers, such as the expression of BH3 domain containing mediators of apoptosis, will be important in fully understanding the impact of these agents.

The largest clinical trial to be conducted among patients with metastatic melanoma is E2603, an ongoing randomized phase III trial comparing sorafenib, carboplatin, and paclitaxel with carboplatin and paclitaxel. In the context of this trial archival tumor blocks are being collected for each participant. Blocks from the most recently resected stage of disease are prioritized for collection, with metastatic lesions favored over lymph nodes removed at the time of staging lymphadenectomy or primary melanomas. A tissue array will be created from these samples for the purpose of performing quantitative immunohistochemistry of proteins known to be involved in MAPK pathway signaling, VEGF signaling, and apoptosis. These categories of markers are derived from the preclinical studies summarized above. This analysis will simultaneously evaluate the predictive value of individual markers or combinations of markers in the setting of chemotherapy treatment alone (on the control arm of E2603) and a sorafenib/

chemotherapy regimen (on the experimental arm). It will be of great interest to see which markers differentiate outcome between the two arms of the trial. This is expected to significantly improve our understanding of sorafenib's mechanism of action when combined with chemotherapy in melanoma. A further correlative analysis is based on the somatic genetic mutations within these tumor specimens. Tumor DNA will be isolated from paraffin-embedded samples and previously described oncogenes and tumor suppressor genes will be assayed for the presence of mutations. Several hypotheses can be addressed with this approach, including the role of *BRAF* mutations in conferring resistance to chemotherapy (among patients on the control arm). With an 800-patient sample size, this analysis will also allow the first-ever categorization of patients on the basis of the full complement of mutations in oncogenes and tumor-suppressor genes known to be mutated in melanoma beyond *BRAF*. It is likely that such an approach will identify discrete subsets of patients for whom chemotherapy alone or the combination of sorafenib with chemotherapy is particularly effective or ineffective. Building such predictive models is an essential component of understanding how molecularly targeted therapies interface with the constellation of aberrant signal transduction pathways elucidated on the past several years.

The central role of *BRAF* mutations in the progression of most melanomas makes it an excellent target for therapy. Early clinical experience with sorafenib suggests that combination therapies need to be developed that incorporate BRAF inhibitors. The optimal drug regimen is still open to debate, but could also involve elements of PI3K/Akt pathway inhibition and/or chemotherapy. The complex interaction of *BRAF*-mutated melanoma cells with their microenvironment requires further investigation and should shed further light on the mechanisms of possible BRAF inhibitor resistance in vivo. The incorporation of pharmacodynamic end points in early drug development and tumor genetic profiling of patients in phase II and phase III trials is a requisite as the translation of MAPK pathway inhibitors in melanoma is still in its infancy.

REFERENCES

1. Davies H, Bignell GR, Cox C, et al. Mutations of the BRAF gene in human cancer. Nature 2002; 417(6892):949–954.
2. Garnett MJ, Marais R. Guilty as charged: B-RAF is a human oncogene. Cancer Cell 2004; 6(4):313–319.
3. Wan PT, Garnett MJ, Roe SM, et al. Mechanism of activation of the RAF-ERK signaling pathway by oncogenic mutations of B-RAF. Cell 2004; 116(6):855–867.
4. Robinson MJ, Cobb MH. Mitogen-activated protein kinase pathways. Curr Opin Cell Biol 1997; 9(2):180–186.
5. Crews CM, Alessandrini A, Erikson RL. The primary structure of MEK, a protein kinase that phosphorylates the ERK gene product. Science 1992; 258(5081):478–480.
6. Kyriakis JM, App H, Zhang XF, et al. Raf-1 activates MAP kinase-kinase. Nature 1992; 358(6385):417–421.

7. Satyamoorthy K, Li G, Gerrero MR, et al. Constitutive mitogen-activated protein kinase activation in melanoma is mediated by both BRAF mutations and autocrine growth factor stimulation. Cancer Res 2003; 63(4):756–759.
8. Padua RA, Barrass NC, Currie GA. Activation of N-ras in a human melanoma cell line. Mol Cell Biol 1985; 5(3):582–585.
9. Padua RA, Barrass N, Currie GA. A novel transforming gene in a human malignant melanoma cell line. Nature 1984; 311(5987):671–673.
10. Brose MS, Volpe P, Feldman M, et al. BRAF and RAS mutations in human lung cancer and melanoma. Cancer Res 2002; 62(23):6997–7000.
11. Curtin JA, Busam K, Pinkel D, et al. Somatic activation of KIT in distinct subtypes of melanoma. J Clin Oncol 2006; 24(26):4340–4346.
12. Sensi M, Nicolini G, Petti C, et al. Mutually exclusive NRASQ61R and BRAF V600E mutations at the single-cell level in the same human melanoma. Oncogene 2006; 25(24):3357–3364.
13. Brazil DP, Park J, Hemmings BA. PKB binding proteins. Getting in on the Akt. Cell 2002; 111(3):293–303.
14. Zhuang L, Lee CS, Scolyer RA, et al. Activation of the extracellular signal regulated kinase (ERK) pathway in human melanoma. J Clin Pathol 2005; 58(11):1163–1169.
15. Pollock PM, Harper UL, Hansen KS, et al. High frequency of BRAF mutations in nevi. Nat Genet 2003; 33(1):19–20.
16. Michaloglou C, Vredeveld LC, Soengas MS, et al. BRAF E600-associated senescence-like cell cycle arrest of human naevi. Nature 2005; 436(7051):720–724.
17. Gray-Schopfer VC, Cheong SC, Chong H, et al. Cellular senescence in naevi and immortalisation in melanoma: a role for p16? Br J Cancer 2006; 95(4):496–505.
18. Wellbrock C, Ogilvie L, Hedley D, et al. V599E B-RAF is an oncogene in melanocytes. Cancer Res 2004; 64(7):2338–2342.
19. Hingorani SR, Jacobetz MA, Robertson GP, et al. Suppression of BRAF(V599E) in human melanoma abrogates transformation. Cancer Res 2003; 63(17):5198–5202.
20. Hoeflich KP, Gray DC, Eby MT, et al. Oncogenic BRAF is required for tumor growth and maintenance in melanoma models. Cancer Res 2006; 66(2):999–1006.
21. Wellbrock C, Marais R. Elevated expression of MITF counteracts B-RAF-stimulated melanocyte and melanoma cell proliferation. J Cell Biol 2005; 170(5):703–708.
22. Sherr CJ. G1 phase progression: cycling on cue. Cell 1994; 79(4):551–555.
23. Bhatt KV, Spofford LS, Aram G, et al. Adhesion control of cyclin D1 and p27Kip1 levels is deregulated in melanoma cells through BRAF-MEK–ERK signaling. Oncogene 2005; 24(21):3459–3471.
24. Persons DL, Yazlovitskaya EM, Cui W, et al. Cisplatin-induced activation of mitogen-activated protein kinases in ovarian carcinoma cells: inhibition of extracellular signal-regulated kinase activity increases sensitivity to cisplatin. Clin Cancer Res 1999; 5(5):1007–1014.
25. Jansen B, Schlagbauer-Wadl H, Eichler HG, et al. Activated N-ras contributes to the chemoresistance of human melanoma in severe combined immunodeficiency (SCID) mice by blocking apoptosis. Cancer Res 1997; 57(3):362–365.
26. Karasarides M, Chiloeches A, Hayward R, et al. B-RAF is a therapeutic target in melanoma. Oncogene 2004; 23(37):6292–6298.
27. Boisvert-Adamo K, Aplin AE. B-RAF and PI-3 kinase signaling protect melanoma cells from anoikis. Oncogene 2006; 25(35):4848–4856.

28. Zhang XD, Borrow JM, Zhang XY, et al. Activation of ERK1/2 protects melanoma cells from TRAIL-induced apoptosis by inhibiting Smac/DIABLO release from mitochondria. Oncogene 2003; 22(19):2869–2881.

29. Eisenmann KM, VanBrocklin MW, Staffend NA, et al. Mitogen-activated protein kinase pathway-dependent tumor-specific survival signaling in melanoma cells through inactivation of the proapoptotic protein bad. Cancer Res 2003; 63(23):8330–8337.

30. Shi YH, Wang YX, Bingle L, et al. In vitro study of HIF-1 activation and VEGF release by bFGF in the T47D breast cancer cell line under normoxic conditions: involvement of PI-3K/Akt and MEK1/ERK pathways. J Pathol 2005; 205(4):530–536.

31. Graells J, Vinyals A, Figueras A, et al. Overproduction of VEGF concomitantly expressed with its receptors promotes growth and survival of melanoma cells through MAPK and PI3K signaling. J Invest Dermatol 2004; 123(6):1151–1161.

32. Bancroft CC, Chen Z, Yeh J, et al. Effects of pharmacologic antagonists of epidermal growth factor receptor, PI3K and MEK signal kinases on NF-kappaB and AP-1 activation and IL-8 and VEGF expression in human head and neck squamous cell carcinoma lines. Int J Cancer 2002; 99(4):538–548.

33. Sharma A, Trivedi NR, Zimmerman MA, et al. Mutant V599E B-Raf regulates growth and vascular development of malignant melanoma tumors. Cancer Res 2005; 65(6):2412–2421.

34. Kumar SM, Yu H, Edwards R, et al. Mutant V600E BRAF increases hypoxia inducible factor-1alpha expression in melanoma. Cancer Res 2007; 67(7):3177–3184.

35. Smalley KS, Brafford PA, Herlyn M. Selective evolutionary pressure from the tissue microenvironment drives tumor progression. Semin Cancer Biol 2005; 15(6):451–459.

36. Montgomery AM, Reisfeld RA, Cheresh DA. Integrin alpha v beta 3 rescues melanoma cells from apoptosis in three-dimensional dermal collagen. Proc Natl Acad Sci U S A 1994; 91(19):8856–8860.

37. Van Belle PA, Elenitsas R, Satyamoorthy K, et al. Progression-related expression of beta 3 integrin in melanomas and nevi. Hum Pathol 1999; 30(5):562–567.

38. Petitclerc E, Stromblad S, von Schalscha TL, et al. Integrin alpha(v)beta3 promotes M21 melanoma growth in human skin by regulating tumor cell survival. Cancer Res 1999; 59(11):2724–2730.

39. Woods D, Cherwinski H, Venetsanakos E, et al. Induction of beta 3-integrin gene expression by sustained activation of the Ras-regulated Raf-MEK-extracellular signal-regulated kinase signaling pathway. Mol Cell Biol 2001; 21(9):3192–3205.

40. Huntington JT, Shields JM, Der CJ, et al. Overexpression of collagenase 1 (MMP-1) is mediated by the ERK pathway in invasive melanoma cells: role of BRAF mutation and fibroblast growth factor signaling. J Biol Chem 2004; 279(32):33168–33176.

41. Ge X, Fu YM, Meadows GG. U0126, a mitogen-activated protein kinase kinase inhibitor, inhibits the invasion of human A375 melanoma cells. Cancer Lett 2002; 179(2):133–140.

42. Benbow U, Tower GB, Wyatt CA, et al. High levels of MMP-1 expression in the absence of the 2G single nucleotide polymorphism is mediated by p38 and ERK1/2 mitogen-activated protein kinases in VMM5 melanoma cells. J Cell Biochem 2002; 86(2):307–319.

43. Sharma A, Tran MA, Liang S, et al. Targeting mitogen-activated protein kinase/extracellular signal-regulated kinase kinase in the mutant (V600E) B-Raf signaling cascade effectively inhibits melanoma lung metastases. Cancer Res 2006; 66(16): 8200–8209.

44. Kono M, Dunn IS, Durda PJ, et al. Role of the mitogen-activated protein kinase signaling pathway in the regulation of human melanocytic antigen expression. Mol Cancer Res 2006; 4(10):779–792.
45. Sumimoto H, Imabayashi F, Iwata T, et al. The BRAF-MAPK signaling pathway is essential for cancer-immune evasion in human melanoma cells. J Exp Med 2006; 203(7):1651–1656.
46. Panka DJ, Wang W, Atkins MB, et al. The Raf inhibitor BAY 43-9006 (Sorafenib) induces caspase-independent apoptosis in melanoma cells. Cancer Res 2006; 66(3): 1611–1619.
47. Wilhelm SM, Carter C, Tang L, et al. BAY 43-9006 exhibits broad spectrum oral antitumor activity and targets the RAF/MEK/ERK pathway and receptor tyrosine kinases involved in tumor progression and angiogenesis. Cancer Res 2004; 64(19): 7099–7109.
48. Smalley KS, Eisen TG. Farnesyl transferase inhibitor SCH66336 is cytostatic, pro-apoptotic and enhances chemosensitivity to cisplatin in melanoma cells. Int J Cancer 2003; 105(2):165–175.
49. King AJ, Patrick DR, Batorsky RS, et al. Demonstration of a genetic therapeutic index for tumors expressing oncogenic BRAF by the kinase inhibitor SB-590885. Cancer Res 2006; 66(23):11100–11105.
50. Smalley KS, Haass NK, Brafford PA, et al. Multiple signaling pathways must be targeted to overcome drug resistance in cell lines derived from melanoma metastases. Mol Cancer Ther 2006; 5(5):1136–1144.
51. Solit DB, Garraway LA, Pratilas CA, et al. BRAF mutation predicts sensitivity to MEK inhibition. Nature 2006; 439(7074):358–362.
52. Tsai J, Lee JT, Wang W, et al. Discovery of a selective inhibitor of oncogenic B-Raf kinase with potent antimelanoma activity. Proc Natl Acad Sci U S A 2008;105(8): 3041–3046.
53. Verhaegen M, Bauer JA, Martin de la Vega C, et al. A novel BH3 mimetic reveals a mitogen-activated protein kinase-dependent mechanism of melanoma cell death controlled by p53 and reactive oxygen species. Cancer Res 2006; 66(23):11348–11359.
54. Rinehart J, Adjei AA, Lorusso PM, et al. Multicenter phase II study of the oral MEK inhibitor, CI-1040, in patients with advanced non-small-cell lung, breast, colon, and pancreatic cancer. J Clin Oncol 2004; 22(22):4456–4462.
55. Lorusso PM, Adjei AA, Varterasian M, et al. Phase I and pharmacodynamic study of the oral MEK inhibitor CI-1040 in patients with advanced malignancies. J Clin Oncol 2005; 23(23):5281–5293.
56. Smalley KS, Herlyn M. Targeting intracellular signaling pathways as a novel strategy in melanoma therapeutics. Ann N Y Acad Sci 2005; 1059:16–25.
57. Smalley KS, Contractor R, Haass NK, et al. Ki67 expression levels are a better marker of reduced melanoma growth following MEK inhibitor treatment than phospho-ERK levels. Br J Cancer 2007; 96(3):445–449.
58. Folkins C, Man S, Xu P, et al. Anticancer therapies combining antiangiogenic and tumor cell cytotoxic effects reduce the tumor stem-like cell fraction in glioma xenograft tumors. Cancer Res 2007; 67(8):3560–3564.
59. Chang DZ, Panageas KS, Osman I, et al. Clinical significance of BRAF mutations in metastatic melanoma. J Transl Med 2004; 2(1):46.
60. Kumar R, Angelini S, Czene K, et al. BRAF mutations in metastatic melanoma: a possible association with clinical outcome. Clin Cancer Res 2003; 9(9):3362–3368.

61. McDaid HM, Horwitz SB. Selective potentiation of paclitaxel (taxol)-induced cell death by mitogen-activated protein kinase kinase inhibition in human cancer cell lines. Mol Pharmacol 2001; 60(2):290–301.

62. Bedogni B, O'Neill MS, Welford SM, et al. Topical treatment with inhibitors of the phosphatidylinositol 3'-kinase/Akt and Raf/mitogen-activated protein kinase kinase/ extracellular signal-regulated kinase pathways reduces melanoma development in severe combined immunodeficient mice. Cancer Res 2004; 64(7):2552–2560.

63. Molhoek KR, Brautigan DL, Slingluff CL Jr. Synergistic inhibition of human melanoma proliferation by combination treatment with B-Raf inhibitor BAY43-9006 and mTOR inhibitor Rapamycin. J Transl Med 2005; 3:39.

64. Lorusso P, Krishnamurthi S, Rinehart JR, et al. A phase 1-2 clinical study of a second generation oral MEK inhibitor, PD 0325901 in 471 patients with advanced cancer. Proc Am Soc Clin Oncol 2005; (abstr 3011).

7

Therapeutic Targeting of the Melanoma Stem Cell Population

Keiran S.M. Smalley

H. Lee Moffitt Cancer Center & Research Institute, Tampa, Florida, U.S.A.

Brijal Desai and Meenhard Herlyn

The Wistar Institute, Philadelphia, Pennsylvania, U.S.A.

MELANOMA THERAPY: THE STATE OF THE ART

Metastatic melanoma is a deadly condition. In a meta-analysis of 83 studies published since 1985, the median survival of patients treated for metastatic disease was 8.9 months (1). The current paradigm for the treatment of cutaneous melanoma largely depends on the stage of the tumor. The official guidelines for staging were developed by the American Joint Committee on Cancer (AJCC) and take into consideration variables such as tumor thickness, ulceration, lymph node involvement, and metastatic disease. The majority of patients present with stage I to IIA disease, and in these patients, surgery is curative in 70% to 90% of cases. In contrast, patients with stage IIB disease, IIC disease, and stage III disease are associated with a 40% to 80% recurrence rate. In these high-risk patients, surgical excision followed by adjuvant interferon-α may be of some use.

Treatment of metastatic melanoma (stage IV disease) remains a challenge and is the focus of intense research. The most successful pharmacological methods to date have been the cytotoxic chemotherapeutic agents dacarbazine (DTIC), platinum analogs, nitrosureas, and microtubular toxins. The most widely used single agent for the treatment of metastatic melanoma is dacarbazine, which has a reported response rate of only 8% to 20% (2,3). DTIC is a DNA-alkylating agent and remains the only cytotoxic drug approved by the FDA for the treatment of patients with metastatic melanoma. However, there are no phase III trial data that demonstrate an overall survival benefit. Temozolomide is an analog of DTIC that can be administered orally and possesses significant CNS penetration. In a head-to-head comparison of temozolomide to DTIC, temozolomide did not show any statistically significant benefits over DTIC and was thus not FDA approved for the treatment of metastatic disease (4). Subsequent trials have been carried out to examine the effects of combining chemotherapeutic agents; however, large phase III trials have not demonstrated an advantage of combination regiments compared with single-agent use of dacarbazine or temozolomide (5).

Targeted Therapy

There is now hope that targeted therapies, as exemplified by imatinib (Gleevec® STI-571) in chronic myeloid leukemia (CML), will be developed for melanoma. These approaches rely upon targeting the key molecular pathways implicated in tumor growth and progression. If tumors are driven by one genetic mutation, such as Bcr-Abl in CML, inhibition of this molecular target can lead to complete disease remission. The best current hope for the melanoma field is targeting of the mitogen-activated protein kinase (MAPK) pathway. Most melanomas have either activating mutations in *BRAF* (approximately 60%) (6), *NRAS* (15%–30%) (7), or *c-Kit* (4%) (8) (see Fig. 1). All of these mutations result in the activation of the MAPK pathway and the induction of proliferative/survival genes such as *MITF* and *cyclin D1* (9). The first putative BRAF inhibitor to be developed was sorafenib (BAY 43-9006) (10). As a monotherapy, sorafenib has only marginal activity; however, when used in combination with other cytotoxic agents the data appears more promising. Following sorafenib, which has many off-target effects, more BRAF selective agents have been developed. One such compound, RAF-265 has recently entered phase I clinical trials for stage III/IV disease. Another targeted inhibitor of mutant BRAF, PLX4032, is currently undergoing phase I evaluation in melanoma. In addition, PD0325901 and AZD6244, agents that target MEK, have shown some efficacy in in vitro models of *BRAF* V600E melanoma.

PTEN is a signal terminator for the PI3 kinase pathway, a pathway that regulates cell survival, growth, apoptosis, and tumor cell chemoresistance [reviewed in (11)]. Its expression is lost in 5% to 20% of late-stage metastatic melanoma, and one of the PI3K effector proteins, Akt, is overexpressed in up to 60% of melanoma (Fig. 1). In addition, loss of PTEN expression in melanoma occurs in association with activating mutations in *BRAF,* but not *NRAS* (12). Biologically, since NRAS can activate both the PI3K and BRAF, the cell would require either NRAS or a mutational loss of combination of PI3K and BRAF for activation of MAPK effectors. The current MAPK pathway and PI3K/Akt compounds being developed in human trials are listed in Table 1.

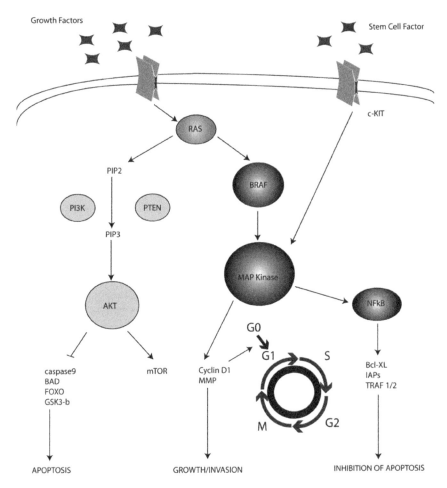

Figure 1 Scheme showing the signaling pathways known to be constitutively active in melanoma and their downstream effectors.

There are many additional signaling pathways currently under investigation for targeted melanoma therapy. Only time will tell whether any of these therapies will provide quantitative benefit in phase III trials. As we have seen from the dismal history of melanoma therapy, it is unlikely that as a monotherapy, any of these agents will prove to be efficacious. Rather, a combination of these targeted therapies with or without cytotoxic agents will more likely yield a successful result. However, it is likely that the activity of most of these compounds will not affect the population of tumor initiator or melanoma stem cells. It is our strong belief that the identification and targeting of the tumor-initiating population is essential for the comprehensive therapy of melanoma.

Table 1 Selected Clinical Trials for Targeted Therapies in Melanoma

Agent	Mechanism of action	Planned/ongoing clinical trials
	RAF	
BAY 43-9006 (sorafenib)	Tyrosine kinase inhibitor	Phase I + perifosine in advanced solid tumors
		Phase I + 17-AAG in advanced solid tumors
		Phase I + temsirolimus in advanced solid tumors
		Phase I + tipifarnib in advanced solid tumors
		Phase I + erlotinib in advanced solid tumors
		Phase I + bortezomib in advanced cancers
		Phase II + bevacizumab in stage III/IV melanoma
		Phase III carboplatin/paclitaxel ± sorafenib in stage III/IV
		Phase I/II + temsirolimus in stage III/IV
		Phase II + tipifarnib or temsirolimus in stage IV
RAF-265	Tyrosine kinase inhibitor	Phase I in stage III/IV
PLX4032	Tyrosine kinase inhibitor	Phase I in advanced solid tumors
	MEK	
CL-1040 (PD0325901)	Tyrosine kinase inhibitor	Phase I/II in advanced melanoma, breast, and colorectal cancer
AZD6244 (ARRY-142886)	Tyrosine kinase inhibitor	Phase II + temozolomide in stage III/IV
	PI3/Akt/PTEN	
Perifosine	Akt inhibitor	Phase I + sorafenib in advanced solid tumors
		Phase I + sunitinib in advanced solid tumors
Temsirolimus	mTOR inhibitor	Phase I + bevacizumab in stage III/IV
		Phase I/II + sorafenib in stage III/IV
		Phase II: temsirolimus or tipifarnib + sorafenib in stage IV
Everolimus	mTOR inhibitor	Phase I + lapatinib in advanced solid tumors
		Phase I + bevacizumab + erlotinib in advanced solid tumors
		Phase II in stage IV

Table 1   Selected Clinical Trials for Targeted Therapies in Melanoma (*Continued*)

Agent	Mechanism of action	Planned/ongoing clinical trials
AP23573	mTOR inhibitor	Phase I + doxorubicin in advanced solid tumors
	c-KIT	
Imatinib	Tyrosine kinase inhibitor	Phase I + capecitabine in advanced solid tumors Phase I/II + bevacizumab in stage III/IV with c-Kit mutations
	Cell cycle inhibitors	
Flavopiridol	CDK inhibitor	Phase I + vorinostat in advanced solid tumors Phase I alone or + chemotherapies in advanced solid tumors
PD0332991	CDK inhibitor	Phase I in Rb-expressing advanced cancer

Clinical trial data obtained from www.clinicaltrials.gov, www.cancer.gov, and www.asco.org.
Abbreviations: CDK, cyclin-dependent kinases; mTOR, mammalian target of rapamycin; Rb, retinoblastoma.

TUMOR-INITIATING CELLS: ARE THEY MALIGNANT STEM CELLS?

Normal Adult Stem Cells

Tumors typically arise in tissues with rapid cell turnover, such as the gastrointestinal tract, the hematopoietic system, and the skin. In these organs, there is a continuous ordered cycle of cell proliferation that replaces the short-lived differentiated cells. This cell proliferation is a highly controlled process whereby a small pool of self-renewing stem cells gives rise to a population of proliferating progenitor cells that undergo limited rounds of cell division before reaching a state of terminal differentiation. In this system, only the stem cells are long-lived, and they have the unique property of being able to undergo self-renewing cell division where at least one of the progeny "daughter cells" remains as a stem cell—a process termed "asymmetric cell division." The daughter cells then either remain as stem cells or undergo a further process of differentiation to become either a multipotent progenitor or a transient amplifying cell. It is through the generation of many transient amplifying cells that stem cells can generate large cell numbers to repopulate entire tissues (Fig. 2). As transient amplifying cells undergo multiple rounds of cell division, their progeny become progressively more differentiated and start losing their potential for further cell proliferation. This delicate balance between self-renewal and differentiation is critical in retaining the size of stem cell pool. Stem cells exist within a

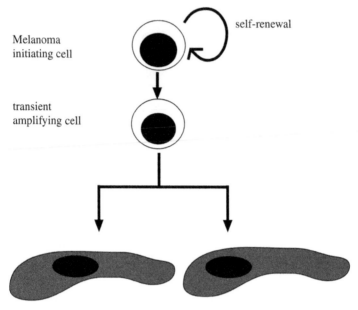

Melanoma
initiating cell

self-renewal

transient
amplifying cell

daughter "non-tumorigenic" melanoma cells

Figure 2 Scheme showing the asymmetrical and symmetrical cell division in the melanoma-initiating cell population. The melanoma-initiating cell can both give rise to more initiating cells through self-renewal and more differentiated transient amplifying cells. The transient amplifying cells are unable to give rise to more stem cells and instead generate large numbers of differentiated non-tumorigenic melanoma cells.

specialized microenvironment termed "the stem cell niche." The niche plays a critical role in maintaining the undifferentiated state of the stem cell pool through the provision of paracrine and extracellular matrix signals.

In both mouse and human skin, melanocyte stem cells reside in the hair follicle bulge of the lower permanent portion of the hair follicle (13,14). The niche is a protective environment for the melanocyte stem cell that serves to keep these cells in a relatively immature, primitive state. During the growth phase of the hair cycle or during tissue repair, signals from the hair bulge niche provide the melanocyte stem cells with signals that drive their proliferation and differentiation. Although the exact nature of the signals required for melanocyte differentiation is poorly defined, work from our own laboratory has revealed a critical role for WNT-3a in the transdifferentiation of embryonic stem cells into melanocytes (15). Whether melanocyte stem cells can only give rise to melanocytes or a full range of skin cells in vivo is unclear. In vitro rather more is known, and human hair follicle cells differentiate into multiple cell lineages, including neuronal, glial, and smooth muscle cells and keratinocytes (16).

A Stem Cell Theory of Cancer

There is a growing body of evidence to suggest that cancers may arise from an oncogenically transformed population of stem cells. The cancer stem cell theory postulates that tumor formation, growth, and metastatic spread are driven by a minority population of tumor-initiating or cancer stem cells. Usefully, this hypothesis helps to explain a number of key observations that have vexed the cancer research community for many years. It has long been known that the majority of tumor cells are actually nontumorigenic and cannot be successfully transplanted into new hosts. This point is well illustrated by the fact that typical mouse xenograft experiments require the injection of one to two million cells to ensure tumor establishment. In a similar vein, the genetic model of cancer predicts that a serial acquisition of oncogenes and inactivation of tumor suppressors is required for oncogenic transformation. This model, which would require a 10- to 30-year time frame, has always been difficult to reconcile with relatively short life span of most somatic cells. The fact that stem cells are the longest-lived cells within the body fits well with the idea of a long-term acquisition of oncogenic mutations.

Most of what we currently know about the tumor-initiating cells comes from a series of pioneering studies on hematopoiesis and leukemia. Early transplantation experiments on lethally irradiated mice, where the native bone marrow was completely eradicated, showed that a minority population of cells (equal to about 0.05% of total bone marrow) were able to completely reconstitute the mouse hematopoietic system (17). Further investigation revealed that these "regenerating cells" were from a very primitive lineage that lacked every known hematopoietic cell surface marker [and were thus termed "lineage marker negative" (Lin neg)]. Subsequent work has shown the hematopoietic system to posses a well-structured cellular hierarchy in which only the stem cells have the ability to self-renew and generate the entire range of differentiated cells. Transplantation of the more differentiated transient-amplifying cell population was unable to reconstitute the hematopoietic system. These early studies on hematopoiesis were rapidly applied to the study of leukemia development. Again, it was found that only a specialized population of acute myeloid leukemic (AML) cells, with the cell surface markers $CD34^+/CD38^-$, were able to transplant the disease into a recipient animal (17). Infusion of more differentiated leukemic cells into similar mice was unable to transplant the AML (17). The leukemia-intiating cells were further shown to have all the important key features of stem cells in that they had the potential for self-renewal, asymmetric cell division, and could differentiate into multiple lineages. This work led to the proposal that leukemia was the result of aberrant hematopoiesis and that the leukemia-initiating cells were, in fact, oncogenically transformed stem cells.

Characterizing the Tumor-Initiating Cells

There are many similarities between stem cells and tumor-initiating cells. Both populations are known to be relatively quiescent and have multiple mechanisms to overcome exogenous genotoxic stimuli through the high expression levels of (ABC) ATP-binding cassette-family drug transporters and an increased capacity for DNA repair. Similarly, both tumor cells and stem cells are able to suppress the activity of p53, following genotoxic insult, leading to reduced levels of apoptosis (18). In addition, both normal stem cells and over 90% of human tumors express the enzyme telomerase, which maintains chromosomal integrity at the chromosome ends, following prolonged rounds of cell proliferation (19).

In addition to leukemia, putative tumor-initiating populations have now also been identified in many solid tumors (20). Tumor-initiating cells share key characteristics of normal stem cells in that they can self-renew and differentiate into multiple cell lineages. They differ from normal stem cells in that they have escaped the physiological growth controls imposed by the niche and proliferate in an uncontrolled manner. Although the tumor-initiating population and the non-tumorigenic population of cancer cells contain similar oncogenic mutations, the nontumorigenic population lack the capacity to self-renew. The first evidence of tumor-initiating cells in a solid tumor came from studies on breast cancer, where it was shown that only a minor subpopulation of tumor cells isolated from patient lesions were able to establish new tumors in mice (21). Again, the tumorigenic cells were distinguished from the nontumorigenic population on the basis of cell surface marker selection and were defined as being $CD24^{-/low}/CD44^+$ (21). Limiting dilution xenograft experiments showed that tumors could be initiated from as little as 100 of the $CD24^{-/low}/CD44^+$ cells. In contrast, injections of tens of thousands of the non-$CD24^{-/low}/CD44^+$ cells were unable to initiate tumor growth in mice. Histological evaluation of the resulting tumors from the $CD24^{-/low}/CD44^+$ mice showed that the full phenotypic heterogeneity of the original breast tumor could be recapitulated by these few tumor-initiating cells. Since this initial ground-breaking work, similar tumor-initiating cell populations have been identified in colon (22), brain (23), and prostate cancer (24), as well as in melanoma (25).

Our group has recently identified a slow-growing, pluripotent melanoma cell population with enhanced tumor-forming ability in severe combined immunode-ficiency (SCID) mice (25). Initial isolation of these cells was based on their ability to grow in embryonic stem cell media. These cells were shown to be $CD20^+$ and to differentiate into multiple cellular lineages, such as adipocytes, chondrocytes, and osteocytes. There is some suggestion that this $CD20^+$ population of melanoma cells may harbor the tumor-initiating population. Although well characterized, these $CD20^+$ cells often have an unstable phenotype in culture, and we have begun the search for more robust stem cell population markers. This discovery marks a radical paradigm shift for the melanoma field and offers new opportunities to readdress the therapeutic targeting of this intractable tumor (Fig. 3).

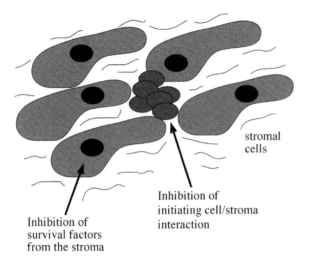

stromal
cells

Inhibition of
initiating cell/stroma
interaction

Inhibition of
survival factors
from the stroma

Figure 3 Possible sites of therapeutic intervention within the melanoma-initiating cell niche. The niche provides important paracrine survival signals and maintains the melanoma-initiating cells in their primitive undifferentiated state. Inhibition of these key survival factors and the physical interaction between the initiating cells and the surrounding matrix and stromal cells is likely to lead to depletion of the initiating cell pool.

TARGETING THE MELANOMA-INITIATING CELLS

The Response of Tumor-Initiating Cells to Therapeutic Intervention

Although the past 40 years have seen many breakthroughs in the treatment of childhood leukemia and testicular cancer, there has been little tangible increase in the survival of patients with most metastatic solid tumors including melanoma, breast, colon, lung, and prostate cancers. The classical approaches to cancer therapy have relied upon killing the rapidly proliferating population of tumor cells through the generation of genotoxic stress, such as chemotherapy/radiation, or by using targeted agents that block the signaling pathways that drive tumor growth (26). The stem cell model posits that as the cancer stem cells cycle very slowly and express multiple drug transporter proteins, they are almost totally resistant to conventional anticancer therapies (27). Although these ideas are widely accepted in the field, data to confirm this hypothesis has only recently become available. It has been recently shown that growth of breast cancer cells under mammosphere culture conditions, which are thought to enrich for the stem cell population, leads to increased radiation resistance and less DNA damage, compared with similar cells grown as adherent cell cultures (28). Intriguingly, radiation treatment actually led to an increase in the percentage of the non-adherent $CD24^{-/low}/CD44^{+}$ cell population, suggesting that radiation treatment increases the size of the tumor-initiating cell pool (28). Similar results were also found in glioma, where the tumor-initiating population is defined through the cell surface expression of CD133$^+$ (29). In these studies, the CD133$^+$ glioma cell population was more resistant to radiation treatment than the CD133$^-$ population. Again, like in the breast cancer studies, it was shown that the CD133$^+$ cell fraction expanded following radiation treatment and that this relatively small increase in the CD133$^+$ population had very profound effects on the tumor growth rate (29). Comparison of DNA damage marker induction following radiation treatment showed that the CD133$^+$ glioma cell population was able to activate the DNA damage checkpoints more efficiently than the CD133$^-$, leading to a more radioresistant phenotype. Hints of a possible strategy to overcome this resistance came when it was shown that inhibition of the DNA damage responsive kinases CHK1 and CHK2 using pharmacological inhibitors sensitized the CD133$^+$ cells to radiation (29).

The marked resistance of tumor-initiating cells to therapeutic intervention also applies to the newer breed of targeted cancer therapies. This is best illustrated by the treatment of CML with the targeted therapy agent imatinib (Gleevec). The progression of CML is driven by a mutation resulting in the splice of the genes encoding for Bcr and the Abl kinase (30). Imatinib works by inhibiting the activity of Bcr-Abl and typically induces a total remission in CML patients. The remission is ultimately followed by disease relapse associated with imatinib resistance, through the acquisition of imatinib-insensitive Bcr-Abl mutations. Recent work has statistically modeled this process on the basis of a cellular hierarchy consisting of terminally differentiated cells, differentiated cells, progenitor cells, and stem cells (31). It showed that during the imatinib treatment there was an initial rapid decline of Bcr-Abl transcript number that correlated with the reduction in the number of differentiated leukemia cells observed. After this treatment there was a prolonged, but slower, reduction in Bcr-Abl transcripts consistent with a depletion of the leukemia progenitor cells. Following treatment cessation or the acquisition of a Bcr-Abl mutation, transcript numbers again began to increase in a manner that was consistent with the failure of imatinib to eradicate the stem cell population (31). At this stage it is not clear whether the failure of the stem cell population to respond to imatinib is a consequence of these cells lacking the Bcr-Abl fusion protein, the lack of Bcr-Abl activity to promote stem cell survival, or whether the niche somehow protects these cells from the deleterious effects of Bcl-Abl inhibition. Taken together, our current understanding of the response of tumor-initiating cells to therapy indicates that most regimens exclusively target the daughter cell or nontumorigenic cell population. Some regimens, such as radiotherapy, may even lead to expansion of the tumor-initiating cell pool, causing rapid tumor regrowth and resistance. Thus, a dual therapeutic approach may be needed, with one drug to target the cancer stem cell population and another drug to target the daughter cell population.

Possible Strategies to Target the Melanoma-Initiating Population

It is becoming clear that neither conventional nor current targeted therapy treatment strategies will deplete the tumor-initiating population in melanoma. To date, most progress in therapeutically targeting tumor-initiating cell populations has focused upon inhibiting the interaction of these cells with their microenvironmental niche. Most progress in this area has been made in studies on leukemia. Recent work has shown that the bone marrow niche provides a protective microenvironment for acute lymphoblastic leukemia (ALL) stem cells, through the stromal cell-derived secretion of asparagine synthetase, an enzyme that is critical for the biosynthesis of the amino acid asparagine (32). Asparaginase, which depletes cells of asparagine, has long been used as an ALL treatment, even though the mechanism of action was unknown. There is a direct correlation between treatment outcome and the intensity of the asparaginase treatment regimen (33). Thus, it was shown that the bone marrow stromal cells produced significantly more asparaginase than the leukemia-initiating cells and that the resistance of the leukemia cells to asparaginase was directly correlated with the expression levels of asparaginase from the bone marrow stromal cells (32).

Another series of leukemia studies demonstrated that the direct targeting of the interaction between the tumor-initiating cells and their niche is a promising future therapeutic strategy. CD44 is a ubiquitously expressed cell surface protein with multiple roles in cell-cell adhesion and cell-matrix adhesion. In the hematopoietic system CD44 is important for leukocyte recruitment to sites of inflammation, and it also seems to play a key role in the adhesion of stem cells to the bone marrow stroma. The possible importance of CD44 in leukemia development was indicated by two recent studies showing that anti-CD44 antibodies prevent leukemia engraftment into immunodeficient mice by preventing migration of the leukemia-initiating cells to the bone marrow (34,35). Blockade of CD44 function also seemed to induce the leukemia-initiating cells to differentiate into a more mature, less stem-like state, leading to substantial reduction in tumor burden (35).

Solid tumor initiating cells do not reside in the bone marrow, and rather less is known about their interactions with the niche. One possible site of the glioma tumor-initiating cell niche is in the vasculature (36). Soluble factors from vascular endothelial cells have been shown to promote self-renewal and inhibit differentiation of neural stem cells, suggesting that this may also be the site of these tumor-initiating cells (37). Evidence for this comes from a recent study showing that the simultaneous targeting of the vascular niche using anti-angiogenic strategies (antivascular endothelial growth factor receptor 2, VEGFR-2 antibodies) in combination with chemotherapy leads to depletion of the tumor-initiating cell compartment (38). Relatively little is known about the niche for melanoma-initiating cells. Previous studies have shown that melanoma cells interact preferentially with both endothelial cells and stromal fibroblasts, and it is possible that these cells may define the melanoma niche (39,40) (Fig. 3). The CD20$^+$ population of melanoma-initiating cells retain the expression of classic melanoma markers such as MCAM (MUC-18) and β3 integrin, suggesting that these adhesion proteins may be involved in the tumor-initiating cell-microenvironmental niche interaction (25). Studies are ongoing to determine the nature of the melanoma-initiating cell niche and whether there are any specific molecules that are amenable to therapeutic targeting.

An alternative therapeutic strategy to deplete the tumor-initiating cell population involves inhibiting the intracellular signaling pathways responsible for regulating stem cell self-renewal and survival (Fig. 3). Preliminary studies have shown that tumor-initiating cells rely more on pathways involved in development, such as Notch, Wnt, and Hedgehog, than normal somatic daughter cells. In pancreatic cancer cells, blockade of the hedgehog signaling pathway using cyclopamine reduces metastatic spread and is associated with a reduced fraction of aldehyde dehydrogenase positive tumor-initiating cells (41). Similarly, studies in glioblastoma show that cyclopamine treatment decreases the self-renewal potential of the tumor-initiating cell population (42). Subsequent intracranial injection of the remaining cyclopamine-treated glioblastoma cells was associated with a complete inhibition of tumor formation, indicating a total depletion of the tumor-initiating cell fraction (42). In melanoma, there is evidence that the Wnt, Notch, and Hedgehog pathways are all involved in cell proliferation and survival (43–45). Notch in particular looks to be important in the metastatic behavior of melanoma, with the overexpression of the Notch converting early-stage nontumorigenic melanomas into those with enhanced potential to form lung metastases (44,45). Under these circumstances, Notch activation involves the activity of β-catenin, suggesting some cross talk between the Notch and Wnt signaling pathways. A number of pharmacological inhibitors of Notch, the γ-secretase inhibitors, are now available for preclinical testing and have been found to reduce melanoma tumorigenecity (46). It remains to be seen whether treatment with γ-secretase inhibitors depletes the melanoma-initiating cell population.

There is a growing realization that any future anticancer treatment will need to target the tumor-initiating population. Ultimately, most solid tumor therapy is associated with eventual relapse and metastatic spread. The successful targeting of the tumor-initiating population is an absolute must to prevent relapse, and it is hoped that the eradication of the cells can reduce most cancers to the level of non-life-threatening chronic diseases. The challenge for the melanoma field is great. At present, we lack even treatments that can impact upon the nontumorigenic cell population, let alone the tumor-initiating population. As most morbidity and mortality from melanoma are the result of metastatic disease, stopping the dissemination of melanoma cells is critical. It is likely that the tumor-initiating cells are the key players in melanoma metastasis, and they should be the major focus of our future studies on melanoma therapy.

REFERENCES

1. Lee ML, Tomsu K, Von Eschen KB. Duration of survival for disseminated malignant melanoma: results of a meta-analysis. Melanoma Res 2000; 10(1):81–92.
2. Atkins MB. The role of cytotoxic chemotherapeutic agents either alone or in combination with biological response modifiers. In: Kirkwood J, ed. Molecular Diagnosis, Prevention & Therapy of Melanoma. New York: Marcel Dekker, 1997:219–225.
3. Houghton AN, Bajorin DF. Chemotherapy for metastatic melanoma. In: Balch CM, Houton AN, Sober AK, et al., eds. Cutaneous Melanoma. Philadelphia, PA: JB Lippincott Company, 1992:498–508.
4. Middleton MR, Grob JJ, Aaronson N, et al. Randomized phase III study of temozolomide versus dacarbazine in the treatment of patients with advanced metastatic malignant melanoma. J Clin Oncol 2000; 18(1):158–166.
5. de Gast GC, Batchelor D, Kersten MJ, et al. Temozolomide followed by combined immunotherapy with GM-CSF, low-dose IL2 and IFN alpha in patients with metastatic melanoma. Br J Cancer 2003; 88(2):175–180.
6. Davies H, Bignell GR, Cox C, et al. Mutations of the BRAF gene in human cancer. Nature 2002; 417(6892):949–954.
7. van Elsas A, Zerp S, van der Flier S, et al. Analysis of N-ras mutations in human cutaneous melanoma: tumor heterogeneity detected by polymerase chain reaction/single-stranded conformation polymorphism analysis. Recent Results Cancer Res 1995; 139:57–67.
8. Curtin JA, Busam K, Pinkel D, et al. Somatic activation of KIT in distinct subtypes of melanoma. J Clin Oncol 2006; 24(26):4340–4346.
9. Smalley KSM. A pivotal role for ERK in the oncogenic behaviour of malignant melanoma? Int J Cancer 2003; 104(5):527–532.
10. Wilhelm SM, Carter C, Tang L, et al. BAY 43-9006 exhibits broad spectrum oral antitumor activity and targets the RAF/MEK/ERK pathway and receptor tyrosine kinases involved in tumor progression and angiogenesis. Cancer Res 2004; 64(19):7099–7109.
11. Wu H, Goel V, Haluska FG. PTEN signaling pathways in melanoma. Oncogene 2003; 22(20):3113–3122.
12. Tsao H, Goel V, Wu H, et al. Genetic interaction between NRAS and BRAF mutations and PTEN/MMAC1 inactivation in melanoma. J Invest Dermatol 2004; 122(2):337–341.
13. Nishimura EK, Granter SR, Fisher DE. Mechanisms of hair graying: incomplete melanocyte stem cell maintenance in the niche. Science 2005; 307(5710):720–724.
14. Tumbar T, Guasch G, Greco V, et al. Defining the epithelial stem cell niche in skin. Science 2004; 303(5656):359–363.
15. Fang D, Leishear K, Nguyen TK, et al. Defining the conditions for the generation of melanocytes from human embryonic stem cells. Stem Cells 2006.
16. Yu H, Fang D, Kumar SM, et al. Isolation of a novel population of multipotent adult stem cells from human hair follicles. Am J Pathol 2006; 168(6):1879–1888.
17. Lapidot T, Sirard C, Vormoor J, et al. A cell initiating human acute myeloid leukaemia after transplantation into SCID mice. Nature 1994; 367(6464):645–648.
18. Inoue A, Seidel MG, Wu W, et al. Slug, a highly conserved zinc finger transcriptional repressor, protects hematopoietic progenitor cells from radiation-induced apoptosis in vivo. Cancer Cell 2002; 2(4):279–288.

19. Blasco MA. Telomeres and human disease: ageing, cancer and beyond. Nat Rev Genet 2005; 6(8):611–622.
20. Dontu G, Al-Hajj M, Abdallah WM, et al. Stem cells in normal breast development and breast cancer. Cell Prolif 2003; 36(suppl 1):59–72.
21. Al-Hajj M, Wicha MS, Benito-Hernandez A, et al. Prospective identification of tumorigenic breast cancer cells. Proc Natl Acad Sci USA 2003; 100(7):3983–3988.
22. Dalerba P, Dylla SJ, Park IK, et al. Phenotypic characterization of human colorectal cancer stem cells. Proc Natl Acad Sci USA 2007; 104(24):10158–10163.
23. Singh SK, Clarke ID, Terasaki M, et al. Identification of a cancer stem cell in human brain tumors. Cancer Res 2003; 63(18):5821–5828.
24. Wicha MS, Liu S, Dontu G. Cancer stem cells: an old idea—a paradigm shift. Cancer Res 2006; 66(4):1883–1890.
25. Fang D, Nguyen TK, Leishear K, et al. A tumorigenic subpopulation with stem cell properties in melanomas. Cancer Res 2005; 65(20):9328–9337.
26. Smalley KS, Herlyn M. Targeting intracellular signaling pathways as a novel strategy in melanoma therapeutics. Ann N Y Acad Sci 2005; 1059:16–25.
27. Dean M, Fojo T, Bates S. Tumour stem cells and drug resistance. Nat Rev Cancer 2005; 5(4):275–284.
28. Phillips TM, McBride WH, Pajonk F. The response of CD24(-/low)/CD44+ breast cancer-initiating cells to radiation. J Natl Cancer Inst 2006; 98(24):1777–1785.
29. Bao S, Wu Q, McLendon RE, et al. Glioma stem cells promote radioresistance by preferential activation of the DNA damage response. Nature 2006; 444(7120): 756–760.
30. Druker BJ, Talpaz M, Resta DJ, et al. Efficacy and safety of a specific inhibitor of the BCR-ABL tyrosine kinase in chronic myeloid leukemia. N Engl J Med 2001; 344(14):1031–1037.
31. Michor F, Hughes TP, Iwasa Y, et al. Dynamics of chronic myeloid leukaemia. Nature 2005; 435(7046):1267–1270.
32. Iwamoto S, Mihara K, Downing JR, et al. Mesenchymal cells regulate the response of acute lymphoblastic leukemia cells to asparaginase. J Clin Invest 2007; 117(4): 1049–1057.
33. Silverman LB, Declerck L, Gelber RD, et al. Results of Dana-Farber Cancer Institute Consortium protocols for children with newly diagnosed acute lymphoblastic leukemia (1981–1995). Leukemia 2000; 14(12):2247–2256.
34. Jin L, Hope KJ, Zhai Q, et al. Targeting of CD44 eradicates human acute myeloid leukemic stem cells. Nat Med 2006; 12(10):1167–1174.
35. Krause DS, Lazarides K, von Andrian UH, et al. Requirement for CD44 in homing and engraftment of BCR-ABL-expressing leukemic stem cells. Nat Med 2006; 12(10): 1175–1180.
36. Calabrese C, Poppleton H, Kocak M, et al. A perivascular niche for brain tumor stem cells. Cancer Cell 2007; 11(1):69–82.
37. Shen Q, Goderie SK, Jin L, et al. Endothelial cells stimulate self-renewal and expand neurogenesis of neural stem cells. Science 2004; 304(5675):1338–1340.
38. Folkins C, Man S, Xu P, et al. Anticancer therapies combining antiangiogenic and tumor cell cytotoxic effects reduce the tumor stem-like cell fraction in glioma xenograft tumors. Cancer Res 2007; 67(8):3560–3564.

39. Smalley KS, Brafford P, Haass NK, et al. Up-regulated expression of zonula occludens protein-1 in human melanoma associates with N-cadherin and contributes to invasion and adhesion. Am J Pathol 2005; 166(5):1541–1554.
40. Li G, Satyamoorthy K, Herlyn M. N-cadherin-mediated intercellular interactions promote survival and migration of melanoma cells. Cancer Research 2001; 61(9): 3819–3825.
41. Feldmann G, Dhara S, Fendrich V, et al. Blockade of hedgehog signaling inhibits pancreatic cancer invasion and metastases: a new paradigm for combination therapy in solid cancers. Cancer Res 2007; 67(5):2187–2196.
42. Bar EE, Chaudhry A, Lin A, et al. Cyclopamine-mediated hedgehog pathway inhibition depletes stem-like cancer cells in glioblastoma. Stem Cells 2007; 25(10): 2524–2533.
43. Stecca B, Mas C, Clement V, et al. Melanomas require HEDGEHOG-GLI signaling regulated by interactions between GLI1 and the RAS-MEK/AKT pathways. Proc Natl Acad Sci USA 2007; 104(14):5895–5900.
44. Balint K, Xiao M, Pinnix CC, et al. Activation of Notch1 signaling is required for beta-catenin-mediated human primary melanoma progression. J Clin Invest 2005; 115(11):3166–3176.
45. Liu ZJ, Xiao M, Balint K, et al. Notch1 signaling promotes primary melanoma progression by activating mitogen-activated protein kinase/phosphatidylinositol 3-kinase-Akt pathways and up-regulating N-cadherin expression. Cancer Res 2006; 66(8):4182–4190.
46. Qin JZ, Stennett L, Bacon P, et al. p53-independent NOXA induction overcomes apoptotic resistance of malignant melanomas. Mol Cancer Ther 2004; 3(8):895–902.

8

Pigmentation Pathways and Microphtalmia-Associated Transcription Factor as New Targets in Melanoma

Rizwan Haq

*Department of Medical Oncology, Dana-Farber Cancer Institute,
Boston, Massachusetts, U.S.A.*

David E. Fisher

*Melanoma Program, Dana-Farber Cancer Institute, Boston,
Massachusetts, U.S.A.*

INTRODUCTION

Skin color is among the most useful predictors of risk of skin cancer including melanoma, squamous cell carcinoma, and basal cell carcinoma (1,2). Darker skin color correlates with reduced incidence of skin cancers, whereas the so-called "red hair color" phenotype of red hair, fair skin, freckling, and inability to tan is associated with a greater risk of cancer. These epidemiologic clues link the pigmentation pathways to the risk and development of melanoma. Here we review the molecular regulation of pigmentation with emphasis on the mechanisms that converge on the microphthalmia-associated transcription factor (MITF), a master regulator of melanocyte development. The ability of these pathways to induce pigmentation and their alteration in melanoma suggests novel rational approaches for the diagnosis, prevention, and therapy of this disease.

REGULATION OF PIGMENTATION

Darker skin results from increased number, size, and altered distribution and composition of pigmentation granules called melanosomes that are produced in melanocytes and transferred to adjacent keratinocytes where most of the pigment resides. Melanosomes contain two types of melanin: yellow-red pheomelanin and brown-black eumelanin. Both are derived from shared biochemical pathways, but the ratio of the two is dependent on the availability of substrates and pigment-enzyme expression (3).

In turn, the biochemical pathways that regulate pigment enzyme production have been revealed by the study of coat color variation in mice. Since the 19th century, more than 100 determinants corresponding to approximately 50 loci have been identified that affect coat color. Among these mutant strains, a series of alleles that "extend" or restrict the amount of eumelanin (with an opposite effect on pheomelanin) were first described in 1968 (4). Whereas wild-type mice have eumelanotic hair, *extension* mice have yellow or pheomelanotic hair. This phenotype was found to result from a point mutation that produces a frameshift in the gene encoding the receptor for melanocyte-stimulating hormone (MSH), known as the melanocortin-1 receptor (*MC1R*) (5). *MC1R* orthologues have been identified in many other species, such as dogs, cats, cattle, birds, bears, fish, amphibians, and reptiles. In humans, geographic differences in pigmentation such as the prevalence of red hair and pale skin in northern European populations are associated with hypomorphic alleles of the *MC1R* gene (6) and increased risk of melanoma (7,8).

MC1R encodes a seven-transmembrane, G-protein-coupled receptor, which, when activated, leads to the generation of adenylate cyclase and the phosphorylation of cyclic adenosine 3',5'-monophosphate (cAMP)-responsive element–binding protein (CREB) (Fig. 1) (9–13). This in turn activates the expression of multiple genes including the one encoding *MITF*, which is required for development of melanocytes and expression of pigment enzymes. As both *MC1R* and *MITF* promote pigmentation, they have not surprisingly been evaluated as targets for melanoma prevention and therapy.

MICROPHTHALMIA TRANSCRIPTION FACTORS

MITF was itself identified as the product of a gene that affects murine coat color (14). Mice lacking all MITF function are devoid of pigment in fur and eyes because of a total absence of melanocytes. These mice also exhibit early-onset deafness, reduced numbers of mast cells, and, for certain mutant alleles, have impairment of secondary bone resorption, leading to an osteopetrotic syndrome (14,15). This phenotype corresponds to the restricted expression pattern of *MITF* in melanocytes, bone, inner ear, and mast cells. Expression can also be detected in cardiac myocytes, which has been hypothesized to be involved in cardiac growth (16). For the purposes of this review, we will limit the discussion to the skin, as reviews of its function in mast cells (17) and bone (18) have been published previously.

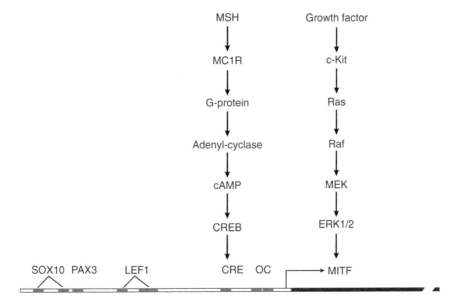

Figure 1 Regulation of MITF via transcriptional and posttranslational mechanisms. *MITF* promoter with key transcriptional regulator-binding sites (*left*). Regulation of MITF through posttranscriptional mechanisms including MSH and ERK/MAPK signaling (*right*). *Abbreviations*: SOX 10, sex-determining region Y box 10; PAX3, paired box region 3; LEF1, lymphoid binding element 1; OC, one-cut; CREB, cAMP-responsive element–binding protein; CRE, CREB-binding element; MC1R, melanocortin-1 receptor; cAMP, cyclic adenosine 3′,5′-monophosphate.

MITF encodes a basic helix-loop-helix leucine zipper (bHLH-ZIP) transcription factor that homo- or heterodimerizes with the related transcription factors, TFEB, TFE3, and TFEC (19) (Fig. 2). These transcription factors, collectively termed the "MiT family of transcription factors," are more ubiquitously expressed and unlike MITF are not essential for melanocytic differentiation (20). Through their basic domains, they bind to DNA target sequences containing the canonical E-box promoter element CACGTC or the nonpalindromic sequence CACATG (21).

Comparisons with other species have identified conservation of regions that are predicted or experimentally shown to regulate MITF expression and activity (22) (Fig. 2). These include the transcription factors CREB (23), *onecut-2* (24), Pax3 (25,26), and targets of the Wnt-signaling pathway, lymphocyte enhancer–binding factor 1/T cell factor (LEF1/TCF) (29–34) and Sox10 (26–28, 35–37). MITF is also regulated by posttranslational modification including phosphorylation, ubiquitination, and SUMOylation. In particular, c-Kit signaling regulates MITF via mitogen-activated protein kinase (MAPK)/extracellular signal–regulated

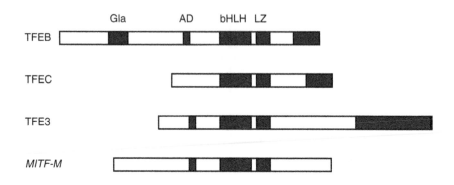

Figure 2 Schematic representation of the micropthalmia family of transcriptional factors. *Abbreviations*: AD, acidic domain; bHLH, basic helix-loop-helix; LZ, leucine zipper domain.

kinase (ERK)-mediated phosphorylation of MITF (38). ERK-dependent phosphorylation leads to the recruitment of the transcriptional coactivators p300/ CREB-binding protein (CBP) and also to ubiquitin-mediated destruction of MITF (9,39,40). MITF is also phosphorylated directly by p38MAPK and glycogen synthase kinases-3β (10,13,41). SUMOylation sites are conserved among vertebrates and invertebrates (22), and SUMOylation by the protein inhibitor of activated signal transducer and activator of transcription 3 (STAT3) differentially affects activation of MITF-responsive promoters (42,43). MITF has a conserved putative site of acetylation, though it has not yet been shown to be acetylated experimentally (22).

When its expression is upregulated in normal melanocytes, MITF initiates a transcriptional program leading to melanocyte differentiation, enhanced cell cycle arrest, survival, and pigmentation (Table 1). It directly regulates the transcription of major pigmentation genes, including tyrosinase (*TYR*) (44–46), tyrosinase-related protein 1 (*TYRP-1*) (47) gene, dopachrome tautomerase (*DCT*)/*TYRP-2* (47,48), quail neuroretina clone 71 (*QNR-71*) (49), *silver* (50,51), and absent in melanoma 1 (*AIM-1*) (52). The antiapoptotic protein Bcl-2 is directly transactivated by MITF and supports the survival of melanocytes since Bcl-2 knockout results in melanocyte death (53). It has also been suggested that MITF may induce cell cycle arrest during melanocytic differentiation, potentially via transcriptional targeting of the cyclin-dependent kinase (CDK) inhibitors *p21*, *CDKN1A* (54), and *CDK4A* (INK4A) (55). Thus, by promoting survival of the melanocyte pool and increasing pigmentation, activation of MITF would be expected to provide cutaneous photoprotection and reduced susceptibility to melanoma.

Table 1 Proposed Direct Targets of MITF in Melanocytes

Pigmentation	References
Tyrosinase (*TYR*)	44–46
Tyrosinase-related protein 1 (*TYRP-1*)	47
Dopachrome tautomerase (*DCT/TYRP-2*)	47,48
Quail neuroretina clone 71(*QNR-71*)	49
Silver homolog (*SILV*)	50,51
Absent in melanoma-1 (*AIM-1*)	52
Melan-A (*MLANA/MART1*)	74
Melanocortin-1 receptor (*MC1R*), α melanocyte–stimulating hormone receptor	75
G-protein-coupled receptor 143 (ocular albinism type 1)	76

Cell cycle control and apoptosis	
Transient receptor potential cation channel, subfamily M, member 1 (melastatin, *TRPM1*)	77
B-cell CLL/lymphoma 2 (*BCL-2*)	53
Cyclin-dependent kinase inhibitor 1A (*CDKN1A*)	54
Cyclin-dependent kinase inhibitor 2A (*CDKN2A*)	55
Cyclin-dependent kinase 2 (*CDK2*)	53
Diaphanous homolog 1 (*DIAPH1*)	78

Invasion and differentiation	
Met proto-oncogene (hepatocyte growth factor receptor, *MET*)	53,70
Bestrophin 1 (*BEST1*), VMD2	79
Hypoxia-inducible factor 1α (*HIF1A*)	80

PIGMENTATION STRATEGIES TO PREVENT MELANOMA

Indeed, a majority of melanomas have diminished levels of *MITF* relative to melanocytes, and high *MITF* expression may in many contexts inhibit proliferation of melanoma cells (56,57). Consistent with its predicted roles in melanocytes, downregulation of *MITF* expression has been associated with worsened overall survival and increased incidence of lymph node metastasis in intermediate-thickness cutaneous malignant melanoma (58). These results suggest that activation of pigmentation pathways might be useful in melanoma prevention.

The feasibility of such an approach was recently suggested using a mouse model with an inactivating mutation of *MC1R* (*MC1R*e/e), recapitulating the red-hair color phenotype in humans. Treatment of these mice with topically delivered forskolin, which directly activates adenylate cyclase and *MITF*, leads to skin darkening and protection from carcinoma and DNA damage after ultraviolet irradiation (59). Alternative strategies to activate MC1R using synthetic mela-notropins or cAMP directly or via topically delivered activators of MSH synthesis have also been evaluated (60–62). As expression of the MSH precursor pro-opiomelanocortin (*POMC*) in keratinocytes is activated by p53 (63), pharmacologic stimulation of the tanning response by augmenting p53 activity without use of DNA-damaging agents is another approach (64). For example, treatment of intact skin with small DNA fragments induced a DNA-damage response in the absence of radiation and may provide photoprotection (65,66). Though there are intensive efforts to activate p53 in a variety of different tumor types, these approaches have a number of caveats, not least of which is activation of senescence in the multiple cell types of the skin. However, the ability to deliver topical therapy may limit systemic toxicity and side effects.

PIGMENTATION STRATEGIES FOR MELANOMA TREATMENT

Despite its role in promoting cutaneous photoprotection, roughly 15% to 20% of melanomas have amplifications of *MITF* (67–69). Integrative genomic analyses of melanomas using high-density single nucleotide polymorphisms have identified *MITF* as an oncogene. In contrast to the studies reported above, dysregulation of *MITF* expression led to decreased cell growth in response to docetaxel or cisplatin (67) and *MITF* overexpression was associated with a decrease in five-year overall survival. Moreover, enforced *MITF* overexpression was shown to cooperate with the common melanoma oncogene *BRAF* (V600E) to transform human melanocytes in which the Rb and p53 pathways had been inactivated. These results indicate that MITF can have either differentiative or pro-tumorigenic effects, depending on the cellular context. Whereas physiologic activation of *Bcl-2* expression may protect melanocytes (for example, from ultraviolet light), its upregulation in the context of melanoma may actually contribute to this cancer's notorious chemoresistance. In the context of melanomas, *MITF* can also activate *CDK2*, which may lead to cell proliferation (53). Diaphanous homolog 1 (*DIAPH1*), a direct target of *MITF*, targets *CDKN1B*, thereby further supporting cell proliferation in melanomas. *MITF* has also been shown to regulate expression of the proto-oncogene *MET*, which may contribute to the invasive nature of melanomas (53,70).

These results suggest that MITF regulates both pigmentation and melanocyte proliferation and survival in a context-dependent manner. Although *MITF* is an amplified oncogene in only a minority of melanomas, its lineage survival role appears to extend to melanomas in which *MITF* is not amplified. For example, melanoma cell lines lacking *MITF* amplification still remain dependent on MITF for proliferation/survival. Whereas elevated MITF expression is generally associated with pigmentation/differentiation within melanocytes, it is unclear how *MITF* amplification in melanoma induces oncogenic transformation and overcomes the potential restraints associated with differentiation. Perhaps inactivation of the Rb or p53 pathway cooperates with *MITF* amplification in driving oncogenesis. Collectively, these observations indicate that in the context of many melanomas, targeting the MITF pathway may offer a therapeutic approach. Given that transcription factors are notoriously difficult to target by chemical biologic approaches, identification of critical upstream or downstream mediators of MITF function in melanomas is an area of intensive evaluation.

FUTURE DIRECTIONS

Melanoma is as much as 500- to 1000-fold more likely to develop in individuals with fair, Caucasian skin (71,72). Therefore, a better understanding of human skin pigmentation may offer improved strategies for melanoma prevention. Given that pigmentation is a major barrier to ultraviolet light, it is tempting to consider potential protective effects of skin tanning (73). Despite the known carcinogenic risk of ultraviolet radiation, alternative nongenotoxic strategies may potentially offer a safer approach. Furthermore, a molecular analysis of the physiologic pathways leading to pigmentation and tanning may be clinically applicable for risk prediction and prognosis. Allied with these approaches, improved screening for early detection would appear likely to have rapid and tangible impact on melanoma mortality. Conversely, improved molecular targeting strategies will also offer novel approaches to disabling the engine driving melanoma growth and survival. MITF is uniquely poised as a regulator of pigmentation (pertinent to melanoma prevention) and proliferation/survival (pertinent to oncogenesis). As the mechanisms governing these divergent activities are more fully elucidated, it is hoped that therapeutic strategies that target MITF will also be identified, both to enhance melanoma prevention and better treat those that have already formed.

ACKNOWLEDGMENTS

The authors gratefully acknowledge research support from the National Institutes of Health. David E. Fisher is a Doris Duke Distinguished Clinical Investigator and Jan and Charles Nirenberg Fellow in Pediatric Oncology at the Dana-Farber Cancer Institute.

REFERENCES

1. Gandini S, Sera F, Cattaruzza MS, et al. Meta-analysis of risk factors for cutaneous melanoma: I. Common and atypical naevi. Eur J Cancer 2005; 41(1):28–44.
2. Xu LY, Koo J. Predictive value of phenotypic variables for skin cancer: risk assessment beyond skin typing. Int J Dermatol 2006; 45(11):1275–1283.
3. Land EJ, Riley PA. Spontaneous redox reactions of dopaquinone and the balance between the eumelanic and phaeomelanic pathways. Pigment Cell Res 2000; 13(4): 273–277.
4. Searle AG. An extension series in the mouse. J Hered 1968; 59(6):341–342.

5. Robbins LS, Nadeau JH, Johnson KR, et al. Pigmentation phenotypes of variant extension locus alleles result from point mutations that alter MSH receptor function. Cell 1993; 72(6):827–834.

6. Valverde P, Healy E, Jackson I, et al. Variants of the melanocyte-stimulating hormone receptor gene are associated with red hair and fair skin in humans. Nat Genet 1995; 11(3):328–330.

7. Box NF, Duffy DL, Chen W, et al. MC1R genotype modifies risk of melanoma in families segregating CDKN2A mutations. Am J Hum Genet 2001; 69(4):765–773.

8. Landi MT, Bauer J, Pfeiffer RM, et al. MC1R germline variants confer risk for BRAF-mutant melanoma. Science 2006; 313(5786):521–522.

9. Wu M, Hemesath T, Takemoto C, et al. c-Kit triggers dual phosphorylations, which couple activation and degradation of the essential melanocyte factor Mi. Genes Dev 2000; 14(3):301–312.

10. Mansky K, Sankar U, Han J, et al. Microphthalmia transcription factor is a target of the p38 MAPK pathway in response to receptor activator of NF-kappa B ligand signaling. J Biol Chem 2002; 277(13):11077–11083.

11. Price ER, Horstmann MA, Wells AG, et al. α-Melanocyte-stimulating hormone signaling regulates expression of microphthalmia, a gene deficient in Waardenburg syndrome. J Biol Chem 1998; 273(49):33042–33047.

12. Takeda K, Takemoto C, Kobayashi I, et al. Ser298 of MITF, a mutation site in Waardenburg syndrome type 2, is a phosphorylation site with functional significance. Hum Mol Genet 2000; 9(1):125–132.

13. Hemesath T, Price E, Takemoto C, et al. MAP kinase links the transcription factor Microphthalmia to c-Kit signalling in melanocytes. Nature 1998; 391(6664):298–301.

14. Hodgkinson C, Moore K, Nakayama A, et al. Mutations at the mouse microphthalmia locus are associated with defects in a gene encoding a novel basic-helix-loop-helix-zipper protein. Cell 1993; 74(2):395–404.

15. Stechschulte DJ, Sharma R, Dileepan KN, et al. Effect of the mi allele on mast cells, basophils, natural killer cells, and osteoclasts in C57Bl/6J mice. J Cell Physiol 1987; 132(3):565–570.

16. Tshori S, Gilon D, Beeri R, et al. Transcription factor MITF regulates cardiac growth and hypertrophy. J Clin Invest 2006; 116(10):2673–2681.

17. Morii E, Oboki K, Ishihara K, et al. Roles of MITF for development of mast cells in mice: effects on both precursors and tissue environments. Blood 2004; 104(6): 1656–1661.

18. Hershey CL, Fisher DE. Mitf and Tfe3: members of a b-HLH-ZIP transcription factor family essential for osteoclast development and function. Bone 2004; 34(4): 689–696.

19. Hemesath TJ, Steingrimsson E, McGill G, et al. Microphthalmia, a critical factor in melanocyte development, defines a discrete transcription factor family. Genes Dev 1994; 8(22):2770–2780.

20. Steingrimsson E, Tessarollo L, Pathak B, et al. Mitf and Tfe3, two members of the Mitf-Tfe family of bHLH-Zip transcription factors, have important but functionally redundant roles in osteoclast development. Proc Natl Acad Sci USA 2002; 99(7): 4477–4482.

21. Aksan I, Goding CR. Targeting the microphthalmia basic helix-loop-helix-leucine zipper transcription factor to a subset of E-box elements in vitro and in vivo. Mol Cell Biol 1998; 18(12):6930–6938.

22. Hallsson JH, Favor J, Hodgkinson C, et al. Genomic, transcriptional and mutational analysis of the mouse microphthalmia locus. Genetics 2000; 155(1):291–300.
23. Lang D, Lu M, Huang L, et al. Pax3 functions at a nodal point in melanocyte stem cell differentiation. Nature 2005; 433(7028):884–887.
24. Jacquemin P, Lannoy VJ, O'Sullivan J, et al. The transcription factor onecut-2 controls the microphthalmia-associated transcription factor gene. Biochem Biophys Res Commun 2001; 285(5):1200–1205.
25. Lang D, Lu MM, Huang L, et al. Pax3 functions at a nodal point in melanocyte stem cell differentiation. Nature 2005; 433(7028):884–887.
26. Potterf SB, Furumura M, Dunn KJ, et al. Transcription factor hierarchy in Waardenburg syndrome: regulation of MITF expression by SOX10 and PAX3. Hum Genet 2000; 107(1):1–6.
27. Huber WE, Price ER, Widlund HR, et al. A tissue-restricted cAMP transcriptional response: SOX10 modulates alpha-melanocyte-stimulating hormone-triggered expression of microphthalmia-associated transcription factor in melanocytes. J Biol Chem 2003; 278(46):45224–45230.
28. Verastegui C, Bille K, Ortonne JP, et al. Regulation of the microphthalmia-associated transcription factor gene by the Waardenburg syndrome type 4 gene, SOX10. J Biol Chem 2000; 275(40):30757–30760.
29. Widlund HR, Horstmann MA, Price ER, et al. Beta-catenin-induced melanoma growth requires the downstream target microphthalmia-associated transcription factor. J Cell Biol 2002; 158(6):1079–1087.
30. Schepsky A, Bruser K, Gunnarsson GJ, et al. The microphthalmia-associated transcription factor Mitf interacts with beta-catenin to determine target gene expression. Mol Cell Biol 2006; 26(23):8914–8927.
31. Saito H, Yasumoto K, Takeda K, et al. Microphthalmia-associated transcription factor in the Wnt signaling pathway. Pigment Cell res 2003; 16(3):261–265.
32. Saito H, Yasumoto K, Takeda K, et al. Melanocyte-specific microphthalmia-associated transcription factor isoform activates its own gene promoter through physical interaction with lymphoid-enhancing factor 1. J Biol Chem 2002; 277(32):28787–28794.
33. Takeda K, Yasumoto K, Takada R, et al. Induction of melanocyte-specific microphthalmia-associated transcription factor by Wnt-3a. J Biol Chem 2000; 275(19): 14013–14016.
34. Dorsky RI, Raible DW, Moon RT. Direct regulation of nacre, a zebrafish MITF homolog required for pigment cell formation, by the Wnt pathway. Genes Dev 2000; 14(2):158–162.
35. Verastegui C, Bille K, Ortonne JP, et al. Regulation of the microphthalmia-associated transcription factor gene by the Waardenburg syndrome type 4 gene, SOX10. J Biol Chem 2000; 275(40):30757–30760.
36. Elworthy S, Lister JA, Carney TJ, et al. Transcriptional regulation of mitfa accounts for the sox10 requirement in zebrafish melanophore development. Development 2003; 130(12):2809–2818.
37. Potterf SB, Furumura M, Dunn KJ, et al. Transcription factor hierarchy in Waardenburg syndrome: regulation of MITF expression by SOX10 and PAX3. Hum Genet 2000; 107(1):1–6.
38. Wu M, Hemesath TJ, Takemoto CM, et al. c-Kit triggers dual phosphorylations, which couple activation and degradation of the essential melanocyte factor Mi. Genes Dev 2000; 14(3):301–12.

39. Sato S, Roberts K, Gambino G, et al. CBP/p300 as a co-factor for the microphthalmia transcription factor. Oncogene 1997; 14(25):3083–3092.
40. Price E, Ding H, Badalian T, et al. Lineage-specific signaling in melanocytes. C-kit stimulation recruits p300/CBP to microphthalmia. J Biol Chem 1998; 273(29): 17983–17986.
41. Khaled M, Larribere L, Bille K, et al. Microphthalmia associated transcription factor is a target of the phosphatidylinositol-3-kinase pathway. J Invest Dermatol 2003; 121(4):831–836.
42. Miller AJ, Levy C, Davis IJ, et al. Sumoylation of MITF and its related family members TFE3 and TFEB. J Biol Chem 2005; 280(1):146–155.
43. Murakami H, Arnheiter H. Sumoylation modulates transcriptional activity of MITF in a promoter-specific manner. Pigment Cell Res 2005; 18(4):265–277.
44. Bentley NJ, Eisen T, Goding CR. Melanocyte-specific expression of the human tyrosinase promoter: activation by the microphthalmia gene product and role of the initiator. Mol Cell Biol 1994; 14(12):7996–8006.
45. Ganss R, Schutz G, Beermann F. The mouse tyrosinase gene. Promoter modulation by positive and negative regulatory elements. J Biol Chem 1994; 269(47):29808–29816.
46. Yasumoto K, Yokoyama K, Takahashi K, et al. Functional analysis of micro-phthalmia-associated transcription factor in pigment cell-specific transcription of the human tyrosinase family genes. J Biol Chem 1997; 272(1):503–509.
47. Bertolotto C, Busca R, Abbe P, et al. Different cis-acting elements are involved in the regulation of TRP1 and TRP2 promoter activities by cyclic AMP: pivotal role of M boxes (GTCATGTGCT) and of microphthalmia. Mol Cell Biol 1998; 18(2):694–702.
48. Yasumoto K, Mahalingam H, Suzuki H, et al. Transcriptional activation of the melanocyte-specific genes by the human homolog of the mouse Microphthalmia protein. J Biochem (Tokyo) 1995; 118(5):874–881.
49. Turque N, Denhez F, Martin P, et al. Characterization of a new melanocyte-specific gene (QNR-71) expressed in v-myc-transformed quail neuroretina. Embo J 1996; 15(13):3338–3350.
50. Baxter LL, Pavan WJ. Pmel17 expression is Mitf-dependent and reveals cranial melanoblast migration during murine development. Gene Expr Patterns 2003; 3(6): 703–707.
51. Du J, Miller AJ, Widlund HR, et al. MLANA/MART1 and SILV/PMEL17/GP100 are transcriptionally regulated by MITF in melanocytes and melanoma. Am J Pathol 2003; 163(1):333–343.
52. Du J, Fisher DE. Identification of Aim-1 as the underwhite mouse mutant and its transcriptional regulation by MITF. J Biol Chem 2002; 277(1):402–426.
53. Reff ME, Davidson RL. Deoxycytidine reverses the suppression of pigmentation caused by 5-BrdUrd without changing the distribution of 5-BrdUrd in DNA. J Biol Chem 1979; 254(15):6869–6872.
54. Carreira S, Goodall J, Aksan I, et al. Mitf cooperates with Rb1 and activates p21Cip1 expression to regulate cell cycle progression. Nature 2005; 433(7027):764–769.
55. Loercher AE, Tank EM, Delston RB, et al. MITF links differentiation with cell cycle arrest in melanocytes by transcriptional activation of INK4A. J Cell Biol 2005; 168(1):35–40.
56. Wellbrock C, Marais R. Elevated expression of MITF counteracts B-RAF-stimulated melanocyte and melanoma cell proliferation. J Cell Biol 2005; 170(5):703–708.

57. Selzer E, Wacheck V, Lucas T, et al. The melanocyte-specific isoform of the microphthalmia transcription factor affects the phenotype of human melanoma. Cancer Res 2002; 62(7):2098–2103.

58. Salti GI, Manougian T, Farolan M, et al. Micropthalmia transcription factor: a new prognostic marker in intermediate-thickness cutaneous malignant melanoma. Cancer Res 2000; 60(18):5012–5016.

59. D'Orazio JA, Nobuhisa T, Cui R, et al. Topical drug rescue strategy and skin protection based on the role of Mc1r in UV-induced tanning. Nature 2006; 443(7109):340–344.

60. Abdel-Malek ZA, Kadekaro AL, Kavanagh RJ, et al. Melanoma prevention strategy based on using tetrapeptide alpha-MSH analogs that protect human melanocytes from UV-induced DNA damage and cytotoxicity. FASEB J 2006; 20(9):1561–1563.

61. Lan EL, Ugwu SO, Blanchard J, et al. Preformulation studies with melanotan-II: a potential skin cancer chemopreventive peptide. J Pharm Sci 1994; 83(8):1081–1084.

62. Levine N, Sheftel SN, Eytan T, et al. Induction of skin tanning by subcutaneous administration of a potent synthetic melanotropin. JAMA 1991; 266(19):2730–2736.

63. Cui R, Widlund HR, Feige E, et al. Central role of p53 in the suntan response and pathologic hyperpigmentation. Cell 2007; 128(5):853–864.

64. Barsh G, Attardi LD. A healthy tan? N Engl J Med 2007; 356(21):2208–2210.

65. Eller MS, Gilchrest BA. Tanning as part of the eukaryotic SOS response. Pigment Cell Res 2000; 13 (suppl 8):94–97.

66. Eller MS, Ostrom K, Gilchrest BA. DNA damage enhances melanogenesis. Proc Natl Acad Sci USA 1996; 93(3):1087–1092.

67. Garraway L, Widlund H, Rubin M, et al. Integrative genomic analyses identify MITF as a lineage survival oncogene amplified in malignant melanoma. Nature 2005; 436(7047):117–122.

68. Stark M, Hayward N. Genome-wide loss of heterozygosity and copy number analysis in melanoma using high-density single-nucleotide polymorphism arrays. Cancer Res 2007; 67(6):2632–2642.

69. Jonsson G, Dahl C, Staaf J, et al. Genomic profiling of malignant melanoma using tiling-resolution arrayCGH. Oncogene 2007; 26(32):4738–4748.

70. Beuret L, Flori E, Denoyelle C, et al. Up-regulation of MET expression by alpha-melanocyte-stimulating hormone and MITF allows hepatocyte growth factor to protect melanocytes and melanoma cells from apoptosis. J Biol Chem 2007; 282(19): 14140–14147.

71. Kollias N, Sayre RM, Zeise L, et al. Photoprotection by melanin. J Photochem Photobiol B 1991; 9(2):135–160.

72. Kaidbey KH, Agin PP, Sayre RM, et al. Photoprotection by melanin—a comparison of black and Caucasian skin. J Am Acad Dermatol 1979; 1(3):249–260.

73. Fitzpatrick TB. The validity and practicality of sun-reactive skin types I through VI. Arch Dermatol 1988; 124(6):869–871.

74. Du J, Miller AJ, Widlund HR, et al. MLANA/MART1 and SILV/PMEL17/GP100 are transcriptionally regulated by MITF in melanocytes and melanoma. Am J Pathol 2003; 163(1):333–343.

75. Aoki H, Moro O. Involvement of microphthalmia-associated transcription factor (MITF) in expression of human melanocortin-1 receptor (MC1R). Life Sci 2002; 71(18):2171–2179.

76. Vetrini F, Auricchio A, Du J, et al. The microphthalmia transcription factor (Mitf) controls expression of the ocular albinism type 1 gene: link between melanin synthesis and melanosome biogenesis. Mol Cell Biol 2004; 24(15):6550–6559.
77. Miller AJ, Du J, Rowan S, et al. Transcriptional regulation of the melanoma prognostic marker melastatin (TRPM1) by MITF in melanocytes and melanoma. Cancer Res 2004; 64(2):509–516.
78. Carreira S, Goodall J, Denat L, et al. Mitf regulation of dia1 controls melanoma proliferation and invasiveness. Genes Dev 2006; 20(24):3426–3439.
79. Esumi N, Kachi S, Campochiaro PA, et al. VMD2 promoter requires two proximal E-box sites for its activity in vivo and is regulated by the MITF-TFE family. J Biol Chem 2007; 282(3):1838–1850.
80. Busca R, Berra E, Gaggioli C, et al. Hypoxia-inducible factor 1{alpha} is a new target of microphthalmia-associated transcription factor (MITF) in melanoma cells. J Cell Biol 2005; 170(1):49–59.

9

Understanding Interferon: Translating Biologic Advances into Clinical Progress

Gregory B. Lesinski

Department of Molecular Virology, Immunology and Medical Genetics, The Ohio State University, Columbus, Ohio, U.S.A.

William E. Carson III

Department of Surgery, The Ohio State University, Columbus, Ohio, U.S.A.

OVERVIEW OF INTERFERON-α IN THE SETTING OF MALIGNANT MELANOMA

More so than most other malignancies, spontaneous regressions of disease have been observed on occasion in patients with advanced malignant melanoma (1,2). Careful histologic evaluations have revealed that this process is associated with the infiltration of tumor tissues by activated lymphocytes (3). Consequently, much effort has centered on the development of immune-based treatments for the therapy of this malignancy, especially in light of the fact that it is a relatively chemoresistant form of cancer (4). Cytokine therapy with interferon-α (IFNα) produced overall response rates in the range of 10% to 15% in the setting of metastatic melanoma, and this cytokine was subsequently evaluated as an adjuvant to the surgical resection of thick primary tumors (>4 mm in Breslow depth) or metastases to regional lymph nodes. Randomized clinical trials have shown that high-dose adjuvant IFNα can increase relapse-free and possibly overall survival after surgery for high-risk lesions and IFNα was therefore approved by the U.S. Food and Drug Administration (FDA) for this indication in 1995 (5). IFNα is the only approved therapy to be used as an adjuvant following surgery; however, as with many cytokine treatments, its use is associated with a unique spectrum of toxicities that limits its acceptance with patients and physicians. Other agents may eventually come into use in the adjuvant setting but it will likely be a decade or more before randomized clinical trials can confirm their superiority to high-dose IFNα therapy. With the new tools that are available for the evaluation of immunologic therapies, it is possible that great strides could be made in our understanding of the mechanisms that underlie the antitumor actions of IFNα. Consequently, it is important that scientists and physicians work together so that rational improvements can be made in the use of IFNα in the clinical setting.

EFFICACY OF IFNα THERAPY IN METASTATIC DISEASE

Recombinant (r) IFNα became available for use in clinical trials in the mid-1980s (6). The available data suggested that IFNα acted to inhibit the proliferation of malignant cells and stimulate immune effectors and might therefore have activity in the setting of advanced disease (7,8). The dosages employed in early phase I and phase II trials ranged from 3 to 100 million units (MU) per square meter (m^2) and would today be considered high-dose regimens. Despite the variety of regimens employed and the variability of the subject populations, response rates consistently ranged between 5% and 30% (9). These results stimulated a great deal of enthusiasm for the immune therapy of cancer, particularly metastatic melanoma. An analysis of selected trials employing rIFNα in patients with malignant melanoma revealed an average overall response rate of 16.7% (10). Complete responses have been encountered most frequently at higher dose levels (10–50 MU/m^2); however, complete responses do occur in response to very low doses of IFNα. The route of administration does not appear to be a critical factor in the induction of objective responses as investigators have reported complete responses following the use of the intravenous (i.v.) or intramuscular routes in sequential trials conducted at the same institution (11). In general, complete responses represent approximately one-third of total responses. More recent reviews of trials employing IFNα have confirmed the role of IFN immunotherapy in the treatment of metastatic melanoma (12). Likewise, the objective response rate and overall survival of metastatic renal cell cancer (RCC) patients treated with IFNα has been investigated in a series of randomized clinical trials (13–15). Investigators have used ''placebo-equivalent'' control arms with agents such as vinblastine or medroxyprogesterone to address the possibility of low compliance in placebo-controlled trials. Under these conditions, an objective response rate of 15% is observed for IFNα therapy of metastatic RCC in conjunction with a modest, but statistically significant, overall survival benefit. Taken together, these studies indicate that administration of IFNα can mediate the regression of disease in a significant number of patients with advanced cancer. Unfortunately, the precise mechanisms that underlie this antitumor activity are not well defined.

ADJUVANT THERAPY OF SURGICALLY RESECTED MELANOMA WITH IFNα

The results obtained with IFNα in the setting of metastatic melanoma prompted investigators to explore the utility of high-dose IFNα for patients who had undergone complete surgical excision of their tumor, yet were at high risk for recurrent disease. Kirkwood et al. conducted a phase III trial in which patients were randomized to receive high-dose IFNα-2b (20 MU/m^2/day) i.v. for one month followed by 10 MU/m^2/thrice weekly subcutaneously for 48 weeks or observation. The results of this trial were reported in 1994 and revealed increased overall survival and relapse-free survival in patients who received IFNα (16). Enthusiasm for this treatment has been tempered by the fact that a confirmatory trial comparing the efficacy of the high-dose and low-dose IFNα regimens (3 MU thrice weekly for two years) in a similar population of surgically treated patients revealed no difference in overall survival for either schedule of IFNα as compared with observation alone, although increased relapse-free survival was observed in patients receiving the higher dose of IFNα (17). Similarly, extended duration low-dose IFNα-2a (3 MU thrice weekly) did not prolong the overall survival or relapse-free survival of high-risk resected patients in a multi-institutional study conducted in the United Kingdom (18). In contrast to this result, an adjuvant trial comparing an antiganglioside vaccine with high-dose IFNα was halted as the result of an early analysis that showed a clear survival advantage to patients in the IFNα arm (19). This development suggested that the effects of IFNα in the adjuvant setting are distinct but perhaps limited to a subgroup of patients (20). Importantly, trials of very low-dose IFNα (i.e., 1 MU/m^2) have not demonstrated significant efficacy in the adjuvant setting (21). Thus, if it were not for the attendant side effects of high-dose IFNα, it is likely that this treatment regimen would be widely employed in high-risk patients. IFNα-2b is the only FDA-approved adjuvant therapy for melanoma patients who have undergone successful surgery for high-risk lesions. There is no alternative therapy that has shown efficacy in randomized trials. Therefore, IFNα will continue as the standard of care for the foreseeable future.

IFNα SIGNALS VIA THE JAK-STAT PATHWAY OF SIGNAL TRANSDUCTION

The cellular events underlying IFNα-induced signal transduction and gene regulation in immune effectors and tumor cells were elucidated, beginning in the early 1990s, and these discoveries have provided important clues as to its mechanism of action as a therapeutic agent for cancer. The receptor for IFNα is widely expressed and has been identified on multiple tumors and cell lines (22).

This receptor consists of two transmembrane chains (IFNAR1 and IFNAR2) that associate with intracellular signaling proteins belonging to the Janus family of kinases, Janus kinase 1 (Jak1) and Tyrosine kinase 2 (Tyk2). The binding of IFNα to its receptor brings the two kinases into close proximity whereupon they become activated via phosphorylation and in turn phosphorylate the cytoplasmic tail of each receptor chain on specific tyrosine residues. These phosphotyrosine residues provide docking sites for cytoplasmic transcription factors belonging to the signal transducer and activator of transcription (STAT) family of proteins. These STAT proteins (STAT1α, STAT2) are phosphorylated by the Jak and subsequently form high-affinity DNA-binding complexes that rapidly translocate to the cell nucleus (23). Here they interact with specific sequences within the promoters of IFNα-responsive genes and initiate transcription (24). The proto-typical IFNα signaling reaction recruits a DNA-binding complex known as the IFN-stimulated gene factor 3 (ISGF3), which consists of STAT1α (or STAT1β), STAT2, and a nonphosphorylated chaperone protein known as p48 or IRF9 (25). ISGF3 binds to a specific DNA sequence known as the IFN-stimulated response element or ISRE (26). Many IFN-responsive genes have been found to contain a region with homology to the ISRE sequence within their promoters (27–29). Some of these genes (e.g., ISG-15, MHC class I, and IP-10) have well-defined functions that could potentially mediate antitumor effects, while the function of most ISGs in mediating the antimelanoma effects of IFNα is only superficially understood. Microarray analysis has only recently been employed in the analysis of the complex cellular response to IFNα in the setting of melanoma, and it is likely that multiple IFN response genes that play a role in the antitumor activities of this cytokine will eventually be identified. Recently, investigators have identified a family of negative regulatory proteins termed suppressors of cyto-kine signaling (SOCS) that are induced by ISGF3 and specifically downregulate Jak-STAT signal transduction (30). Jak-STAT activation is also negatively regulated by other mechanisms including protein inhibitors of activated STATs (PIAS), SHP-1 and SHP-2 (SH2 domain-containing tyrosine phosphatases that dephosphorylate activated receptors), and truncated STAT isoforms (31–33). Recent published reports have indicated that sodium stibogluconate (SSG), an inhibitor of SHP-1 and SHP-2, can synergize with IFNα to inhibit growth of melanoma cells in vitro and in vivo (34,35). Future investigations into the clinical importance of these negative regulatory pathways may lead to further strategies for augmenting the antitumor effects of IFNα.

STAT1 MODIFICATIONS IN RESPONSE TO IFNα

The critical role of STAT1 phosphorylation on tyrosine residue 701 (Tyr[701]) for the induction of gene expression in response to IFNα has been well documented, but it is clear that other STAT1 modifications occur following IFNα stimulation (36–38). STAT1 undergoes serine phosphorylation at residue 727 (Ser[727]) in response to a variety of stimuli and signaling pathways, including members of the mitogen-activated protein kinase (MAPK) family (39,40). Cells treated with type I and type II IFNs undergo phosphorylation at both Tyr^{701} and Ser^{727} (41), however, reconstitution of a STAT1-deficient cell line with a modified STAT1 protein (serine→alanine at residue 727) largely restored biological responses to IFNα (but not IFN-γ) (42). The precise role of STAT1 serine phosphorylation in the antitumor effects of IFNα remains to be explored, although it appears that this modification serves largely to prime the STAT1 protein for increased transcriptional activity in response to IFN-γ. Methylation of STAT1 on Arg^{31} by an arginine methyltransferase (PRMT1) is also required for IFNα-induced gene transcription, and inhibition of STAT1 methylation impairs STAT1 DNA binding because of its association with the STAT inhibitor, PIAS-1 (43). Somewhat unexpectedly, the DNA demethylating nucleoside analog 5-AZA-2'-deoxycytidine (5-AZA-dC) has been shown to synergistically augment the antiproliferative and proapoptotic effects of IFNα in vitro and inhibit the growth of human melanoma xenografts in a mouse model (44).

POTENTIAL ROLE OF OTHER SIGNALING PATHWAYS IN MEDIATING THE ANTITUMOR EFFECTS OF IFNα

STAT proteins are also known to interact with several coactivator molecules within the nucleus that aid in regulating transcription via mechanisms including chromatin remodeling and histone deacetylase activity (45). In addition, CRKL (a member of the CRK family of adaptor proteins) interacts with Tyk2 and is tyrosine phosphorylated in response to IFNα. CRKL can then activate RAP1, a small GTPase that is related to RAS (46), or bind to STAT5 and translocate to the cell nucleus (47). Activation of the RAP1 pathway thereby regulates a broad spectrum of biological activities, including cell proliferation, differentiation, and adhesion (48). RAP1 has also been shown to regulate the activation of MAPK signaling cascades, including the p38 pathway (49,50), which transmits signals that are essential for the generation of IFNα-mediated antiproliferative activity. The phosphatidyl-inositol 3-kinase (PI3K) signaling pathway has been shown to be activated by IFNα in a STAT1-independent manner (51,52), leading to regulation of apoptosis, mRNA translation, and nuclear factor kappa-B (NF-κB) signal transduction (53). Finally, it has also been demonstrated that the presence of phosphorylated STAT3 can inhibit the responsiveness of cells to IFNα (54,55). The involvement of these additional signaling systems demonstrates the complexity of IFN signal transduction, the central role of the Jak-STAT pathway, and the potential for significant downstream amplification of the IFNα signal.

POTENTIAL MECHANISMS UNDERLYING THE ACTIONS OF IFNα: IMMUNOSTIMULATORY EFFECTS

It has been difficult to determine the optimal dose of IFNα for cancer patients or devise strategies to enhance its antitumor effects because its cellular target(s) and mechanism of action are unknown. In theory, an exogenously administered cytokine might exert an antitumor effect via stimulation of the host immune system or by a direct effect on the tumor cell or its immediate environment (56). The type I IFNs (IFNα and IFN-β) exert multiple effects on T cells and natural killer (NK) cells that enhance their ability to recognize and destroy malignant cells, thus linking the innate immune response with the more sustained adaptive-immune response (57). IFNα induces NK cell–mediated cytotoxicity and proliferation in vivo and regulates either directly or indirectly the activity of numerous chemokines and cytokines including IFN-γ, interleukin (IL)-1, IL-2, IL-3, IL-6, IL-8, IL-12, IL-13, and IL-15, tumor necrosis factor-alpha (TNF-α), granulocyte macrophage colony stimulating factor (GM-CSF), IFN-inducible protein 10 (IP-10), and IFN-stimulated gene 15 (ISG-15) as well as the cell-surface expression or soluble expression of numerous cytokine receptor components (56). IFNα elicits lymphocyte-activated killer (LAK) activity in vivo and also exerts a profound effect on cytotoxic T cell responses by stimulating the proliferation, generation, and activation of existing memory $CD8^+$ cytotoxic T cells (56,57). It is to be noted that there is evidence that IFNα/β can elicit expression of IL-15 in peripheral blood monocytes and cultured dendritic cells (DC), which has been theorized to contribute to the proliferation and survival of NK cells and CD8-positive T cells (57). IFNα also strongly upregulates tumor cell expression of MHC class I and class II antigens and adhesion molecules such as intercellular adhesion molecule-1 (ICAM-1) and L-selectin, which are critical for the recognition and destruction of malignant cells by cytotoxic T cells (58,59). Data from clinical trials have demonstrated a correlation between therapy relapse and melanoma cell expression of nonclassical human leukocyte antigen (HLA) molecules such as HLA-G (60). This suggests that resistance to IFNα therapy might be a result of altered NK cell immunosurveillance. These data support the analysis of the T cell and NK cell compartments following IFNα therapy. Interestingly, recent reports indicate that patients who develop autoantibodies and clinical manifestations of autoimmunity during the course of adjuvant IFNα therapy are less likely to experience disease recurrence. In a study by Gogas et al., autoantibodies were detected in 52 melanoma patients following adjuvant IFNα therapy (26%). Univariate and multivariate regression analyses indicated that autoimmunity was an independent prognostic marker for improved relapse-free survival and overall survival ($p < 0.001$) (61). The development of autoimmunity may signify that exogenous IFNα can break the tolerance of host T lymphocytes to host antigens as well as melanoma-associated antigens and further suggests that its mechanism of antitumor action is largely immunologic in nature.

POTENTIAL MECHANISMS UNDERLYING THE ACTIONS OF IFNα: DIRECT ANTITUMOR EFFECTS

The direct antitumor effects of IFNα may be roughly classified as antiproliferative, anti-angiogenic, or proapoptotic in nature (62–65). The precise mechanism of growth inhibition remains a topic of investigation but likely involves the modulation of several major cell cycle–regulatory proteins. Sangfelt et al. showed that the activity of the G_1 cyclin-dependent kinases (which promote the passage of cells through the cell cycle) was inhibited by IFNα and that this event was preceded by the rapid induction of p15 and p21 (and later p27), which are important inhibitors of the cyclin-dependent kinases (66). Recently, Xiao et al. found that IFNα induces the expression of RIG-G, which in turn mediates increased expression of p21 and p27 (67). The ability of IFNα to inhibit the formation of new blood vessels is probably due to its ability to inhibit the release of fibroblast growth factor (FGF) by tumor cells. Reports of its efficacy in the therapy of life-threatening hemangiomas of infancy (which are dependent on autocrine FGF production) are evidence for the importance of the latter pathway (68,69). In general, the proapoptotic effects of IFNα are modest, however, under certain circumstances, it can exert measurable apoptotic effects on cancer cells. Studies investigating IFNα-induced apoptosis performed in the Daudi cell line, multiple myeloma, and SV-40-transformed keratinocytes have shown that apoptosis occurs via activation of caspases-1, -2, -3, -8, and -9 and that this activation was a critical event (70,71). Interestingly, IFNα has also been reported to activate the mitochondrial pathway of apoptosis through the release of cytochrome c in renal cancer cell lines (72). Recent studies conducted in the U266 multiple myeloma cell line further suggested that the proapoptotic proteins Bak and Bax may play a key role in IFNα-induced apoptosis, and that IFNα treatment leads to caspase-8-mediated cleavage of Bid (BH3 interacting domain death agonist, a proapoptotic member of the Bcl-2 protein family) to its active form, tBid (73). Other studies in bladder cancer and basal cell carcinoma cell lines have shown that IFNα can stimulate Fas-mediated apoptosis and autocrine secretion of TNF-α and TNF-related apoptosis–inducing ligand (TRAIL) (74,75). These studies demonstrate that IFNα has many different effects on melanoma cells and that the relative importance of any one pathway may be difficult to determine.

EVIDENCE AGAINST A DIRECT EFFECT OF IFNα ON MELANOMA CELLS IN THE ADJUVANT SETTING

Most cancer cells (including melanoma tumors) routinely express functional IFNα receptors and their growth is inhibited by physiologic concentrations of this cytokine (76,77). We have previously demonstrated that ex vivo treatment of patient tumors with clinically relevant concentrations of IFNα consistently led to activation of STAT1 and STAT2 (78). It was also shown that some IFNα-resistant human melanoma cell lines exhibit defects in specific Jak-STAT intermediates, which when reversed, led to the recovery of in vitro sensitivity to IFNα (79–81). Of note, the most common defect appeared to be the loss of STAT1. These findings suggested that IFNα administration might help to prevent tumor recurrence via a direct effect on tumor cells. However, we recently reported that tumor expression of STAT1 and STAT2 did not correlate with effectiveness of adjuvant IFNα. We identified a large cohort of high-risk patients with loss of STAT1 in their tumor, which exhibited prolonged survival in response to adjuvant IFNα, while other patients, who had normal expression of Jak-STAT proteins, recurred after just a few months of IFN therapy (82). These results have recently been confirmed by a second group, who showed that while phosphorylation of STAT1 at Tyr^{701} and Ser^{727} was not inducible in 63% of patient tumors, STAT1 activation defects showed no correlation with disease outcome or response to IFNα-2b immunotherapy as indicated by progression-free survival (83). Recent studies from our laboratory have also shown that patient melanoma cells exhibit low levels of STAT1 activation in response to IFNα (as compared with immune cells from the same patient), even when all the major components of the Jak-STAT signaling pathway were present (55). Thus, the direct effects of IFNα on melanoma tumor cells, while measurable and distinct, may not be a key determinant of IFN responsiveness at the clinical level.

THE ANTITUMOR EFFECTS OF EXOGENOUS IFNα ARE ABROGATED IN A STAT1-DEFICIENT MOUSE

The fact that STAT1-deficient ($STAT1^{-/-}$) mice manifest severe deficiencies in IFN-mediated antiviral immunity suggested that the antitumor effects of IFNα might proceed primarily via immunologic mechanisms (84). To investigate the contribution of STAT1-mediated gene regulation within the tumor, our group generated a STAT1-deficient murine melanoma cell line, AGS-1 (85,86). STAT1 was reconstituted within AGS-1 cells by retroviral gene transfer. The resulting cell line ($AGS-1^{STAT1}$) showed normal regulation of IFNα-stimulated genes (H2k, ISG-54) as compared with AGS-1 cells infected with the empty vector ($AGS-1^{MSCV}$). However, mice challenged with the AGS-1, $AGS-1^{STAT1}$, and $AGS-1^{MSCV}$ cell lines exhibited nearly identical survival in response to IFNα treatment, indicating that restored STAT1 signaling within the tumor did not augment the antitumor activity of IFNα. In contrast, $STAT1^{-/-}$ mice could not utilize exogenous IFNα to inhibit the growth of $STAT1^{+/+}$ melanoma cells in either an intraperitoneal tumor model or in the adjuvant setting (Fig. 1). The survival of tumor-bearing $STAT1^{-/-}$ mice was identical regardless of whether they received IFNα or phosphate-buffered saline (PBS) (Fig. 1b). $STAT1^{-/-}$ mice exhibited normal levels of circulating immune effector cells, but spleno-cytes from $STAT1^{-/-}$ mice exhibited a 90% to 95% reduction in cytotoxic activity against the NK-sensitive YAC1 cell line in a ^{51}Cr-release assay. Thus, STAT1-mediated gene regulation within immune effectors (but not tumor cells) was necessary for mediating the antitumor effects of IFNα in this experimental system (85). These experiments provide compelling evidence that the immu-nostimulatory effects of IFNα are a critical component of its mechanism of action. IFNα can activate transcription via alternate signaling pathways that do no not employ Jak-STAT signaling intermediates (e.g., p38 MAP kinase, phosphatidylinositol 3-kinase [PI3K], NF-κB, and double-stranded RNA-activated serine-threonine protein kinase) (40,87–90). However, if activation of STAT1-independent signaling pathways within the host, the tumor, or the tumor

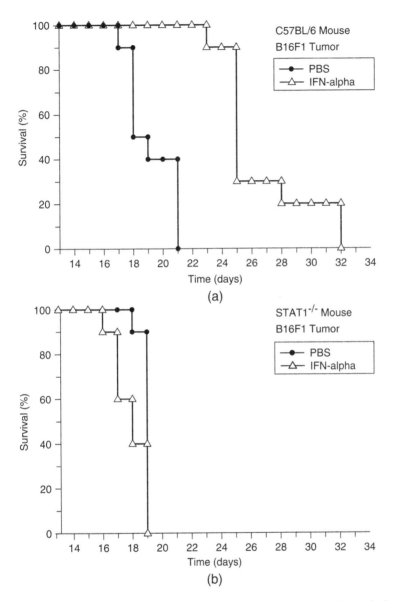

Figure 1 Absence of STAT1 in the host results in decreased survival following tumor challenge. STAT1$^{-/-}$ and C57BL/6 mice ($n = 10$ mice/group) were injected i.p. with 1×10^6 B16F1 melanoma cells. Compared with PBS-treated controls (—●—), IFNα treatment (2×10^4 U/d) (—△—) prolonged the survival of C57BL/6 mice but not STAT1$^{-/-}$ mice challenged with B16F1 melanoma cells (**a** and **b**). *Abbreviations*: STAT, signal transducer and activator of transcription; PBS, phosphate-buffered saline; i.p., intraperitoneally. *Source*: From Ref. 85.

microenvironment were critically important to the antitumor effects of IFNα, then administration of this cytokine should have prolonged the survival of STAT1-deficient mice bearing the parental B16 melanoma cell line. More recently, our group has explored the role of a class of proteins known as SOCS, which we hypothesized might inhibit IFNα-induced signal transduction, gene regulation, and antitumor activity of immune effector cells (91). As predicted, the induction of P-STAT1 and the subsequent transcription of ISGs in IFNα-treated splenocytes were significantly greater in SOCS1- and SOCS3-deficient mice than in splenocytes from their respective wild-type counterparts ($p < 0.05$). SOCS1-deficient mice bearing a murine melanoma tumor exhibited prolonged survival in response to treatment with IFNα as compared with wild-type mice, and mice that survived this challenge were able to reject subsequent tumor challenges. Importantly, depletion of $CD8^+$ T cells abrogated the antitumor effects of IFNα in tumor-bearing SOCS-deficient mice. Thus, cytotoxic T cells appear to play an important role in the elimination of melanoma tumor cells in this model. Taken together, these results indicate that STAT1-mediated signal transduction within host immune effector cells, but not tumor cells, is critical to the antitumor action of exogenously administered IFNα.

A NOVEL FLOW CYTOMETRIC ASSAY FOR PHOSPHORYLATED STAT1 REVEALS DOSE-DEPENDENT ACTIVATION

The use of phosphorylation state–specific antibodies for intracellular flow cytometry has unique potential for the evaluation of signaling events in immune effectors following the administration of immunomodulatory cytokines. A flow cytometric technique has been developed for the detection of phosphorylated (P) STAT1 within immune effector subsets that is rapid, highly quantitative, and extremely sensitive (92). Representative data obtained using this methodology and its validation via fluorescent microscopy are illustrated in Figure 2. Our group has used this method to examine the peripheral blood mononuclear cell (PBMC) response to IFN in vitro and in patient PBMCs following IFNα immunotherapy. As a result of this work, we have made the following discoveries: (*i*) Jak-STAT signal transduction is rapidly (<15 minutes) stimulated within all the major immune cell subsets; (*ii*) The P-STAT1 response to IFNα is most vigorous in T lymphocytes and monocytes; (*iii*) Optimal signal transduction is obtained at relatively low doses of IFNα (10^2–10^3 U/mL); (*iv*) The P-STAT1 response to high dose IFNα varies significantly from patient to patient; and (*v*) Flow cytometry for P-STAT1 can potentially be used to optimize Jak-STAT signal transduction in response to IFNα therapy on an individual basis. Until the precise molecular determinants of IFNα responsiveness are identified, it seems reasonable to use signal transduction within immune effector cells as a surrogate marker of IFNα action in patients undergoing immunotherapy. Other groups have utilized this methodology to examine the IFNα responsiveness of patient immune cells and have demonstrated reduced generation of P-STAT1 in

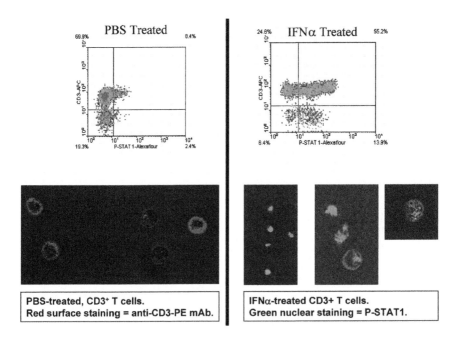

Figure 2 Flow cytometric analysis and fluorescent microscopy of phosphorylated STAT1 (P-STAT1) in peripheral blood mononuclear cells treated with PBS (vehicle; *Left Panel*) or IFNα (10^4 U/mL; 15 minutes; *Right Panel*). Cells were also costained with an antibody targeting CD3. *Abbreviations*: STAT, signal transducer and activator of transcription; PBS, phosphate-buffered saline (*See Color Insert*).

patient T cells after in vitro IFNα stimulation as compared with T cells from normal donors (93).

COMPARISON OF IFNα-INDUCED SIGNAL TRANSDUCTION AND GENE REGULATION IN PATIENT PBMCS FOLLOWING ADMINISTRATION OF ESCALATING DOSES OF IFNα-2B

Our group has shown that intermediate doses of IFNα were most effective in activating STAT1 and inducing the expression of IFN-stimulated gene in patient PBMCs in vitro (92). We therefore hypothesized that intermediate doses of IFNα might be just as effective as higher doses in activating Jak-STAT signal transduction and inducing the transcription of ISGs in immune cells. We studied samples obtained from patients with metastatic melanoma who were enrolled in a clinical trial of bevacizumab in combination with IFNα-2b. Escalating doses of IFNα-2b (5 MU/m^2 for two weeks and then 10 MU/m^2 thereafter) were employed. PBMCs were procured from patient peripheral blood ($n = 11$) just prior to therapy and again one hour after the administration of IFNα-2b and were analyzed for the presence of native STAT1 and activated STAT1 by intracellular flow cytometric analysis and the induction of ISG transcripts by real-time polymerase chain reaction (PCR). Activation of STAT1 in response to IFNα at 5 MU/m^2 was greater or equivalent to the 10 MU/m^2 dose of IFNα for 10 of 11 of the patients studied. Within individual patients, overall levels of unphosphorylated STAT1 did not diminish greatly over time following administration of IFNα for two weeks. In fact, in most patients, levels of STAT1 were actually higher at the time that the 10 MU/m^2 dose was administered as compared with baseline. Similarly, the induction of ISGs within PBMCs at a dose of 5 MU/m^2 IFNα was greater or statistically equivalent to that observed for 10 MU/m^2 IFNα for the majority of the patients. In addition, microarray analysis was performed on four patients with metastatic melanoma undergoing immunotherapy with escalating doses of IFNα-2b (95). Analysis of the gene-expression profile within PBMCs from these patients revealed that a total of 33 genes (e.g., *IFIT1, IFIT3, IFIT5, IFI44, CXCL10, OAS1, MX1, STAT1*) were induced to an equivalent extent with 5 MU/m^2 as compared with 10 MU/m^2 IFNα-2b (fold induction ≥2). Because of the trial design, it is not known whether the reduced IFN responsiveness (at the level of STAT1 phosphorylation) would have been observed following continued administration of the lower dose of IFNα (i.e., the drop in P-STAT1 was a time-dependent effect rather than a dose-dependent effect). These results suggest that lower doses of IFNα-2b may be just as effective as higher doses with respect to the induction of Jak-STAT signal transduction and ISGs within immune effector cells and support further studies of IFNα signal transduction and gene regulation in patients receiving IFNα therapy.

MICROARRAY ANALYSIS OF THE IMMUNE RESPONSE TO IFNα THERAPY

We hypothesized that microarray analysis could be utilized to identify candidate molecular targets important for mediating the antitumor effect of exogenously administered IFNα. To identify the STAT1-dependent genes regulated by IFNα, the gene expression profile of splenocytes from wild-type and STAT1-deficient mice was characterized (94). This analysis identified 30 genes that required STAT1 signal transduction for optimal expression in response to IFNα ($p < 0.001$). These genes include granzyme b (*GZMB*), interferon regulatory factor 7 (*IRF7*), Fas death domain–associated protein (*DAXX*), and lymphocyte antigen 6 complex, locus C (*LY6C*). The expression of 20 genes was found to be suppressed in the presence of STAT1 including chemokine ligand 2 (*CCL2*), *CCL5*, and *CCL7*. Nineteen genes were significantly upregulated in murine splenocytes following treatment with IFNα regardless of the presence of STAT1 including *CD86*, lymphocyte antigen 6 complex, locus A (*LY6A*), and Tap-binding protein (*TAPBP*). The expression of representative IFN-responsive genes was confirmed at the transcriptional level by real-time PCR.

This report is the first to investigate the profile of STAT1-dependent gene expression in murine immune cells following treatment with IFNα.

Our group has also employed microarray analysis to identify the genes that are regulated by IFNα therapy in human immune cells. The gene expression profiles of PBMCs obtained from melanoma patients receiving their first dose of adjuvant IFNα (20 MU/m^2 i.v.) was examined. Twenty-three genes (e.g., *IFIT3, ISG20,* and *IRF7*) were found to be upregulated by greater than twofold ($p < 0.001$). This report was the first to characterize the transcriptional profiles of PBMCs from melanoma patients undergoing IFNα immunotherapy. Future studies will examine the gene expression profiles of specific immune cell subsets, such as NK cells and CD8-positive T cells, and will correlate gene expression patterns with clinical outcome.

CONCLUSIONS

IFNα exhibits antimelanoma activity in vitro, in murine models, and in clinical trials. Its mechanism of action is complex and, in humans, may involve both the ability to activate host immune cells as well as direct effects on tumor cells. Utilization of novel technologies such as microarray analysis in the clinical setting will help to identify patient populations that are most likely to benefit from IFNα administration.

REFERENCES

1. Papac RJ. Spontaneous regression of cancer. Cancer Treat Rev 1996; 22:395–423.
2. Glaspy JA. Therapeutic options in the management of renal cell carcinoma. Semin Oncol 2002; 29(3 suppl 7):41–46
3. Schneeberger A, Koszik F, Stingl G. Immunologic host defense in melanoma: delineation of effector mechanisms involved and of strategies for the augmentation of their efficacy. J Invest Dermatol 1995; 105:110S–116S.
4. Balch CM, Reintgen DS, Kirkwood JM. Cutaneous Melanoma. In: DeVita VT, Hellman S, Rosenberg SA, eds. Principles and Practice of Oncology. Philadelphia, PA: Lipincott, Williams & Wilkens, 2001: 1499–1547.
5. Moschos S, Kirkwood JM. Present role and future potential of type I interferons in adjuvant therapy of high-risk operable melanoma. Cytokine Growth Factor Rev 2007; 18(5–6):451–458.
6. Dorr RT. Interferon-alpha in malignant and viral diseases: a review. Drugs 1993; 45:177–211.
7. Bart RS, Porzio NR, Kopf AW, et al. Inhibition of growth of B16 murine malignant melanoma by exogenous interferon. Cancer Res 1980; 40:614–619.
8. Gresser I, De Maeyer-Guignard J, Tovey MG, et al. Electrophoretically pure mouse interferon exerts multiple biologic effects. Proc Natl Acad Sci USA 1979; 76: 5308–5312.
9. Chapman PB, Parkinson DR, Kirkwood JM. Biologic Therapy. In: Balch CM, Houghton AN, Sober AJ, et al., eds. Cutaneous Melanoma. St. Louis, MO: Quality Medical Publishing, 1998:419–436.

10. Legha SS. Interferons in the treatment of malignant melanoma. A review of recent trials. Cancer 1986; 57:1675–1677.
11. Kirkwood JM, Ernstoff MS, Davis CA, et al. Comparison of intramuscular and intravenous recombinant alpha-2 interferon in melanoma and other cancers. Ann Intern Med 1985; 103:32–36.
12. Agarwala S. Improving survival in patients with high-risk and metastatic melanoma: Immunotherapy leads the way. Am J Clin Dermatol 2003; 4:333–346.
13. Steineck G, Strander H, Carbin BE, et al. Recombinant leukocyte interferon alpha-2a and medroxyprogesterone in advanced renal cell carcinoma. A randomized trial. Acta Oncol 1990; 29:155–162.
14. Interferon-alpha and survival in metastatic renal carcinoma: early results of a randomised controlled trial. Medical Research Council Renal Cancer Collaborators. Lancet 1999; 353:14–17.
15. Pyrhönen S, Salminen E, Ruutu M, et al. Prospective randomized trial of interferon alfa-2a plus vinblastine versus vinblastine alone in patients with advanced renal cell cancer. J Clin Oncol 1999; 17:2859–2867.
16. Kirkwood JM, Strawderman MH, Ernstoff MS, et al. Interferon alpha-2b adjuvant therapy of high-risk resected cutaneous melanoma: The Eastern Cooperative Oncology Group Trial EST 1684. J Clin Oncol 1996; 14:7–17.
17. Kirkwood JM, Ibrahim JG, Sondak VK, et al. High- and low-dose interferon alfa-2b in high-risk melanoma: first analysis of intergroup trial E1690/S9111/C9190. J Clin Oncol 2000; 18:2444–2458.
18. Hancock BW, Wheatley K, Harris S, et al. Adjuvant interferon in high-risk melanoma: the AIM HIGH study–United Kingdom Coordinating Committee on cancer research randomized study of adjuvant low-dose extended duration interferon alfa-2a in high-risk resected malignant melanoma. J Clin Oncol 2004; 22:53–61.
19. Kirkwood JM, Ibrahim JG, Sosman JA, et al. High-dose interferon alfa-2b significantly prolongs relapse-free and overall survival compared with the GM2-KLH/QS-21 vaccine in patients with resected stage IIB-III melanoma: results of intergroup trial E1694/S9512/C509801. J Clin Oncol 2001; 19:2370–2380.
20. Kirkwood JM, Manola J, Ibrahim J, et al. A pooled analysis of Eastern Cooperative Oncology Group and intergroup trials of adjuvant high-dose interferon for melanoma. Clin Cancer Res 2004; 10:1670–1677.
21. Schuchter LM. Adjuvant interferon therapy for melanoma: high-dose, low-dose, no dose, which dose? J Clin Oncol 2004; 22:7–10.
22. Kim SH, Cohen B, Novick D, et al. Mammalian type I interferon receptors consists of two subunits: IFNaR1 and IFNaR2. Gene 1997; 196:279–286.
23. Haque SJ, Williams BR. Signal transduction in the interferon system. Semin Oncol 1998; 25:14–22.
24. Ransohoff RM. Cellular responses to interferons and other cytokines: the JAK-STAT paradigm. N Engl J Med 1998; 338:616–618.
25. Darnell JE, Kerr IM, Stark GR. Jak-STAT pathways and transcriptional activation in response to IFNs and other extracellular signaling proteins. Science 1994; 264:1415–1421.
26. Levy DE, Kessler DS, Pine R, et al. Interferon-induced nuclear factors that bind a shared promoter element correlate with positive and negative control. Genes Dev 1988; 2:383–393.

27. Meraro D, Gleit-Kielmanowicz M, Hauser H, et al. IFN-stimulated gene 15 is synergistically activated through interactions between the myelocyte/lymphocyte-specific transcription factors, PU.1, IFN regulatory factor-8/IFN consensus sequence binding protein, and IFN regulatory factor-4: characterization of a new subtype of IFN-stimulated response element. J Immunol 2002; 168:6224–6231.

28. Hatina VJ, Kralova J, Jansa P. Identification of an intragenic interferon-stimulated response element sequence of the mouse class I MHC complex H-2Kb gene. Exp Clin Immunogene 1996; 13:55–60.

29. Ohmori Y, Hamilton TA. The interferon-stimulated response element and a kappa B site mediate synergistic induction of murine IP-10 gene transcription by IFN-gamma and TNF-alpha. J Immunol 1995; 154:5235–5244.

30. Alexander WS. Suppressors of cytokine signaling (SOCS) in the immune system. Nat Rev Immunol 2002; 2:410–416.

31. Liu B, Liao J, Rao X, et al. Inhibition of Stat1-mediated gene activation by PIAS1. Proc Natl Acad Sci USA. 1998; 95:10626–10631.

32. You M, Yu DH, Feng GS. Shp-2 tyrosine phosphatase functions as a negative regulator of the interferon-stimulated Jak/STAT pathway. Mol Cell Biol 1999; 19:2416–2424.

33. Kile BT, Nicola NA, Alexander WS. Negative regulators of cytokine signaling. Int J Hematol 2001; 73:292–298.

34. Li J, Lindner DJ, Farver C, et al. Efficacy of SSG and SSG/IFNalpha2 against human prostate cancer xenograft tumors in mice: a role for direct growth inhibition in SSG anti-tumor action. Cancer Chemother Pharmacol 2007; 60(3):341–349.

35. Yi T, Pathak MK, Lindner DJ, et al. Anticancer activity of sodium stibogluconate in synergy with IFNs. J Immunol 2002; 169(10):5978–5985.

36. O'Shea JJ, Gadina M, Schreiber RD. Cytokine signaling in 2002: new surprises in the Jak/Stat pathway. Cell 2002; 109(suppl):S121–S131.

37. Nusinzon I, Horvath CM. Interferon-stimulated transcription and innate antiviral immunity require deacetylase activity and histone deacetylase 1. Proc Natl Acad Sci USA 2003; 100:14742–14747.

38. Wesemann DR, Qin H, Kokorina N, et al. TRADD interacts with STAT1-alpha and influences interferon-gamma signaling. Nat Immunol 2004; 5:199–207.

39. Decker T, Kovarik P. Serine phosphorylation of STATs. Oncogene 2000; 19: 2628–2637.

40. Uddin S, Majchrzak B, Woodson J, et al. Activation of the p38 mitogen-activated protein kinase by type I interferons. J Biol Chem 1999; 274:30127–30131.

41. Kovarik P, Mangold M, Ramsauer K, et al. Specificity of signaling by STAT1 depends on SH2 and C-terminal domains that regulate Ser727 phosphorylation, differentially affecting specific target gene expression. EMBO J 2001; 20:91–100.

42. Horvath CM, Darnell JE Jr. The antiviral state induced by alpha interferon and gamma interferon requires transcriptionally active Stat1 protein. J Virol 1996; 70:647–650.

43. Mowen KA, Tang J, Zhu W, et al. Arginine methylation of STAT1 modulates IFNalpha/beta-induced transcription. Cell 2001; 104:731–741.

44. Reu FJ, Bae SI, Cherkassky L, et al. Overcoming resistance to interferon-induced apoptosis of renal carcinoma and melanoma cells by DNA demethylation. J Clin Oncol 2006; 24(23):3771–3779.

45. Huang M, Qian F, Hu Y, et al. Chromatin-remodelling factor BRG1 selectively activates a subset of interferon-alpha-inducible genes. Nat Cell Biol 2002; 4(10): 774–781.
46. Feller SM. Crk family adaptors-signalling complex formation and biological roles. Oncogene 2001; 20(44):6348–6371.
47. Fish EN, Uddin S, Korkmaz M, et al. Activation of a CrkL-stat5 signaling complex by type I interferons. J Biol Chem 1999; 274(2):571–573.
48. Bos JL, de Rooij J, Reedquist KA. Rap1 signalling: adhering to new models. Nat Rev Mol Cell Biol 2001; 2(5):369–377.
49. Stork PJ. Does Rap1 deserve a bad Rap? Trends Biochem Sci 2003; 28(5):267–275.
50. Platanias LC. Mechanisms of type-I- and type-II-interferon-mediated signalling. Nat Rev Immunol 2005; 5(5):375–386.
51. Uddin S, Fish EN, Sher D, et al. The IRS-pathway operates distinctively from the Stat-pathway in hematopoietic cells and transduces common and distinct signals during engagement of the insulin or interferon-alpha receptors. Blood 1997; 90(7): 2574–2582.
52. Uddin S, Lekmine F, Sharma N, et al. The Rac1/p38 mitogen-activated protein kinase pathway is required for interferon alpha-dependent transcriptional activation but not serine phosphorylation of Stat proteins. J Biol Chem 2000; 275(36):27634–27640.
53. Thyrell L, Hjortsberg L, Arulampalam V, et al. Interferon alpha-induced apoptosis in tumor cells is mediated through the phosphoinositide 3-kinase/mammalian target of rapamycin signaling pathway. J Biol Chem 2004; 279(23):24152–24162.
54. Wang W, Edington HD, Rao UN, et al. Modulation of signal transducers and activators of transcription 1 and 3 signaling in melanoma by high-dose IFNalpha2b. Clin Cancer Res 2007; 13(5):1523–1531.
55. Lesinski GB, Trefry J, Brasdovich M, et al. Melanoma cells exhibit variable signal transducer and activator of transcription 1 phosphorylation and a reduced response to IFN-alpha compared with immune effector cells. Clin Cancer Res 2007; 13(17): 5010–5019.
56. Brassard DL, Grace MJ, Bordens RW. Interferon-alpha as an immunotherapeutic protein. J Leukoc Biol 2002; 71:565–581.
57. Biron CA. Interferons alpha and beta as immune regulators–a new look. Immunity 2001; 14:661–664.
58. Von Stamm U, Brocker EB, Von Depka Prondzinski M, et al. Effects of interferon-alpha (IFN-alpha) on the antigenic phenotype of melanoma metastases. EORTC melanoma group cooperative study No. 18852. Melanoma Res 1993; 3:173–180.
59. Martin-Henao GA, Quiroga R, Sureda A, et al. L-selectin expression is low on CD34+ cells from patients with chronic myeloid leukemia and interferon-α up-regulates this expression. Haematologica 2000;85(2):139–146.
60. Wagner SN, Rebmann V, Willers CP, et al. Expression analysis of classic and non-classic HLA molecules before interferon alfa-2b treatment of melanoma. Lancet 2000; 356:220–221.
61. Gogas H, Ioannovich J, Dafni U, et al. Prognostic significance of autoimmunity during treatment of melanoma with interferon. N Engl J Med 2006; 354(7):709–718.
62. Chin YE, Kitagawa M, Su WC, et al. Cell growth arrest and induction of cyclin-dependent kinase inhibitor p21 WAF1/CIP1 mediated by STAT1. Science 1996; 272:719–722.

63. Huang S, Bucana CD, Van Arsdall M, et al. Stat1 negatively regulates angiogenesis, tumorigenicity and metastasis of tumor cells. Oncogene 2002; 21:2504–2512.
64. Selleri C, Sato T, Del Vecchio L, et al. Involvement of Fas-mediated apoptosis in the inhibitory effects of interferon-alpha in chronic myelogenous leukemia. Blood 1997; 89:957–964.
65. Baker PK, Pettitt AR, Slupsky JR, et al. Response of hairy cells to IFN-alpha involves induction of apoptosis through autocrine TNF-alpha and protection by adhesion. Blood 2002; 100:647–653.
66. Sangfelt O, Erickson S, Castro J, et al. Molecular mechanisms underlying interferon-alpha-induced G0/G1 arrest: CKI-mediated regulation of G1 Cdk-complexes and activation of pocket proteins. Oncogene 1999; 18(18):2798–2810.
67. Xiao S, Li D, Zhu HQ, et al. RIG-G as a key mediator of the antiproliferative activity of interferon-related pathways through enhancing p21 and p27 proteins. Proc Natl Acad Sci USA 2006; 103(44):16448–16453.
68. Dinney CP, Bielenberg DR, Perrotte P, et al. Inhibition of basic fibroblast growth factor expression, angiogenesis, and growth of human bladder carcinoma in mice by systemic interferon-alpha administration. Cancer Res 1998; 58:808–814.
69. Ezekowitz RA, Mulliken JB, Folkman J. Interferon alfa-2a therapy for life-threatening hemangiomas of infancy. N Engl J Med 1992; 326:1456–1463.
70. Thyrell L, Erickson S, Zhivotovsky B, et al. Mechanisms of interferon-alpha induced apoptosis in malignant cells. Oncogene 2002; 21:1251–1262.
71. Thyrell L, Hjortsberg L, Arulampalam V, et al. Interferon alpha-induced apoptosis in tumor cells is mediated through the phosphoinositide 3-kinase/mammalian target of rapamycin signaling pathway. J Biol Chem 2004; 279:24152–24162.
72. Kelly JD, Dai J, Eschwege P, et al. Downregulation of Bcl-2 sensitises interferon-resistant renal cancer cells to Fas. Br J Cancer 2004; 91:164–170.
73. Panaretakis T, Pokrovskaja K, Shoshan MC, et al. Interferon-alpha-induced apoptosis in U266 cells is associated with activation of the proapoptotic Bcl-2 family members Bak and Bax. Oncogene 2003; 22:4543–4556.
74. Li C, Chi S, He N, et al. IFNalpha induces Fas expression and apoptosis in hedgehog pathway activated BCC cells through inhibiting Ras-Erk signaling. Oncogene 2004; 23:1608–1617.
75. Papageorgiou A, Lashinger L, Millikan R, et al. Role of tumor necrosis factor-related apoptosis-inducing ligand in interferon-induced apoptosis in human bladder cancer cells. Cancer Res 2004; 64:8973–9.
76. Morell-Quadreny L, Fenollosa-Entrena B, Clar-Blanch F, et al. Expression of type I interferon receptor in renal cell carcinoma. Oncol Rep 1999; 6:639–642.
77. Johns TG, Mackay IR, Callister KA, et al. Antiproliferative potencies of interferons on melanoma cell lines and xenografts: higher efficacy of interferon beta. J Natl Cancer Inst 1992; 84:1185–1190.
78. Carson WE. IFN-alpha-induced activation of STAT proteins in malignant melanoma. Clin Cancer Res 1998; 4:2219–2228.
79. Kaplan DH, Shankaran V, Dighe AS, et al. Demonstration of an interferon gamma-dependent tumor surveillance system in immunocompetent mice. Proc Natl Acad Sci USA 1998; 95:7556–7561.
80. Wong LH, Hatzinisiriou I, Devenish RJ, et al. IFN-gamma priming up-regulates IFN-stimulated gene factor 3 (ISGF3) components, augmenting responsiveness of IFN-resistant melanoma cells to type I IFNs. J Immunol 1998; 160:5475–5484.

81. Pansky A, Hildebrand P, Fasler-Kan E, et al. Defective Jak-STAT signal transduction pathway in melanoma cells resistant to growth inhibition by interferon-alpha. Int J Cancer 2000; 85:720–725.
82. Lesinski GB, Valentino D, Hade EM, et al. Expression of STAT1 and STAT2 in malignant melanoma does not correlate with response to interferon-alpha adjuvant therapy. Cancer Immunol Immunother 2005; 54(9):815–825.
83. Boudny V, Kocak I, Lauerova L, et al. Interferon inducibility of STAT 1 activation and its prognostic significance in melanoma patients. Folia Biol (Praha) 2003; 49:142–146.
84. Durbin JE, Hackenmiller R, Simon MC, et al. Targeted disruption of the mouse Stat1 gene results in compromised innate immunity to viral disease. Cell 1996; 84:443–450.
85. Lesinski GB, Anghelina M, Zimmerer J, et al. The anti-tumor effects of interferon-alpha are abrogated in a STAT1-deficient mouse. J Clin Invest 2003; 112(2):170–180.
86. Badgwell B, Lesinski GB, Magro C, et al. The anti-tumor effects of interferon-alpha are maintained in a STAT1-deficient murine melanoma cell line. J Surg Res 2004; 116(1):129–136.
87. Gil MP, Bohn E, O'Guin AK, et al. Biologic consequences of Stat1-independent IFN signaling. Proc Natl Acad Sci USA 2001; 98:6680–6685.
88. Uddin S, Fish EN, Sher DA, et al. Activation of the phosphatidylinositol 3-kinase serine kinase by IFN-alpha. J Immunol 1997; 158:2390–2397.
89. Yang CH, Murti A, Pfeffer SR, et al. IFNalpha/beta promotes cell survival by activating NF-kappa B. Proc Natl Acad Sci USA 2000; 97:13631–13636.
90. Ramana CV, Grammatikakis N, Chernov M, et al. Regulation of c-myc expression by IFN-gamma through Stat1-dependent and -independent pathways. EMBO J 2000; 19:263–272.
91. Zimmerer JM, Lesinski GB, Kondadasula SV, et al. IFN-alpha-induced signal transduction, gene expression, and anti-tumor activity of immune effector cells are negatively regulated by suppressors of cytokine signaling proteins. J Immunol 2007; 178:4832–4845.
92. Lesinski GB, Kondadasula SV, Crespin T, et al. Multiparametric flow cytometric analysis of inter-patient variation in STAT1 phosphorylation following interferon alfa immunotherapy. J Natl Cancer Inst 2004; 96:1331–1342.
93. Critchley-Thorne RJ, Yan N, Nacu S, et al. Down-regulation of the interferon signaling pathway in T lymphocytes from patients with metastatic melanoma. PLoS Med 2007; 4(5):E176.
94. Zimmerer JM, Lesinski GB, Radmacher MD, et al. STAT1-dependent and STAT1-independent gene expression in murine immune cells following stimulation with interferon-alpha. Cancer Immunol Immunother 2007; 56(11):1845–1852.
95. Zimmerer JM, Lehman A, Ruppert A, et al. Interferon-alpha-2b induced signal transduction and gene regulation in patient immune cells is not enhanced by a dose increase from 5 MU/m^2 to 10 MU/m^2. Clin Cancer Res 2008; 14(5):1438–1445.

10

Predicting and Increasing Response of Melanoma to Interferon Therapy

Helen Gogas

First Department of Internal Medicine, University of Athens, Athens, Greece

John M. Kirkwood

University of Pittsburgh Cancer Institute, Hillman Cancer Center, Pittsburgh, Pennsylvania, U.S.A.

INTRODUCTION

Interferon alpha (IFNα) was the first cytokine to demonstrate antitumor activity when administered systemically to patients with advanced melanoma. Objective tumor response rates of up to 20% were observed in phase I and phase II trials for metastatic disease (1,2).

IFNα has been widely tested as adjuvant therapy of melanoma in patients with intermediate (American Joint Committee on Cancer [AJCC] stage IIA) and higher risk for recurrence melanoma (AJCC stage IIB and III). A variety of regimens utilizing low, intermediate, and high doses of IFNα and administered at a variety of schedules for various periods of short and more extended intervals have been evaluated (Table 1).

In 1995, IFNα-2b (Intron A, Schering Corporation, Kenilworth, New Jersey, U.S.) became the first immunotherapy approved for adjuvant treatment of patients with stage IIB/III melanoma by the U.S. Food and Drug Administration (FDA). To this day, it remains the only agent approved for adjuvant therapy of patients who are at intermediate or high risk of recurrence and death from

Table 1 Trials of Adjuvant Interferon for Melanoma

Trial (refs.)	Year	No. of patients	Dose	Treatment duration
ECOG E1684 (3)	1984–1989	287	A. 20 MU/m^2 IV daily 5/7 day/wk then	4 wk
			10 MU/m^2 SC t.i.w.	48 wk
			B. Observation	
North Central Cancer Treatment Group 83-7052 (4)	1984–1989	262	A. 20 MU/m^2 IM t.i.w. B. Observation	12 wk
World Health Organization 16 (5,6)	1990–1993	444	A. 3 MU SC t.i.w. B. Observation	36 mo
Southwest Oncology Group 8642 (7)	1988–1989	134	A. IFNγ 0.2 mg SC daily B. Observation	12 mo
French Cooperative Group on Melanoma (8)	1990–1994	499	A. 3 MU SC t.i.w. B. Observation	18 mo
Austrian Malignant Melanoma Cooperative Group (9)	1990–1994	311	A. 3 MU SC t.i.w. B. Observation	12 mo
ECOG E1690 (10)	1990–1995	642	A. 20 MU/m^2 IV daily 5/7 day/wk then	4 wk
			10 MU/m^2 SC t.i.w.	48 wk
			B. 3 MU SC t.i.w. (LDI)	24 mo
			C. Observation	
ECOG E1694 (11)	1995–1998	880	A. 20 MU/m^2 IV daily 5/7 day/wk then	4 wk
			10 MU/m^2 SC t.i.w.	48 wk
			B. GMK SC once weekly	4 wk
			then once every 3 mo	92 wk
European Organization for Research and Treatment of Cancer (EORTC) 18871 (12)	1987–1994	800	A. 1 MU every other day B. IFNγ 0.2 mg SC every other day C. Observation	1 yr 1 yr
EORTC 18952 (13)	1995–2000	1388	A. 10 MU SC daily 5/7 followed by	4 wk
			10 MU SC t.i.w.	52 wk
			B. 10 MU SC daily 5/7 followed by	4 wk
			5 MU SC t.i.w.	104 wk
			C. Observation	
AIM HIGH (14)	1995–2000	675	A. 3 MU t.i.w. B. Observation	2 yr

Abbreviations: SC, subcutaneously; t.i.w., three times a week; LDI, low-dose interferon; GMK, ganglioside GM2 conjugated to keyhole limpet hemocyanin.

operable thick primary or regionally metastatic melanoma (3). The value of adjuvant high-dose IFNα-2b (HDI) therapy for the treatment of intermediate and high-risk melanoma has been evaluated in three cooperative group studies (3,10,11). These studies have shown that HDI consistently and durably reduced the risk of recurrence to a statistically significant degree. Two of these studies also demonstrated a significant improvement in overall survival compared with observation, or with a vaccine comparator (the GMK vaccine, Progenics, Tarry-town, New York, U.S.) (15). However, the tolerability of this regimen has been an issue because of the frequent occurrence of flu-like symptoms, fatigue, anorexia, and occasional depression.

This regimen is currently the standard of care for adjuvant therapy of high-risk melanoma patients treated off-protocol and the reference standard for evaluation of alternative modalities such as newer cytokines, combinations, and vaccines in current U.S. cooperative group trials.

Attempts to identify patients who benefit from adjuvant treatment with IFNα-2b have been undertaken almost from the point of the discovery of IFN's benefits, but to date, the results of these efforts have largely been dis-appointing. Analyses of individual studies suggest that the benefit of HDI therapy might be restricted to certain subgroups of patients, as these have been evaluated on the basis of the number of melanoma-involved lymph nodes, but no consistent overall pattern has been observed. There are no clinical or demographic features of the patient population that is benefited by this therapy that can presently be used in the clinic to distinguish patients who are likely to benefit from HDI therapy from those who ultimately do not. However, as reviewed below, early insights into the features of populations benefited by this therapy are emerging, which may be the basis of more widely applicable tests to distinguish subsets of patients who are capable of benefiting from HDI. These developments will be of keen interest to patients and physicians alike over the next few years.

There is a critical need for greater understanding of the immunological and disease-related variables that predict clinical benefit from IFNα-2b. The iden-tification of predictive markers that permit selection of patients who are most likely to benefit would allow us to avoid the toxicity of treatment that is not associated with benefit, in more than half of the patients who are now offered this therapy. Notably, immunotherapies that have shown a benefit in advanced melanoma have also been shown to induce the collateral appearance of auto-immunity to normal tissues, including the thyroid and skin melanocytes, resulting in thyroid dysfunction and depigmentation. In this chapter, these facets of adjuvant therapy are discussed in the context of the recently concluded U.S. Intergroup trials of IFNα-2b as well as translational research studies that are ongoing. These may provide insight into the mechanism of therapeutic action for IFNα-2b and permit the more precise identification of patients who are most likely to benefit from this therapy.

DISEASE STAGE AND THERAPEUTIC RESPONSE IN PREVIOUS RANDOMIZED CONTROLLED TRIALS (SUBGROUP ANALYSES)

In all previously conducted randomized controlled trials, patients were stratified according to clinical and/or pathological features at randomization to assure balance in the distribution of risk factors between the groups assigned to treatment with IFN versus observation or vaccination. These stratification factors have not been identical over time, as the assessment of risk has evolved over time (e.g., the E1684 trial was originally designed using a three-stage system). Additionally, in some trials patients were not required to undergo lymphadenectomy in the absence of clinical evidence of lymph node metastasis (e.g., E1690, and the French and the Austrian studies) or were stratified according to the presence of microscopic or macroscopic lymph node involvement (e.g., EORTC 18952). However, the statistical analysis to compare efficacy between treatment arms in each of these trials has been performed as specified in the original protocols, on the basis of eligible and total (intent-to-treat [ITT]) populations. Subgroup analyses were not prespecified in these trials and have generally not been appropriate as the statistical power of the studies was based on the original overall trial analysis. The performance of subgroup analyses has nonetheless been pursued within and across trials as it has been of interest to try to determine whether the effects of treatment might be confined to one or another subgroup. These subgroup analyses are at least hypothesis generating, and we commence with this discussion as the topic remains one that has and will continue to be discussed and debated in relation to the various adjuvant therapeutic regimens at our disposal.

E1684

Analysis of the effects of treatment according to the four risk groups originally defined in this study shows differences in the impact of therapy on relapse-free survival (RFS) among the four stage groups. Among the small number of CS1/PS1 patients, no impact of therapy is apparent, but this subset of 31 patients was too small to be interpreted on its own in this trial. This group showed an imbalance in the presence of primary tumor ulceration that may bear on the outcome, and numbers precluded further analysis. In the pathologically proven microscopically involved node-positive group of 34 patients (without clinically apparent lymphadenopathy), striking differences between the IFN-treated and observed groups were detected. The apparent difference in outcome between IFN-treated and observation arm populations in this relatively small subgroup suggests effects of IFN treatment on microscopic metastatic disease that may be worthy of further evaluation. The largest accrual to this trial occurred in the higher risk groups with clinically apparent nodal metastasis at presentation ($n = 41$) or at recurrence ($n = 174$). The difference observed between relapses among treated and observed groups with gross clinically apparent disease in these groups was accompanied by suppression of estimated hazard functions for relapse in each subgroup. The hazard functions for relapse demonstrate the largest reduction of the hazard of relapse among patients with microscopic involvement of regional lymph nodes detected during elective lymphadenectomy and in patients treated at initial presentation with lymph node metastasis (3).

E1690

The impact of HDI on RFS compared with the observation arm (OBS) was calculated for each stratification group of this trial by testing HDI, low-dose IFNα (LDI), and observation on the basis of stage of disease and number of involved lymph nodes. Differences were not observed in the benefit of HDI for the subsets of node-negative and node-positive patients. Subset analyses did achieve statistical significance for the benefit of HDI for the subset of patients with two to three positive nodes (hazard ratio [HR] 1.92; $p_2 = 0.02$, $p_1 = 0.01$). These patients had an estimated five-year RFS rate of 50% in the HDI arm compared with only 28% in the OBS arm. In contrast, HDI did not seem to have an impact on RFS among the subset of patients with only one positive node (HR 1.0) (10).

E1694

Analysis of the hazard of relapse and death in each stratification group was performed according to the number of positive lymph nodes and demonstrated the superiority of IFNα-2b over a ganglioside vaccine (GMK) in all subsets according to nodal disease. In this trial, patients with no nodal metastasis ($n = 202$) had the greatest reduction in the risk of relapse and death. A two-sided log-rank test adjusting for number of positive nodes demonstrated that node-negative patients treated with IFNα-2b had a statistically significant RFS benefit compared with patients treated with GMK ($p_2 = 0.015$ for eligible patients and $p_2 = 0.012$ in the ITT analysis). The two-sided log-rank analysis also demonstrated a significant overall survival (OS) benefit for IFNα-2b over GMK ($p_2 = 0.046$) in the eligible node-negative population (11).

EORTC 18952

In this trial comparing two regimens in which intermediate dosages of IFNα were administered over one or two years with observation, exploratory analyses suggested that the higher the stage, the smaller the difference associated with IFNα treatment. Subgroup analyses by tumor stage were performed, and in the stage IIB subgroup, adjustment for sex, tumor site, and ulceration yielded significant treatment-associated differences between the two-year treatment group and observation (HR 0.54). The investigators concluded that the effect of adjuvant IFNα was greater among those patients with earlier stages of disease, with two years of treatment with IFNα having a borderline significant effect on relapse among patients with stage IIB, some effect on stage III N1 (microscopic disease) but no effect on relapse or mortality among patients with stage III N2 (gross disease with palpable nodal involvement). In this trial, the staging convention used was that of the EORTC in which N1 comprised patients with nonenlarged microscopically involved lymph nodes on sentinel node biopsy and N2 comprised those with palpable or grossly involved nodes (13).

AIM HIGH Study

Subgroup analysis for age, sex, and disease stage did not show any conclusive evidence of a difference between the IFN-treated and control groups either in RFS or OS. In patients younger than 50 years, RFS was significantly better with IFN with a 30% reduction in the risk of disease recurrence ($p = 0.02$) and evidence of heterogeneity between age groups ($p = 0.03$). However, there was no significant survival benefit for IFN therapy at the doses tested, even in the younger age subgroup ($p = 0.1$). It is probable that the subset findings are false positives, because of inappropriate subgroup analysis as there were multiple endpoints (24 total) tested, of which at least one endpoint would be likely to be statistically significant at the $p = 0.05$ level by chance (14).

WHO 16

In an early WHO report on this trial, it was suggested that there was survival benefit with IFN therapy for younger females and older males. This early report contrasts with the formal analysis at maturity for this trial in which the subgroup analysis for age and sex showed no significant differences in outcome between the treatment arms. This demonstrates the dangers of subgroup analysis compounded by early and immature data, and as for all such analyses, it suggests that findings should be interpreted with caution and require confirmation in independent studies (5,6).

TRANSLATIONAL RESEARCH STUDIES

Hypotheses: Mechanisms Relevant to Antitumor Action

The mechanism by which IFNα-2b exerts an antitumor effect has long been debated. IFNα-2b is a highly pleiotropic cytokine with potent immunoregulatory, antiproliferative, differentiation-inducing, proapoptotic, and anti-angiogenic effects that have been observed in relation to a variety of malignancies (16). The pleiotropic actions of the IFNs may be separated into categories that are useful in analyzing preclinical and clinical data, including the direct (tumor cell–inhibiting), composite (tumor cell antigen–modulating), and indirect (immune as well as vascular) effects. Direct effects of the IFNs include antiproliferative and differentiating effects that may be demonstrated against fresh melanoma tissues or cultured cell lines in vitro. Effects have been designated as composite that result in alterations in tumor cell surface antigen expression without any direct effect on tumor cell growth, invasion, and metastasis. These effects may permit host recognition and response in vivo. The indirect effects of the IFNs include those that are mediated by the host immune system, including natural killer (NK) cells, dendritic cells, T and B cells (17). Relevant to this category of antitumor activity, IFNα induces STAT1 activation in the host and inhibits STAT3 activation that is constitutively induced in the tumor, and this pathway is one of the principal pathways that have been shown to play a role in the indirect IFNα-mediated antitumor effects in preclinical murine model systems (18,19). Furthermore, the relevance of IFNα-induced changes in Janus kinase–signal transducer and activator of transcription (JAK-STAT) signaling is reflected in the following observations: (*i*) IFNα-resistant melanoma cell lines frequently exhibit defects in JAK-STAT signaling (20) and (*ii*) STAT3 is constitutively activated in a variety of tumors, including melanoma and squamous cell carcinoma, where the resulting induction of transforming growth factor-β (TGFβ), interleukin-10 (IL-10), and vascular endothelial growth factor (VEGF) lead to immunological tolerance (21,22).

Immunomodulatory

The immunomodulatory effects of high-dose and low-dose IFNα-2b in patients with high-risk melanoma were originally evaluated in the E2690 laboratory corollary trial of E1690. Peripheral blood lymphocyte phenotypic and functional assays that were performed prestudy and at 3 months and 12 months were analyzed according to the treatment dosage to which patients were assigned and correlated with outcome. Immunological data were obtained for 143 patients who enrolled in this trial, and 20 of these patients contributed lymph node tumor samples. For the phenotypic analysis, the following monoclonal antibodies were used: anti-CD3, CD4, CD8, HLA-DR, CD11a, CD56, CD45RO, CD45RA, CD19, p75, IL-2RA, and CD16. Baseline blood phenotypic and functional assays did not predict disease outcome; however, modulation of these immunological assays by IFNα-2b treatment was observed and was associated with IFNα-2b dosage. Tumor cell class II major histocompatibility antigen expression (HLA-DR) and adhesion molecule expression (ICAM-1) were modulated by exposure to IFNα-2b in a dose-dependent manner. Blood NK cell function, T cell function, and T cell subset distribution were modulated early by patients treated on the HDI arm and were affected only later by treatment on the LDI arm. None of the variables tested predicted RFS (23).

In 20 patients, HDI was investigated in the neoadjuvant setting (24). Immunohistochemical (IHC) analysis of tumor tissue revealed that HDI did not appear to influence the tumor cell phenotype, proliferation rate, or apoptotic fraction of cells in tumor biopsies and did not significantly affect tumor vasculature, irrespective of clinical response. In contrast, IHC analysis of immunological markers including T lymphocytes (CD3, CD4, and CD8), NK cells (CD56), and dendritic cells (CD11c, CD83, and CD86) showed that clinical response to HDI was consistently associated with augmented numbers of mononuclear immune cells infiltrating the tumor, but not those in the peritumoral or perivascular cellular compartments. These changes exhibited strong trends approaching nominal significance regarding CD3 and CD11c as well as CD83/86-positive populations.

IHC analysis did not demonstrate significant alterations of the number of mononuclear cells infiltrating the tumor in general, but rather showed changes in the endotumoral compartment. This has been previously shown in patients with metastatic melanoma treated with IFNα (25–27). As no changes in the expression of lineage or other antigens of melanoma with IFN were observed, it was suggested that the primary antitumor mechanism of HDI is an indirect immuno-modulatory mechanism, rather than a direct and/or cytotoxic mechanism.

Proinflammatory and Anti-angiogenic Effects

In 86 high-risk melanoma patients who participated in E1694, serum concentrations of IL-1α, IL-1β, IL-6, IL-8, IL-12p40, IL-13 granulocyte colony-stimulating factor, monocyte chemoattractant protein 1 (mcp-1), macrophage inflammatory protein (MIP)-1α, MIP-1β, IFNα, tumor necrosis factor (TNF)-α, epidermal growth factor, VEGF, and TNF receptor II were found to be circulating at significantly higher levels in the serum of patients with resected high-risk melanoma as compared with healthy controls. IFNα-2b therapy resulted in a significant decrease of serum levels of immunosuppressive and tumor angiogenic/growth stimulatory factors (VEGF, epidermal growth factor, and hepatocyte growth factor) and increased levels of anti-angiogenic IFN-γ inducible protein 10 (IP-10) and IFN-1. Pretreatment levels of proinflammatory cytokines IL-1β, IL-1α, IL-6, TNF-α, and chemokines MIR-1α and MIR-1β were found to be significantly higher in the serum of patients with longer RFS values of 1 to 5 and more than five years when compared with patients with shorter RFS of less than one year (28).

Autoimmunity

All immunotherapies that have been demonstrated to confer a survival benefit in patients with advanced melanoma have also been shown to induce the collateral appearance of autoimmunity to nontumor tissue antigens, particularly in relation to the thyroid. Hypothyroidism, hyperthyroidism, and the antiphospholipid-antibody syndrome, as well as vitiligo-like depigmentation (often referred to as vitiligo but technically not identical to this spontaneous development of auto-immune depigmentation), have been correlated to benefit in relation to high-dose IL-2 therapy (29–35). For example, the development of vitiligo after therapy with high-dose IL-2 has consistently been associated with clinical response to therapy ($p < 0.001$) (33,35), and in at least one study, the appearance of vitiligo was associated with improved overall survival. In a study of 49 patients with metastatic melanoma receiving IL-2 and GM-CSF, patients developing vitiligo ($n = 21$) had a median overall survival of 18.2 months compared with 8.5

months for patients without vitiligo ($p = 0.027$) (36). Indeed, the appearance of paraneoplastic and presumably autoimmune vitiligo was considered a favorable prognostic factor in patients with melanoma even before the advent of IL-2 therapy. In case-control studies published in the 1980s, the appearance of vitiligo in patients with metastatic melanoma was associated with a longer survival than expected, and it was suggested that the mechanisms that inhibit or destroy normal melanocytes may also slow the growth of melanoma, a malignant disease of melanocytic origin. These patients in which vitiligo-like depigmentation was observed were not necessarily cured of their tumor, and many have ultimately still succumbed to metastatic disease (37–41).

In patients receiving adjuvant therapy with HDI, autoimmune phenomena have also been reported. In a substudy analysis from a large randomized trial of HDI in patients with stage IIB/III melanoma, 26% of 200 patients studied developed antithyroid autoantibodies or other autoimmune manifestations (40). Notably, the appearance of autoantibodies or clinical manifestations of auto-immunity was associated with significant improvements in RFS and OS ($p <$ 0.001). Only 7 (13%) of 52 patients with autoantibodies or clinical manifes-tations of autoimmunity had a relapse and only 4% had died compared with a 73% relapse rate and 54% death rate among 148 patients without autoimmunity (40). This relation between autoimmunity and outcome was demonstrated in univariate as well as multivariate Cox proportional hazards models, and in an analysis of disease stage (according to the current AJCC staging criteria) among patients with evidence of autoimmunity and those without it. Models in which autoantibody formation was used as a time-dependent variable yielded similar results. Additionally, landmark analyses at 3, 6, 9, and 12 months of RFS and OS according to the autoimmunity status reached the same conclusion. It was sug-gested that the induction of autoimmunity could be a surrogate marker for monitoring the efficacy of IFN therapy. However, as autoimmunity was observed only after a median of three months—and in some instances, more than a year from the start of IFNα-2b therapy, the development of autoimmunity per se did not appear to be useful as a criterion for selecting patients for the therapy. In a retrospective analysis of autoantibody induction in patients receiving HDI compared with vaccine-only controls of two ECOG and Intergroup U.S. studies (E2696 and E1694), RFS and OS of the groups with and without serological evidence of autoimmunity were compared (41). In the E2696 study, autoanti-body responses were found to be induced among 25% of patients (significantly greater numbers of subjects developed autoimmunity on HDI arms compared to control arm, $p_2 = 0.029$), while 20% of the E1694 study population demonstrated serological evidence of autoimmunity following IFN ($p_2 < 0.001$). In E2696, RFS was improved among HDI recipients with autoantibodies, but with the limited numbers in this phase II trial, this trend did not achieve statistical significance. In 691 patients studied from the E1694 trial, HDI patients who developed autoantibodies tended to have improved RFS and OS, but these did not achieve statistical significance ($p = 0.178$ for RFS and $p = 0.091$ for OS).

These findings were corroborated by landmark analysis at one year, so lead time bias is unlikely to play a part in the results. In a retrospective analysis of the EORTC study 18952 involving 278 patients, seroconversion was observed among 36% of patients treated for 13 months with IFN and 42% treated for 25 months with IFN (42). RFS was evaluated using three statistical models. Comparing RFS of autoantibody-positive patients with antibody-negative patients, the HR for RFS was 0.50 ($p = 0.0002$ with the usual Cox model), 0.63 ($p = 0.02$ with a time-dependent Cox model), and 0.87 ($p = 0.48$ with a time-dependent Cox model using the latest positive antibody value). Differences among the results of these three studies were potentially attributed to the differences in IFN regimens, the monitoring of clinical and laboratory endpoints, the diverse time points and different sensitivity of the tests employed, as well as to the inclusion of patients with unknown pretreatment autoantibody status, differing genetic backgrounds, and finally the use of different statistical models. In the simple Cox model, the sample is divided in two groups, one that has the characteristic of interest (positive) and another that does not (negative). This model is considered as irrelevant when the characteristic appears. In the time-dependent Cox model, the individual changes group at the time that the characteristic appears for the first time (from negative to positive) and stays in this group (positive) from then on. But in the time-dependent Cox model using the latest positive antibody value, the individual changes group every time the characteristic changes (from negative to positive or from positive to negative). In the previous two studies cited, a time-dependent Cox model was used, while in the EORTC series all statistical models were employed but the time-dependent model using the latest positive antibody value was considered the most appropriate model and was used as the basis of their conclusion that antibody status was not statistically significantly correlated with outcome. Further research and understanding of both the biological processes at work here and the statistical methodologies most appropriate to analyze them are clearly needed.

Although the development of autoimmunity during adjuvant therapy with IFN appears to have importance in both Hellenic and U.S. cooperative group–based studies, as well as in the EORTC study in some statistical models, the development of autoimmunity as a treatment-associated phenomenon cannot help with the initial selection of patients for therapy. Tests are needed that can define patients with the propensity for induction of autoimmunity, for whom treatment with IFN may be most effective. Multiple genes are involved in autoimmune diseases (e.g., HLA haplotypes, CTLA-4 polymorphisms, and FOXP3 mutations) (43–47) and should be investigated in prospective trials for predisposition to the development of HDI-induced autoimmunity. It is noteworthy that the subset analyses in the E2690 study by HLA-A2 status produced an unexpected result. Among patients in the HLA-A2 positive subset, outcome in the E1690 trial was improved, and there was no evidence of an IFNα-2b treatment benefit—and in fact a negative impact on RFS ($p = 0.02$)—compared with the observation arm; among HLA-A2 negative patients, the disease outcome appeared to be worse untreated but RFS benefit was observed with IFNα-2b. The test for interaction between treatment and HLA-A2 status was marginally significant ($p = 0.06$) (23). This apparent interaction may be the result of a statistical artifact, as there was no a priori reason to believe that IFNα-2b treatment would be less effective or deleterious for HLA-A2 positive patients. Moreover, in a larger study of 289 patients that received adjuvant IFN and were genotyped for HLA class I and class II, no statistically significant differences were seen between patients free of recurrence and those who recurred. However, statistically significant differences were seen according to typing for HLA-A, HLA-C, HLA-DRB1, and HLA-DQB1 alleles between patients developing autoimmunity and those with no evidence of autoimmunity (48). CTLA-4 (Cytotoxic T-Lymphocyte–Associated protein-4) gene is a member of the immunoglobulin superfamily and encodes a protein that transmits an inhibitory signal to T cells (49). Several polymorphisms have been found within the CTLA-4 gene and have been shown to have an association with Graves' disease, type 1 diabetes, Addison's disease (44,45,50) (e.g., GG allele of the +49 A/G polymorphism is associated with decreased expression of CTLA-4 on T cell activation and thus a higher proliferation of T cells). Additionally, in a phase I study of 19 patients receiving anti-CTLA-4 monoclonal antibody with multiple melanoma peptides and montanide ISA 51, three of four (75%) patients with the low-expression CTLA-4 allele JO30 (GG) developed autoimmune symptoms, while only two of the four (50%) experienced disease relapse. Of the remaining 15 patients expressing either the AA or AG alleles, only five (33%) developed autoimmune symptoms and 10 (67%) experienced disease relapse (51).

Therefore, a greater understanding of the dynamic interaction between melanoma and the immune system is likely to lead to the identification of new targets for more effective treatment and to aid in the development of newer and more effective immunotherapies. As the factors that define the capacity of a particular patient to benefit from IFNα-2b therapy are defined, we may look forward to the development of a more selective approach in which only patients who are more likely to benefit from therapy may be treated and to the development of therapies that build on the current regimen of high-dose IFNα-2b to achieve greater specificity and less toxicity than is currently the case.

REFERENCES

1. Kirkwood JM, Ernstoff M. Melanoma: therapeutic options with recombinant interferons. Semin Oncol 1985; 12:7–12.
2. Kirkwood JM, Ernstoff MS, Davis CA, et al. Comparison of intramuscular and intravenous recombinant alpha-2 interferon in melanoma and other cancers. Ann Intern Med 1998; 103:32–36.
3. Kirkwood JM, Strawderman MH, Ernstoff MS, et al. Interferon alfa-2b adjuvant therapy of high-risk resected cutaneous melanoma: the Eastern Cooperative Oncology Group Trial EST 1684. J Clin Oncol 1996; 14:7–17.

4. Creagan ET, Dalton RJ, Ahmann DL, et al. Randomized, surgical adjuvant clinical trial of recombinant interferon alfa-2a in selected patients with malignant melanoma. J Clin Oncol 1998; 13:2776.
5. Cascinelli N, Bufalino R, Morabito A, et al. MacKie R. Results of adjuvant interferon study in WHO melanoma programme. Lancet 1994; 343:913.
6. Cascinelly N, Belli F, MacKie RM, et al. Effect of long-term adjuvant therapy with interferon alpha-2a in patients with regional node metastases from cutaneous melanoma: a randomized trial. Lancet 2001; 358:866–869.
7. Meyskens FL Jr., Kopecky KJ, Taylor CW, et al. Randomized trial of adjuvant human interferon gamma versus observation in high-risk cutaneous melanoma: a Southwest Oncology Group study. J Natl Cancer Inst 1995; 87:1710–1713.
8. Grob JJ, Dreno B, de la Salmoniere P, et al. Randomised trial of interferon α-2a as adjuvant therapy in resected primary melanoma thicker than 1.5 mm without clinically detectable node metastases. Lancet 1998; 351:1905–1910.
9. Pehamberger H, Soyer HP, Steiner A, et al. Adjuvant interferon alfa-2a treatment in resected primary stage II cutaneous melanoma. Austrian Malignant Melanoma Cooperative Group. J Clin Oncol 1998; 16:1425–1429.
10. Kirkwood JM, Ibrahim JG, Sondak VK, et al. High- and low-dose interferon alfa-2b in high-risk melanoma: first analysis of intergroup trial E1690/S9111/C9190. J Clin Oncol 2000; 18:2444–2458.
11. Kirkwood JM, Ibrahim JG, Sosman JA, et al. High-dose interferon alfa-2b significantly prolongs relapse-free and overall survival compared with the GM2-KLH/QS-21 vaccine in patients with resected stage IIB-III melanoma: results of intergroup trial E1694/S9512/C509801. J Clin Oncol 2001; 19:2370–2380.
12. Kleeberg UP, Suciu S, Brocker EB, et al. Final results of the EORTC 18871/DKG 80-1 randomised phase III trial. rIFN-alpha2b versus rIFN-gamma versus ISCADOR M versus observation after surgery in melanoma patients with either high-risk primary (thickness >3 mm) or regional lymph node metastasis. Eur J Cancer 2004; 40:390–402.
13. Eggermont AMM, Suciu S, Macki R, et al. Post-surgery adjuvant therapy with intermediate doses of interferon alfa 2b versus observation in patients with stage IIb/III melanoma (EORTC 18952): randomized controlled trial. Lancet 2005; 366:1189–1196.
14. Hancock BW, Wheatley K, Harris S, et al. Adjuvant interferon in high-risk melanoma: The AIM HIGH Study-United Kingdom Coordinating Committee on Cancer Research Randomized Study of adjuvant low-dose extended-duration interferon alfa-2a in high-risk resected malignant melanoma. J Clin Oncol 2004; 22(1):53–61.
15. Kirkwood JM, Manola J, Ibrahim J, et al. A pooled analysis of Eastern Cooperative Oncology Group and intergroup trials of adjuvant high-dose interferon for melanoma. Clin Cancer Res 2004; 10:1670–1677.
16. Kirkwood J. Cancer immunotherapy: the interferon-alpha experience. Semin Oncol 2002; 29:18–26.
17. Ernstoff MS, Fusi S, Kirkwood JM. Parameters of interferon action: II. immunological effects of recombinant leukocyte interferon (IFN alpha-2) in phase I/II trials. J Biol Resp Mod 1983; 2:540.
18. Pestka S. The interferon receptors. Semin Oncol 1997; 24:S9-18–S19-40.
19. Lesinski GB, Anghelina M, Zimmerer J, et al. The antitumor effects of IFN-alpha are abrogated in a STAT1-deficient mouse. J Clin Invest 2003; 112:170–180.

20. Pansky A, Hildebrand P, Fasler-Kan E, et al. Defective Jak-STAT signal transduction pathway in melanoma cells resistant to growth inhibition by interferon-alpha. Int J Cancer 2000; 85:720–725.
21. Kirkwood JM, Farkas DL, Chakraborty A, et al. Systemic interferon-alpha (IFN-alpha) treatment leads to Stat3 inactivation in melanoma precursor lesions. Mol Med 1999; 5:11–20.
22. Wang T, Niu G, Kortylewski M, et al. Regulation of the innate and adaptive immune responses by Stat-3 signaling in tumor cells. Nat Med 2004; 10:48–54.
23. Kirkwood JM, Richards T, Zarour H, et al. Immunomodulatory effects of high-dose and low-dose interferon α2b in patients with high-risk resected melanoma: the 2690 laboratory corollary of Intergroup adjuvant trial E1690. Cancer 2002; 95:1101–1112.
24. Moschos SJ, Edington HD, Land SR, et al. Neoadjuvant treatment of regional stage IIIB melanoma with high-dose interferon alfa-2b induces objective tumor regression in association with modulation of tumor infiltrating host cellular immune responses. J Clin Oncol 2006; 24:3164–3171.
25. Mihm MC Jr., Clemente CG, Cascineli N. Tumor infiltrating lymphocytes in lymph node melanoma metastases: a histopathologic prognostic indicator and an expression of local immune response. Lab Invest 1996; 74:43–47.
26. Hakansson A, Gustafsson B, Krysander I, et al. Tumor-infiltrating lymphocytes in metastatic malignant melanoma and response to interferon alpha treatment. Br J Cancer 1996; 74:670.
27. Hakansson A, Gustafsson B, Krysander L, et al. Effect of IFN-alpha on tumor-infiltrating mononuclear cells and regressive changes in metastatic malignant melanoma. J Interferon Cytokine Res 1998; 18:33–39.
28. Yurkovetsky ZR, Kirkwood JM, Edington HD, et al. Multiplex analysis of serum cytokines in melanoma patients treated with interferon-a2b. Clin Cancer Res 2007; 13(8):2422–2428.
29. Atkins MB, Mier JW, Parkinson DP, et al. Hypothyroidism after treatment with interleukin-2 and lymphokine-acivated killer cells. N Engl J Med 1988; 318:1557–1562.
30. Weijl NI, Van Der Harst D, Brand A, et al. Hypothyroidism during immunotherapy with interleukin-2 is associated with antithyroid antibodies and response to treatment. J Clin Oncol 1993; 11:1376–1383.
31. Scalzo S, Gengaro A, Boccoli G, et al. Primary hypothyroidism associated with interleukin-2 and interferon alpha-2 therapy of melanoma and renal carcinoma. Eur J Cancer 1990; 26:1152–1156.
32. Krouse RS, Royal RE, Heywood G, et al. Thyroid dysfunction in 281 patients with metastatic melanoma in renal carcinoma treated with interleukin-2 alone. J Immunother Emphasis Tumor Immunol 1995; 18:272–278.
33. Phan GQ, Attia P, Steinberg SM, et al. Factors associated with response to high-dose interleukin-2 in patients with metastatic melanoma. J Clin Oncol 2001; 19:477–3482.
34. Becker JC, Winkler B, Klingert S, et al. Antiphospholipid syndrome associated with immunotherapy for patients with melanoma. Cancer 1994; 73:1621–1624.
35. Rosenberg SA, White DE. Vitiligo in patients with melanoma: normal tissue antigens can be targets for cancer immunotherapy. J Immunother Emphasis Tumor Immunol 1996; 19:81–84.
36. Boasberg PD, Hoon DS, Piro LD, et al. Enhanced survival associated with vitiligo expression during maintenance biotherapy for metastatic melanoma. J Invest Dermatol 2006; 126:2658–2663.

37. Nordlund JJ, Kirkwood JM, Forget BM, et al. Vitiligo in patients with metastatic melanoma: a good prognostic sign. J Am Acad Dermatol 1983; 9:689–696.
38. Bystryn JC, Rigel D, Friedman RJ, et al. Prognostic significance of hypopigmentation in malignant melanoma. Arch Dermatol 1987; 123:1053–1055.
39. Schallreuter KU, Levenig C, Berger J. Vitiligo and cutaneous melanoma. A case study. Dermatologica 1991; 183:239–245.
40. Gogas H, Ioannovich J, Dafni U, et al. Prognostic significance of autoimmunity during treatment of melanoma with interferon. N Engl J Med 2006; 354:709–718.
41. Stuckert II JJ, Tarhini AA, Lee S, et al. Interferon alfa-induced autoimmunity and serum S100 levels as predictive and prognostic biomarkers in high risk melanoma in the ECOG-intergroup phase II trial E2696. Proc Am Soc Clin Oncol 2007; 25:S473 (abstr 8506).
42. Bouwhuis M, Suciu S, Kruit W, et al. Prognostic value of autoantibodies (auto-AB) in melanoma patients (pts) in the EORTC 18952 trial of adjuvant interferon (IFN) compared to observation (obs). Proc Am Soc Clin Oncol 2007; 25:S473 (abstr 8507).
43. Shiina T, Iniko H, Kulski JK. An update of the HLA genomic region, locus information and disease associations: 2004. Tissue Antigens 2004; 64(6):631–649.
44. Kristiansen OP, Larsen ZM, Pociot F. CTLA-4 in autoimmune diseases—a general susceptibility gene to autoimmunity? Genes Immun 2000; 1(3):170–184.
45. Thompson CB, Allison JP. The emerging role of CTLA-4 as an immune attenuator. Immunity 1997; 7(4):445–550.
46. Bennet L, Christie J, Ransdell F, et al. The immune dysregulation, polyendocrinopathy, enteropathy, X-linked syndrome (IPEX) is caused by mutations of FOXP3. Nat Genet 2001; 27(1):21–21.
47. Hori S, Nomura T, Sakaquchi S. Control of regulatory T cell development by the transcription factor Foxp3. Science 2003; 299(5609):1057–1061.
48. Gogas H. Molecular HLA typing and outcome. Session IV. Presented at: The Imedex-sponsored conference on Perspectives in Melanoma XI; October 3–4, 2007; Huntington Beach, CA.
49. Brunet JF, Denizot F, Luciani MF, et al. A new member of the immunoglobulin superfamily-CTLA-4. Nature 1987; 328(6127):267–270.
50. Ueda H, Howson JMM, Esposito L, et al. Association of the T-cell regulatory gene CTLA4 with susceptibility to autoimmune disease. Nature 2003; 423:506–511.
51. Sanderson K, Scotland R, Lee P, et al. Autoimmunity in a phase I trial of a fully human anti-cytotoxic T-lymphocyte antigen-4 monoclonal antibody with multiple melanoma peptides and montanide ISA 51 for patients with resected stages III and IV melanoma. J Clin Oncol 2005; 23:741–750.

11

New Approaches for Optimizing Melanoma Vaccines

Nasreen Vohra

H. Lee Moffitt Cancer Center and Department of Surgery, University of South Florida College of Medicine, Tampa, Florida, U.S.A.

Shari Pilon-Thomas and James J. Mulé

H. Lee Moffitt Cancer Center, Tampa, Florida, U.S.A.

Jeffrey Weber

H. Lee Moffitt Cancer Center and the Department of Oncologic Sciences, University of South Florida College of Medicine, Tampa, Florida, U.S.A.

INTRODUCTION

Vaccination against infectious diseases has led to great improvements in human health. A better understanding of the molecular basis of adaptive immunity, including the activation and regulation of $CD8^+$ cytotoxic T cell (CTL) responses, has resulted in the development of immunotherapies for a wide range of diseases, including cancer. Advanced melanoma, a deadly disease with few nonsurgical treatment options, has been the malignancy most targeted for active immunotherapy. This emphasis on melanoma as an immunogenic tumor is the result of a variety of observations, which includes the occurrence of rare spontaneous remissions in melanoma patients, believed to be immune-mediated (1). In addition, tumor-specific T cells can be measured in the peripheral blood as well as infiltrating primary tumors of melanoma patients. These T cells are capable of responding to melanoma antigens from the same patient in vitro. Finally, therapy with interleukin-2 (IL-2) that leads to T cell expansion and prevents lymphocyte apoptosis results in durable complete responses in a relatively small proportion of patients with metastatic melanoma (2,3). Together, these observations have led to the development of novel immunotherapies for the treatment of advanced melanoma.

MECHANISM OF IMMUNITY INDUCED BY ANTIMELANOMA VACCINES

The frequency of precursor T cells with antitumor activity is low in patients with advanced cancers, and those cells often have a naïve phenotype (4). The goal of current vaccination strategies against melanoma is to activate and expand tumor-reactive T cells as an effective means of immunity. Activation of tumor-specific T cells requires presentation of peptides derived from melanoma-associated antigens. Most melanoma-associated antigens such as tyrosinase, gp100, and MART-1 are nonmutated proteins expressed exclusively by melanocytes. For a vaccine to be effective, antigens must be taken up by professional antigen presenting cells (APC), such as dendritic cells (DC). Immature DC, which reside mainly in peripheral tissues, are characterized by the ability to efficiently internalize and process antigen, but demonstrate low T cell stimulatory capacity. The captured antigens are targeted either to the proteasome or endocytic pathway where they are degraded into peptides. The resulting peptides are bound to major histocompatibility complex (MHC) class I molecules and presented to $CD8^+$ CTL or MHC class II molecules and presented to $CD4^+$ helper T cells. As immature DC acquire antigens at the vaccination site, they may also come in contact with vaccine-associated bacterial DNA or viral vectors, immune-stimulating adjuvants, or activated T cells. These interactions lead to DC maturation and migration to the draining lymph nodes. The process of DC maturation results in diminished antigen uptake, downregulation of chemokine receptor expression, and the enhanced ability to interact with naïve T lymphocytes through upregulation of MHC class I and class II and costimulatory molecules such as CD80 and CD86. After antigen uptake and migration to secondary lymphoid tissues, DC educate naïve T cells for the induction of effective primary immune responses and immunologic memory. Terminal maturation of the DC is completed by reciprocal interactions with activated T cells via cognate surface receptors such as 4-1BB/4-1BBL, CD40/CD40L, and OX40/OX40L (5–7).

CURRENT STATE OF AFFAIRS FOR MELANOMA VACCINES

Immunotherapies incorporating melanoma antigens in the form of peptides, whole tumor cells, DNA or viral vectors, alone or in combination with in vitro-generated DC, have been explored (Fig. 1) (8–10). These vaccine strategies have been successful in some cases at inducing tumor-specific T cell responses in patients with melanoma. Unfortunately, to date, these T cell responses have not translated into meaningful clinical responses for the vast majority of melanoma patients. Rosenberg et al. analyzed 440 patients with metastatic cancer, mainly melanoma, treated with 541 different vaccines over a nine-year period at the

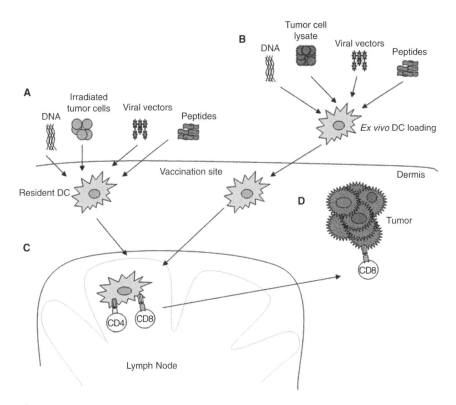

Figure 1 Tumor-specific T cell responses induced by vaccination. (**A**) Direct intradermal injection of melanoma antigens, in the form of naked DNA, peptide, killed tumor cells, or encoded by viral vectors, leads to uptake by resident DC in the skin. (**B**) Melanoma antigens, such as tumor cell lysates or peptides, are pulsed onto ex vivo-derived DC. Alternatively, DC are transduced with DNA or viral vectors encoding melanoma antigens. DC are injected intradermally. (**C**) DC migrate from the injection site to the regional lymph node. Peptides derived from melanoma antigens are presented on MHC class II molecules to CD4$^+$ T cells and on MHC class I molecules to CD8$^+$ T cells. (**D**) Activated CD8$^+$ T cells migrate from the lymph node to the site of tumor. CD8$^+$ T cells recognize melanoma antigens presented by MHC class I molecules on the tumor cells. *Abbreviations*: DC, dendritic cells; MHC, major histocompatibility complex.

National Cancer Institute (11). Using conventional oncologic-response criteria, the overall response rate was only 2.6%, without a correlation with immune response. This low clinical response rate indicates the necessity for additional strategies to enhance tumor rejection in melanoma patients.

COULD MELANOMA VACCINES ACTUALLY BE HARMFUL?

Recently, results of several large randomized vaccine trials have raised the question of whether certain vaccine strategies in cancer and HIV disease may actually induce a worse outcome compared with control groups. In two recent adjuvant clinical trials of a cell-based melanoma vaccine, Canvaxin, conducted in resected stage III and stage IV melanoma patients, the control group receiving placebo plus BCG survived longer than the group randomized to receive Canvaxin plus BCG (12). In the resected stage IV population, five-year survival was 44 months in the control cohort compared with 39 months for the vaccine-treated group ($p = $ NS); median survival showed a similar trend in favor of the control group. For stage III patients, the results were 67 and 59 months, respectively ($p = 0.04$), with a similar effect for median survival. Did the vaccine actually result in a worse outcome in both populations? Equally worrisome data were shown in a randomized phase III HIV vaccine trial using an adenoviral type 5 vector–encoding multiple HIV epitopes (13). That trial was stopped because there was a worsening in numbers of infections in the patients in the vaccinated group compared with controls, and there was no evidence of a reduction in viral load in vaccinated patients. How are we to interpret these data? Could the vaccines have actually induced T regulatory cells that suppressed any endogenous immune responses, resulting in a less favorable outcome in the above trials (14)? One reasonable conclusion is that no approach with a vaccine alone will be successful in cancer or HIV, rather combination approaches that incorporate elimination of T regulatory cells, induction of long-lived memory cells, overcoming of T regulatory circuits, and priming and boosting strategies will be required for future trials to be successful.

STRATEGIES TO ENHANCE ANTI-MELANOMA VACCINE RESPONSES

Despite modest numbers of clinical responses in patients with advanced melanoma, vaccination with DC pulsed with peptides or whole tumor lysate remains a promising approach (15,16). Some current approaches to optimize DC-based vaccines are described in Table 1. As DC are the most potent inducer of primary and memory T cell responses, strategies are being explored to achieve a more

Table 1   Augmenting DC Immunotherapy

Obstacle	Strategy	References
T cell responses to multiple antigens not induced	Pulse DC with multiple peptides to induce both CD4$^+$ and CD8$^+$ T cells	102
Inefficient antigen processing/ presentation by DC	Manipulation of antigen processing pathways in DC (i.e. block immunoproteosome; antigen targeting via cell-surface receptors)	17–19
Inadequate DC maturation/ activation	Optimize DC maturation cocktails Co-injection of adjuvants such as CpG	20–23
DC do not interact with T cells	Transduction of DC with chemokine-expressing adenovirus	28,29

Abbreviation: DC, dendritic cells.

efficient and multiepitope-directed immune response against melanoma. Clinical trials are currently under way to examine whether immunization with DC pulsed with multiple peptides, rather than a single peptide, leads to activation of tumor-specific CD4$^+$ and CD8$^+$ T cells and heightened clinical responses in melanoma patients. To further optimize the processing and presentation of melanoma antigens, preclinical strategies to deliver tumor cells or lysates to DC via cell surface receptors, such as Fcγ receptors, have been shown to enhance the activation of tumor-specific CD8$^+$ T cells (17,18). Another approach to enhance CD8$^+$ T cell activation involves downmodulating immunoproteasomes in DC. While DC process antigens through the immunoproteasome, tumor cells express a constitutive form of proteasome. It is possible that T cells, activated by DC presenting tumor antigens processed by the immunoproteasome, will not recognize tumor cells. In a preclinical model, disabling the immunoproteasome resulted in antigen processing through the constitutive proteasome in DC and led to the induction of antitumor CD8$^+$ T cells (19).

It has been suggested that vaccination with mature DC pulsed with tumor antigens leads to a significantly higher clinical response rate in patients with melanoma but this has yet to be convincingly confirmed (20). Mature DC are characterized by expression of high levels of MHC class II and costimulatory molecules and secrete cytokines required for antitumor immune responses. Strategies to optimize DC maturation with cocktails containing Th1-polarizing cytokines have been shown to induce strong anti-melanoma T cell responses in preclinical models (21,22). Alternatively, approaches targeting toll-like receptors on the surface of DC using adjuvants such as CpG that potentiate cell-mediated immunity are also being tested (23).

Optimizing DC-T cell interactions is another strategy that is being explored to improve vaccine efficacy. It is known that ex vivo-derived DC administered intradermally do not efficiently migrate from the vaccination site to the regional lymph nodes (24,25). As direct interaction between T cells and DC in the lymph node is pivotal for the initiation of antitumor T cell responses, a failure thereof may contribute to the low clinical response rate for patients treated with DC-based immunotherapy. To improve DC-T cell interactions at the site of vaccination, the use of CCL21-SLC (Secondary Lymphoid-Tissue Chemokine) modified DC is being explored. CCL21 is a chemokine expressed in the high endothelial venules and the T cell zones of the spleen and lymph nodes. This chemokine is required for homing of CCR7$^+$ naïve T cells and mature DC to lymphoid organs. In murine models of melanoma, transduction of tumor lysate-pulsed DC with the *CCL21* gene and its expression has led to T cell stimulation at the site of vaccination, bypassing the requirement of lymph node involvement (26). Direct injection of DC expressing the *CCL21* gene into an established melanoma led to an influx of tumor-specific T cells as well as a systemic antitumor immune response capable of inhibiting growth of metastatic lesions (27). In preclinical models, transduction of human monocyte–derived DC with an adenovirus expressing the *CCL21* gene leads to enhanced migration of DC and T cells and priming of MART-1-specific T cell responses in vitro (28,29). A phase I trial testing *CCL21* gene–modified lysate-pulsed DC in melanoma patients is pending.

BARRIERS TO EFFECTIVE MELANOMA VACCINES

Current vaccine trials have included late-stage melanoma patients with large tumor burdens and metastatic disease. It is possible that use of cancer vaccines in the adjuvant setting to prevent disease recurrence will demonstrate more benefit to cancer patients. Peoples et al. have provided some of the strongest evidence to date that vaccines might have a role in preventing relapse in solid tumors, albeit in a non-randomized trial (30). Twenty-four breast cancer patients with HER2/nue-expressing tumors who were HLA-A2+ received a vaccine consisting of an HLA-A2-restricted immunogenic peptide from the HER2/neu protein plus GM-CSF, while 29 HLA-A2- breast cancer patients were observed as a concurrent control arm. At 22 months of follow-up, 85.7% of patients treated with the vaccine were disease-free, compared with 59.8% of patients not receiving the vaccine. To demonstrate a benefit of melanoma vaccines in patients with advanced disease, many potential barriers would need to be overcome. As tumors progress, there is an increase in overall immune suppression in cancer patients (31,32). Large tumor burdens have been linked to great heterogeneity in antigen expression, making it more likely that tumors can escape immune surveillance (33). Loss of class I MHC molecules and β-2 microglobulin has been observed in a variety of cancers, particularly melanoma, and is associated with metastatic disease burden (34,35). Mechanisms employed by the immune system to downregulate and inhibit ongoing T cell responses can prevent the induction of robust antitumor T cells. Factors in the tumor micro-environment, such as IL-10, TGF-β, and arginase, may limit the ability of T cells to respond to tumor cells (36). The presence of regulatory T cells and myeloid-derived cells that inhibit autoreactive T cell responses can also suppress antitumor immune responses (14). New approaches to target these suppressive mechanisms as well as immune regulatory pathways will now be discussed.

IMMUNE REGULATION IN MELANOMA PATIENTS

Increased appreciation of the importance of both negative and positive cos-timulatory pathways in the regulation of T cell responses has allowed the development of new strategies for immunotherapy of cancer by manipulation of these pathways to either enhance or terminate immune responses. Counter-regulatory molecules like cytotoxic T lymphocyte antigen 4 (CTLA-4) and programmed death 1 (PD-1) have been shown to attenuate T cell activity and are implicated in the induction of immune tolerance (37,38). By blocking these molecules using novel antibodies, the ultimate goal is to break tolerance to self-antigens and augment T cell activity against self tumor antigens to achieve regression of established tumor or prevent recurrence in patients with high risk of relapse after cancer resection. In the sections to follow, we aim to briefly describe the biochemistry of some of these molecules, summarize the important preclinical murine and in vitro data about CTLA-4 and PD-1, as well as give a detailed description of the clinical experience with two human CTLA-4 antibodies that are already in use in several early-phase clinical trials.

CTLA-4 BLOCKADE

As shown in Figure 2, T cell activation requires at least two signals: stimulation via the T cell receptor (TCR)–antigen-MHC (signal 1) and an additional signal (signal 2) by engagement of costimulatory receptors on the surface of T cell with ligands expressed by APC (39). Two such critical T cell immunoregulatory molecules are CD28 and CTLA-4 (CD152) whose ligands on DC are CD80 and CD86 (40,41). Although CD28 and CTLA-4 are closely related members of the Ig superfamily, they function antagonistically whereby CD28 is the stimulatory receptor and CTLA-4 an inhibitory receptor (40,42–44). CD28 is constitutively expressed on the surface of T cells, whereas CTLA-4 is rapidly upregulated following T cell activation. Binding of the CD80/CD86 ligands to the CTLA-4 receptor leads to delivery of a negative signal to the T cell via Akt signaling, resulting in shutting down of the activated state with inhibition of IL-2 synthesis and termination of T cell expansion (45–47). The overall T cell response is determined by the sum total of all responses, stimulatory and inhibitory. Because CTLA-4 plays a pivotal role in T cell-dependent tolerance by downregulating

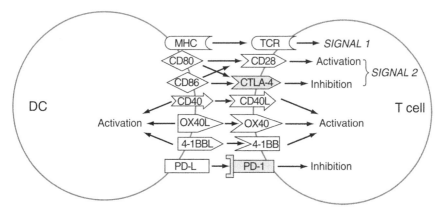

Figure 2 Schematic representation of stimulatory and inhibitory ligands on DC and T cells. To become activated, T cells must recognize peptides via TCR/MHC interactions (signal 1). A second signal (signal 2) is received through ligation of CD80/CD86 with CD28. Alternatively, ligation of CTLA-4, a competitor of CD28, leads to inhibition of T cell activation. If activated, T cell activity can be modulated by additional stimulatory signals through CD40, OX40, or 4-1BB or inhibitory signals through PD-1. Activated T cells can also send stimulatory signals to DC through CD40, OX40, and 4-1BB, enhancing the ability of DC to induce T cell-mediated immune responses. *Abbreviations*: DC, dendritic cells; MHC, major histocompatibility complex; TCR, T cell receptor; CTLA-4, cytotoxic T lymphocyte antigen 4; PD-1, programmed death 1.

immune responses, CTLA-4 blockade with anti-CTLA-4 monoclonal antibodies (mAb) has been used in murine models of immunotherapy. Initial murine experiments showed that treatment with an anti-CTLA-4 antibody resulted in enhanced antitumor immunity when used alone to treat immunogenic tumors or in combination with vaccines for the therapy of poorly immunogenic tumors (48,49). In addition, tumor rejection in mice treated with anti-CTLA-4 antibody was accompanied by depigmentation, suggesting that the antitumor response was at least in part directed to melanocyte differentiation antigens (50).

A number of early-phase clinical trials employing CTLA-4 blockade with two different anti-CTLA-4 mAbs in the treatment of patients with metastatic melanoma have yielded some encouraging results. CP-675,206 (tremelimumab, Pfizer Inc., New York, New York, U.S.) is a fully human IgG2 mAb with high CTLA-4 specificity. Ribas et al. reported the results of a dose escalation, phase I clinical trial of a single intravenous infusion of CP-675,206 in 34 patients with stage IV melanoma. There were four objective responses, two of which were complete and two with partial responses, all sustained over 25 months without further therapy. Four other patients had stable disease at the end of the study evaluation (51).

Because of compelling preclinical data indicating that the combination of CTLA-4 antibody blockade and cancer vaccination induced greater levels of antitumor immunity than either approach alone, several clinical trials were undertaken to test the biologic activity of anti-CTLA-4 in conjunction with other vaccines. Seven previously vaccinated metastatic melanoma patients were given a single dose of anti-CTLA-4 (MDX-010, ipilimumab, Medarex, Princeton, New Jersey, U.S.) in a phase I trial. No significant toxicity was observed, although all seven patients developed an asymptomatic grade I rash with skin biopsies showing perivascular T cell infiltrates. No patients had objective cancer regression, but three patients had evidence of tumor necrosis at biopsied sites (52). Another phase I clinical trial involved MDX-010 given repeatedly in conjunction with tumor-specific peptide vaccinations in patients with progressive stage IV melanoma. This blockade of CTLA-4 induced grade III/IV autoimmune manifestations or immune breakthrough events (IBEs) in six patients (43%), including dermatitis, enterocolitis, hepatitis, and hypophysitis, and mediated objective cancer regression in three (21%; 2 complete and 1 partial responses) of the 14 patients that were enrolled (53). Sanderson and colleagues reported a phase I study where 19 patients with high-risk resected stage III and IV melanoma were immunized with three tumor antigen epitope peptides from gp100, MART-1, and tyrosinase emulsified with adjuvant Montanide ISA 51 in combination with MDX-010 in three cohorts that received escalating doses of ipilimumab (54). Dose-related autoimmune adverse events, predominantly skin and gastrointestinal toxicities, were generally self-limited or medically manageable using steroids. IBEs were associated with the clinical endpoint of time to relapse. In addition, significant immune responses were measured by enzymelinked immunosorbent spot (ELISPOT) assays against gp100 and MART-1, indicating an antigen-specific immune response.

In a recent phase I/II clinical trial, the biologic and immunomodulatory effects of CTLA-4 blockade in patients with advanced malignant melanoma receiving tremelimumab were investigated and correlated with clinical responses (55). Four of 12 patients with immune-related adverse events attained an objective antitumor response, whereas only 1 of 18 patients without immune-related adverse events had a clinical response. Patients with immune-related adverse events and antitumor responses after treatment with tremelimumab had a significant reduction in $CD4^+CD25^{hi}$ T regulatory cells that was associated with a reduction in constitutive IL-10 secretion in resting peripheral blood mono-nuclear cell (PBMC) cultures and increase in IL-2 production by activated T cells. These early clinical trials demonstrate the promise of antibody-mediated CTLA-4 blockade as a safe and powerful strategy for the enhancement of T cell responses and induction of clinical benefit in tumor immunotherapy.

THERAPEUTIC MANIPULATION OF THE PD-L: PD-1 PATHWAY

Another way to utilize T cell regulatory pathways for tumor immunotherapy is by modulation of PD-1, an inhibitory receptor belonging to the CD28 family that has been found to play a critical role in tumor immune escape (56). PD-1 expressed on activated T and B cells negatively regulates antigen receptor–signaling on engagement with ligands PD-L1 (B7-H1) and PD-L2 (B7-DC) (57–62). PD-L1 is expressed on T cells, B cells, macrophages, DC, and some nonimmune cells such as tumors, whereas PD-L2 is regulated more tightly and is expressed mainly on activated macrophages and DC (63,64). The role of PD-1 in the establishment and maintenance of immunologic self-tolerance was first revealed when PD-1-deficient mice spontaneously developed autoimmune manifestations such as glomerulonephritis, arthritis, and dilated cardiomyopathy (65,66). It was speculated that a PD-1 antagonist would augment immune responses and may be useful in cancer therapy. This has led to several animal studies in different cancer models. The use of PD-1 antibody in murine meta-static melanoma resulted in inhibition of hematogenous spread to the liver by enhanced recruitment of effector T cells (67). In addition, work done by Wong and colleagues showed that postvaccine and endogenous prevaccine CTL specific for antigens MART-1 and gp100 from melanoma patients are increased in function and avidity as well as in number by 3- to 30-fold after exposure to PD-1 antibody in vitro (68). Interestingly, in a recent clinical trial using CTLA-4 antibody in advanced melanoma patients, a positive correlation in gene expression of CTLA-4 and PD-1 was seen in those who did not have any anti-tumor responses (54). This observation may account for the lack of antitumor response, as PD-1 can bind with PD-L1 on APC or on tumor cells to attenuate the generation of CTL (69).

Another way in which tumors can be targeted using the PD-1/PD-L1 pathway is through the blockade of PD ligands. Analysis of clinical specimens of several different human tumors including melanoma has shown the overexpression of PD-L1 and less frequently that of PD-L2 (60). Recently, a strong correlation between PD-L1 expression on tumor cells and negative prognosis has been demonstrated for human cancer patients (70). It is tempting to speculate that PD-1:PD-L1–dependent inhibition is exploited by tumor cells to evade the host immune system. In fact, several different murine studies have shown that PD-L1 expressed on tumor cells plays a role in immune escape and that its blockade potentiates antitumor immunity (71,72). Clinical trials targeting this pathway alone and in combination with cancer vaccines are in progress.

SUPPRESSOR CELL POPULATIONS IN CANCER PATIENTS

Myeloid-Derived Suppressor Cells

Myeloid-derived suppressor cells (MDSC), formerly referred to as immature myeloid suppressor cells, infiltrate solid tumors and inhibit T cell function. In mice, these MDSC express both CD11b and Gr1. In humans, MDSC are defined by expression of CD34 and CD33, the common myeloid marker, but lack markers of mature myeloid or lymphoid cells and do not express MHC class II (73). MDSC are increased in the peripheral blood of mice and patients with tumors and can induce immune suppression through multiple mechanisms. Production of reactive nitrogen and oxygen species by MDSC has been shown to block T cell activation and proliferation (74). MDSC can inhibit IFN-γ production by CD8$^+$ T cells in response to peptide, prevent CTL development, and induce CTL tolerance (75). In addition, MDSC produce high levels of arginase, depriving T cells of the essential nutrient arginine and preventing effective T cell-mediated immunity (76–78). Since depletion of myeloid cells with anti-Gr1 antibodies led to tumor regression in murine models, strategies to eliminate MDSC are being studied (79). Differentiation agents, such as all-trans-retinoic acid (ATRA), induce the maturation of MDSC into DC, macrophages, and granulocytes (80). In cancer patients, treatment with ATRA resulted in the differentiation of MDSC and enhanced tetanus vaccine–induced T cell responses, suggesting the potential for the use of ATRA in combination with melanoma immunotherapies (81). The chemotherapeutic drug gemcitabine has also been shown to reduce the total number of Gr1$^+$ cells in tumor-bearing mice, leading to enhanced antitumor CD8$^+$ T cell responses and a reversal of immune suppression in the tumor microenvironment (82,83).

Regulatory/Suppressor T cells

Thymic-derived CD4$^+$ regulatory (T$_{reg}$) T cells are characterized by the expression of both the high-affinity IL-2 receptor α chain, CD25, and the transcription factor FOXP3. These cells play an important role in peripheral T cell tolerance and control of autoimmunity by inhibiting self-reactive T cells (84–87). T$_{reg}$ cells have also been implicated in the impairment of T cell responses directed against autoantigens expressed by tumor cells. Regulatory $CD4^+CD25^+$ $Foxp3^+$ T cells can be measured in human melanoma metastases and have been shown to suppress the activation of tumor-specific $CD8^+$ T cells in patients with cancer (84,88,89). Strategies to deplete or inactivate regulatory T cells as a means of enhancing immunity induced by cancer vaccines have been explored. The use of the chemotherapeutic drug cyclophosphamide has been shown to decrease the number of regulatory T cells in tumor-bearing mice (90). But, even at low doses, cyclophosphamide is nonspecific and depletes other T cell subsets, limiting its usefulness for vaccination strategies (91). Targeted therapy against CD25 is also being explored. As activated T cells also express CD25, it remains to be determined whether this approach will be successful. In murine models, depletion of $CD25^+$ T cells prior to vaccination leads to enhancement of anti-tumor T cell responses and rejection of established tumors (92). Denileukin diftitox (ONTAK) is a fusion protein composed of diphtheria toxin fused to IL-2 that is designed to target T cells expressing CD25. It has a half-life of 58 minutes and can potentially be combined with vaccine-based immuno-therapies to target CD25-expressing T_{reg} cells (93). In patients with cancer, treatment with ONTAK has led to transient depletion of $CD25^+$ T_{reg} cells from the circulation (94–96). Another study, however, reported only a modest reduction in FOXP3 mRNA expression in circulating $CD4^+$ T cells (97). In renal cell carcinoma patients, treatment with ONTAK prior to DC vaccination significantly improved antitumor T cell responses (95). Together these data provide evidence that depletion of T_{reg} cells prior to vaccination can lead to enhanced priming of antitumor T cells. It remains to be seen whether this strategy will translate into a clear clinical benefit.

FUTURE DIRECTIONS

Even though tremendous progress has been made in the field of tumor immu-nology over the past two decades, there has been little definitive headway made in developing clinically effective vaccine-based immunotherapies for advanced melanoma. Clinical response rates to multiple different vaccine types have been exceedingly low in spite of often observed immunologic responses, but it is through these approaches that we have gained valuable insight and knowledge about tumor immunology. With advances in our understanding of immunology at the molecular level and development of sensitive techniques such as tetramer or ELISPOT assays, investigators are now able to measure surrogate endpoints like lymphocytic infiltration of tumors and tumor-specific T cells in a more rigorous manner than ever before. However, it is generally accepted that such immuno-logic endpoints do not often correlate with objective cancer regression and clinical benefit. The lack of clinical effectiveness of cancer vaccines thus far should not mean that vaccine approaches should be abandoned. Rather it should emphasize the need for changes in the application of these approaches for the treatment of melanoma. Some exciting immunotherapeutic strategies, including the blockade of regulatory and suppressive mechanisms, as well as adoptive immunotherapy using a patient's autologous peripheral blood lymphocytes (98,99) or tumor-infiltrating lymphocytes (100,101) are in development. Future success is likely to lie in using a combination of immunologic approaches for the successful induction of tumor-specific T cell responses and inhibition of suppressive mechanisms.

REFERENCES

1. King M, Spooner D, Rowlands DC. Spontaneous regression of metastatic malignant melanoma of the parotid gland and neck lymph nodes: a case report and a review of the literature. Clin Oncol (R Coll Radiol) 2001; 13(6):466–469.
2. Atkins MB, Lotze MT, Dutcher JP, et al. High-dose recombinant interleukin 2 therapy for patients with metastatic melanoma: analysis of 270 patients treated between 1985 and 1993. J Clin Oncol 1999; 17(7):2105–2116.
3. Quan W, Ramirez M, Taylor WC, et al. High-dose continuous infusion plus pulse interleukin-2 and famotidine in melanoma. Cancer Biother Radiopharma 2004; 19(6): 770–775.
4. Pittet MJ, Valmori D, Dunbar PR, et al. High frequencies of naive Melan-A/MART-1-specific CD8(+) T cells in a large proportion of human histocompatibility leukocyte antigen (HLA)-A2 individuals. J Exp Med 1999; 190(5):705–715.
5. Futagawa T, Akiba H, Kodama T, et al. Expression and function of 4-1BB and 4-1BB ligand on murine dendritic cells. Int Immunol 2002; 14(3):275–286.
6. Grewal IS, Flavell RA. The role of CD40 ligand in costimulation and T cell activation. Immunol Rev 1996; 153:85–106.
7. Ohshima Y, Tanaka Y, Tozawa H, et al. Expression and function of OX40 ligand on human dendritic cells. J Immunol 1997; 159(8):3838–3848.
8. Sondak VK, Sabel MS, Mulé JJ. Allogeneic and autologous melanoma vaccines: where have we been and where are we going? Clin Cancer Res 2006; 12(7 pt 2): 2337s–2341s.
9. Slingluff CL Jr., Engelhard VH, Ferrone S. Peptide and dendritic cell vaccines. Clin Cancer Res 2006; 12(7 Pt 2):2342s–2345s.
10. Cross D, Burmester JK. Gene therapy for cancer treatment: past, present and future. Clin Med Res 2006; 4(3):218–227.
11. Rosenberg SA, Yang JC, Restifo NP. Cancer immunotherapy: moving beyond current vaccines. Nat Med 2004; 10(9):909–915.
12. Morton DL, Mozzilo N, Thompson JF, et al. MMAIT Clinical Trials Group. An international, randomized, phase III trial of bacillus Calmette-Guerin (BCG) plus allogeneic melanoma vaccine (MCV) or placebo after complete resection of melanoma metastatic to regional or distant sites. Proceedings of American Society of Clinical Oncology Part I. J Clin Oncol, 2007; 25(suppl 18S) (abstr 8508).
13. Editorial. Cold Shower for AIDS Vaccines. Nat Med 2007; 13:12.
14. Vieweg J, Su Z, Dahm P, et al. Reversal of tumor-mediated immunosuppression. Clin Cancer Res 2007; 13(2 Pt 2):727s–732s.
15. Chang AE, Redman BG, Whitfield JR, et al. A phase I trial of tumor lysate-pulsed dendritic cells in the treatment of advanced cancer. Clin Cancer Res 2002; 8(4): 1021–1032.

16. Nestle FO, Alijagic S, Gilliet M, et al. Vaccination of melanoma patients with peptide- or tumor lysate-pulsed dendritic cells. Nat Med 1998; 4(3):328–332.
17. Pilon-Thomas S, Verhaegen M, Kuhn L, et al. Induction of anti-tumor immunity by vaccination with dendritic cells pulsed with anti-CD44 IgG opsonized tumor cells. Cancer Immunol Immunother 2006; 55(10):1238–1246.
18. Dhodapkar KM, Krasovsky J, Williamson B, et al. Antitumor monoclonal antibodies enhance cross-presentation of cellular antigens and the generation of myeloma-specific killer T cells by dendritic cells. J Exp Med 2002; 195(1):125–133.
19. Dannull J, Lesher DT, Holzknecht R, et al. Immunoproteasome down-modulation enhances the ability of dendritic cells to stimulate anti-tumor immunity. Blood 2007; 110(13):4341–4350.
20. McIlroy D, Gregoire M. Optimizing dendritic cell-based anticancer immunotherapy: maturation state does have clinical impact. Cancer Immunol Immunother 2003; 52(10):583–591.
21. Mailliard RB, Wankowicz-Kalinska A, Cai Q, et al. α-type-1 polarized dendritic cells: a novel immunization tool with optimized CTL-inducing activity. Cancer Res 2004; 64(17):5934–5937.
22. Wesa A, Kalinski P, Kirkwood JM, et al. Polarized type-1 dendritic cells (DC1) producing high levels of IL-12 family members rescue patient TH1-type anti-melanoma CD4+ T cell responses in vitro. J Immunother 2007; 30(1):75–82.
23. Pilon-Thomas S, Li W, Briggs JJ, et al. Immunostimulatory effects of CpG-ODN upon dendritic cell-based immunotherapy in a murine melanoma model. J Immunother 2006; 29(4):381–387.
24. Eggert AA, Schreurs MW, Boerman OC, et al. Biodistribution and vaccine efficiency of murine dendritic cells are dependent on the route of administration. Cancer Res 1999; 59(14):3340–3345.
25. Morse MA, Coleman RE, Akabani G, et al. Migration of human dendritic cells after injection in patients with metastatic malignancies. Cancer Res 1999; 59(1):56–58.
26. Kirk CJ, Hartigan-O'Connor D, Mulé JJ. The dynamics of the T cell antitumor response: chemokine-secreting dendritic cells can prime tumor-reactive T cells extranodally. Cancer Res 2001; 61(24):8794–8802.
27. Kirk CJ, Hartigan-O'Connor D, Nickoloff BJ, et al. T cell-dependent antitumor immunity mediated by secondary lymphoid tissue chemokine: augmentation of dendritic cell-based immunotherapy. Cancer Res 2001; 61(5):2062–2070.
28. Terando A, Roessler B, Mulé JJ. Chemokine gene modification of human dendritic cell-based tumor vaccines using a recombinant adenoviral vector. Cancer Gene Ther 2004; 11(3):165–173.
29. Riedl K, Baratelli F, Batra RK, et al. Overexpression of CCL-21/secondary lymphoid tissue chemokine in human dendritic cells augments chemotactic activities for lymphocytes and antigen presenting cells. Mol Cancer 2003; 2:35.
30. Peoples GE, Gurney JM, Hueman MT, et al. Clinical trial results of a HER2/neu (E75) vaccine to prevent recurrence in high-risk breast cancer patients. J Clin Oncol 2005; 23(30):7536–7545.
31. Gabrilovich DI, Corak J, Ciernik IF, et al. Decreased antigen presentation by dendritic cells in patients with breast cancer. Clin Cancer Res 1997; 3(3):483–490.
32. Celis E. Overlapping human leukocyte antigen class I/II binding peptide vaccine for the treatment of patients with stage IV melanoma: evidence of systemic immune dysfunction. Cancer 2007; 110(1):203–214.

33. Riker A, Cormier J, Panelli M, et al. Immune selection after antigen-specific immunotherapy of melanoma. Surgery 1999; 126(2):112–120.
34. Ferrone S, Marincola FM. Loss of HLA class I antigens by melanoma cells: molecular mechanisms, functional significance and clinical relevance. Immunol Today 1995; 16(10):487–494.
35. Chang CC, Campoli M, Restifo NP, et al. Immune selection of hot-spot beta 2-microglobulin gene mutations, HLA-A2 allospecificity loss, and antigen-processing machinery component down-regulation in melanoma cells derived from recurrent metastases following immunotherapy. J Immunol 2005; 174(3):1462–1471.
36. Rabinovich GA, Gabrilovich D, Sotomayor EM. Immunosuppressive strategies that are mediated by tumor cells. Annu Rev Immunol 2007; 25:267–296.
37. Blattman JN, Greenberg PD. PD-1 blockade: rescue from a near-death experience. Nat Immunol 2006; 7(3):227–228.
38. Egen JG, Kuhns MS, Allison JP. CTLA-4: new insights into its biological function and use in tumor immunotherapy. Nat Immunol 2002; 3(7):611–618.
39. Bretscher P, Cohn M. A theory of self-nonself discrimination. Science (New York, NY) 1970; 169(950):1042–1049.
40. Linsley PS, Brady W, Urnes M, et al. CTLA-4 is a second receptor for the B cell activation antigen B7. J Exp Med 1991; 174(3):561–569.
41. Linsley PS, Brady W, Grosmaire L, et al. Binding of the B cell activation antigen B7 to CD28 costimulates T cell proliferation and interleukin 2 mRNA accumulation. J Exp Med 1991; 173(3):721–730.
42. Brunet JF, Denizot F, Luciani MF, et al. A new member of the immunoglobulin superfamily–CTLA-4. Nature 1987; 328(6127):267–270.
43. Aruffo A, Seed B. Molecular cloning of a CD28 cDNA by a high-efficiency COS cell expression system. Proc Natl Acad Sci USA 1987; 84(23):8573–8577.
44. Gross JA, St John T, Allison JP. The murine homologue of the T lymphocyte antigen CD28. Molecular cloning and cell surface expression. J Immunol 1990; 144(8):3201–3210.
45. Brunner MC, Chambers CA, Chan FK, et al. CTLA-4-Mediated inhibition of early events of T cell proliferation. J Immunol 1999; 162(10):5813–5820.
46. Alegre ML, Shiels H, Thompson CB, et al. Expression and function of CTLA-4 in Th1 and Th2 cells. J Immunol 1998; 161(7):3347–3356.
47. Lee KM, Chuang E, Griffin M, et al. Molecular basis of T cell inactivation by CTLA-4. Science (New York, NY) 1998; 282(5397):2263–2266.
48. Leach DR, Krummel MF, Allison JP. Enhancement of antitumor immunity by CTLA-4 blockade. Science (New York, NY) 1996; 271(5256):1734–1736.
49. van Elsas A, Sutmuller RP, Hurwitz AA, et al. Elucidating the autoimmune and antitumor effector mechanisms of a treatment based on cytotoxic T lymphocyte antigen-4 blockade in combination with a B16 melanoma vaccine: comparison of prophylaxis and therapy. J Exp Med 2001; 194(4):481–489.
50. van Elsas A, Hurwitz AA, Allison JP. Combination immunotherapy of B16 melanoma using anti-cytotoxic T lymphocyte-associated antigen 4 (CTLA-4) and granulocyte/macrophage colony-stimulating factor (GM-CSF)-producing vaccines induces rejection of subcutaneous and metastatic tumors accompanied by autoimmune depigmentation. J Exp Med 1999; 190(3):355–366.

51. Ribas A, Camacho LH, Lopez-Berestein G, et al. Antitumor activity in melanoma and anti-self responses in a phase I trial with the anti-cytotoxic T lymphocyte-associated antigen 4 monoclonal antibody CP-675,206. J Clin Oncol 2005; 23(35): 8968–8977.
52. Phan GQ, Yang JC, Sherry RM, et al. Cancer regression and autoimmunity induced by cytotoxic T lymphocyte-associated antigen 4 blockade in patients with metastatic melanoma. Proc Natl Acad Sci USA 2003; 100(14):8372–8377.
53. Hodi FS, Mihm MC, Soiffer RJ, et al. Biologic activity of cytotoxic T lymphocyte-associated antigen 4 antibody blockade in previously vaccinated metastatic melanoma and ovarian carcinoma patients. Proc Natl Acad Sci USA 2003; 100(8): 4712–4717.
54. Sanderson K, Scotland R, Lee P, et al. Autoimmunity in a phase I trial of a fully human anti-cytotoxic T-lymphocyte antigen-4 monoclonal antibody with multiple melanoma peptides and Montanide ISA 51 for patients with resected stages III and IV melanoma. J Clin Oncol 2005; 23(4):741–750.
55. Reuben JM, Lee BN, Li C, et al. Biologic and immunomodulatory events after CTLA-4 blockade with ticilimumab in patients with advanced malignant melanoma. Cancer 2006; 106(11):2437–2444.
56. Okazaki T, Maeda A, Nishimura H, et al. PD-1 immunoreceptor inhibits B cell receptor-mediated signaling by recruiting src homology 2-domain-containing tyrosine phosphatase 2 to phosphotyrosine. Proc Natl Acad Sci USA 2001; 98(24): 13866–3871.
57. Agata Y, Kawasaki A, Nishimura H, et al. Expression of the PD-1 antigen on the surface of stimulated mouse T and B lymphocytes. Int Immunol 1996; 8(5):765–772.
58. Ishida Y, Agata Y, Shibahara K, et al. Induced expression of PD-1, a novel member of the immunoglobulin gene superfamily, upon programmed cell death. EMBO J 1992; 11(11):3887–3895.
59. Tseng SY, Otsuji M, Gorski K, et al. B7-DC, a new dendritic cell molecule with potent costimulatory properties for T cells. J Exp Med 2001; 193(7):839–846.
60. Freeman GJ, Long AJ, Iwai Y, et al. Engagement of the PD-1 immunoinhibitory receptor by a novel B7 family member leads to negative regulation of lymphocyte activation. J Exp Med 2000; 192(7):1027–1034.
61. Dong H, Zhu G, Tamada K, et al. B7-H1, a third member of the B7 family, co-stimulates T cell proliferation and interleukin-10 secretion. Nat Med 1999; 5(12): 1365–1369.
62. Liang SC, Latchman YE, Buhlmann JE, et al. Regulation of PD-1, PD-L1, and PD-L2 expression during normal and autoimmune responses. Eur J Immunol 2003; 33(10): 2706–2716.
63. Ishida M, Iwai Y, Tanaka Y, et al. Differential expression of PD-L1 and PD-L2, ligands for an inhibitory receptor PD-1, in the cells of lymphohematopoietic tissues. Immunol Lett 2002; 84(1):57–62.
64. Latchman Y, Wood CR, Chernova T, et al. PD-L2 is a second ligand for PD-1 and inhibits T cell activation. Nat Immunol 2001; 2(3):261–268.
65. Nishimura H, Nose M, Hiai H, et al. Development of lupus-like autoimmune diseases by disruption of the PD-1 gene encoding an ITIM motif-carrying immunoreceptor. Immunity 1999; 11(2):141–151.
66. Nishimura H, Okazaki T, Tanaka Y, et al. Autoimmune dilated cardiomyopathy in PD-1 receptor-deficient mice. Science (New York, NY) 2001; 291(5502):319–322.
67. Iwai Y, Terawaki S, Honjo T. PD-1 blockade inhibits hematogenous spread of poorly immunogenic tumor cells by enhanced recruitment of effector T cells. Int Immunol 2005; 17(2):133–144.

68. Wong RM, Scotland RR, Lau RL, et al. Programmed death-1 blockade enhances expansion and functional capacity of human melanoma antigen-specific CTLs. Int Immunol 2007; 19(10):1223–1234.

69. Dong H, Strome SE, Salomao DR, et al. Tumor-associated B7-H1 promotes T cell apoptosis: a potential mechanism of immune evasion. Nat Med 2002; 8(8): 793–800.

70. Hamanishi J, Mandai M, Iwasaki M, et al. Programmed cell death 1 ligand 1 and tumor-infiltrating CD8+ T lymphocytes are prognostic factors of human ovarian cancer. Proc Natl Acad Sci USA 2007; 104(9):3360–3365.

71. Hirano F, Kaneko K, Tamura H, et al. Blockade of B7-H1 and PD-1 by monoclonal antibodies potentiates cancer therapeutic immunity. Cancer Res 2005; 65(3):1089–1096.

72. Iwai Y, Ishida M, Tanaka Y, et al. Involvement of PD-L1 on tumor cells in the escape from host immune system and tumor immunotherapy by PD-L1 blockade. Proc Natl Acad Sci USA 2002; 99(19):12293–2297.

73. Almand B, Clark JI, Nikitina E, et al. Increased production of immature myeloid cells in cancer patients: a mechanism of immunosuppression in cancer. J Immunol 2001; 166(1):678–689.

74. Kusmartsev SA, Li Y, Chen SH. Gr-1+ myeloid cells derived from tumor-bearing mice inhibit primary T cell activation induced through CD3/CD28 costimulation. J Immunol 2000; 165(2):779–785.

75. Kusmartsev S, Nagaraj S, Gabrilovich DI. Tumor-associated CD8+ T cell tolerance induced by bone marrow-derived immature myeloid cells. J Immunol 2005; 175(7): 4583–4592.

76. Rodriguez PC, Quiceno DG, Zabaleta J, et al. Arginase I production in the tumor microenvironment by mature myeloid cells inhibits T cell receptor expression and antigen-specific T cell responses. Cancer Res 2004; 64(16):5839–5849.

77. Bronte V, Serafini P, De Santo C, et al. IL-4-induced arginase 1 suppresses alloreactive T cells in tumor-bearing mice. J Immunol 2003; 170(1):270–278.

78. Liu Y, Van Ginderachter JA, Brys L, et al. Nitric oxide-independent CTL suppression during tumor progression: association with arginase-producing (M2) myeloid cells. J Immunol 2003; 170(10):5064–5074.

79. Pekarek LA, Starr BA, Toledano AY, et al. Inhibition of tumor growth by elimination of granulocytes. J Exp Med 1995; 181(1):435–440.

80. Kusmartsev S, Cheng F, Yu B, et al. All-trans-retinoic acid eliminates immature myeloid cells from tumor-bearing mice and improves the effect of vaccination. Cancer Res 2003; 63(15):4441–4449.

81. Mirza N, Fishman M, Fricke I, et al. All-trans-retinoic acid improves differentiation of myeloid cells and immune response in cancer patients. Cancer Res 2006; 66(18): 9299–9307.

82. Suzuki E, Kapoor V, Jassar AS, et al. Gemcitabine selectively eliminates splenic Gr-1+/CD11b+ myeloid suppressor cells in tumor-bearing animals and enhances antitumor immune activity. Clin Cancer Res 2005; 11(18):6713–6721.

83. Sinha P, Clements VK, Bunt SK, et al. Cross-talk between myeloid-derived suppressor cells and macrophages subverts tumor immunity toward a type 2 response. J Immunol 2007; 179(2):977–983.

84. Sakaguchi S. Naturally arising Foxp3-expressing CD25+CD4+ regulatory T cells in immunological tolerance to self and non-self. Nat Immunol 2005; 6(4):345–352.

85. Shevach EM, McHugh RS, Piccirillo CA, et al. Control of T cell activation by CD4+ CD25+ suppressor T cells. Immunol Rev 2001; 182:58–67.
86. Shevach EM. Certified professionals: CD4(+)CD25(+) suppressor T cells. J Exp Med 2001; 193(11):F41–F46.
87. Sakaguchi S. The origin of FOXP3-expressing CD4+ regulatory T cells: thymus or periphery. J Clin Invest 2003; 112(9):1310–1312.
88. Viguier M, Lemaitre F, Verola O, et al. Foxp3 expressing CD4+CD25(high) regulatory T cells are overrepresented in human metastatic melanoma lymph nodes and inhibit the function of infiltrating T cells. J Immunol 2004; 173(2):1444–1453.
89. Cesana GC, DeRaffele G, Cohen S, et al. Characterization of CD4+CD25+ regulatory T cells in patients treated with high-dose interleukin-2 for metastatic melanoma or renal cell carcinoma. J Clin Oncol 2006; 24(7):1169–1177.
90. Lutsiak ME, Semnani RT, De Pascalis R, et al. Inhibition of CD4(+)25+ T regulatory cell function implicated in enhanced immune response by low-dose cyclophosphamide. Blood 2005; 105(7):2862–2868.
91. Zhang H, Chua KS, Guimond M, et al. Lymphopenia and interleukin-2 therapy alter homeostasis of CD4+CD25+ regulatory T cells. Nat Med 2005; 11(11):1238–1243.
92. Onizuka S, Tawara I, Shimizu J, et al. Tumor rejection by in vivo administration of anti-CD25 (interleukin-2 receptor alpha) monoclonal antibody. Cancer Res 1999; 59(13):3128–3133.
93. Foss FM. DAB(389)IL-2 (ONTAK): a novel fusion toxin therapy for lymphoma. Clin Lymphoma 2000; 1(2):110–116.
94. Barnett B, Kryczek I, Cheng P, et al. Regulatory T cells in ovarian cancer: biology and therapeutic potential. Am J Reprod Immunol 2005; 54(6):369–377.
95. Dannull J, Su Z, Rizzieri D, et al. Enhancement of vaccine-mediated antitumor immunity in cancer patients after depletion of regulatory T cells. J Clin Invest 2005; 115(12):3623–3633.
96. Mahnke K, Schonfeld K, Fondel S, et al. Depletion of CD4+CD25+ human regulatory T cells in vivo: kinetics of Treg depletion and alterations in immune functions in vivo and in vitro. Int J Cancer 2007; 120(12):2723–2733.
97. Attia P, Maker AV, Haworth LR, et al. Inability of a fusion protein of IL-2 and diphtheria toxin (Denileukin Diftitox, DAB389IL-2, ONTAK) to eliminate regulatory T lymphocytes in patients with melanoma. J Immunother 2005; 28(6): 582–592.
98. Powell DJ Jr., Dudley ME, Hogan KA, et al. Adoptive transfer of vaccine-induced peripheral blood mononuclear cells to patients with metastatic melanoma following lymphodepletion. J Immunol 2006; 177(9):6527–6539.
99. Morgan RA, Dudley ME, Wunderlich JR, et al. Cancer regression in patients after transfer of genetically engineered lymphocytes. Science (New York, NY) 2006; 314(5796):126–129.
100. Hussein MR. Tumour-infiltrating lymphocytes and melanoma tumorigenesis: an insight. Br J Dermatol 2005; 153(1):18–21.
101. Dudley ME, Wunderlich JR, Yang JC, et al. Adoptive cell transfer therapy following non-myeloablative but lymphodepleting chemotherapy for the treatment of patients with refractory metastatic melanoma. J Clin Oncol 2005; 23(10): 2346–2357.
102. Slingluff CL Jr., Chianese-Bullock KA, Bullock TN, et al. Immunity to melanoma antigens: from self-tolerance to immunotherapy. Adv Immunol 2006; 90:243–295.

12

Adoptive T Cell Immunotherapy

Susan Tsai and Alfred E. Chang

Department of Surgery, University of Michigan, Ann Arbor, Michigan, U.S.A.

HISTORICAL PERSPECTIVE

Adoptive T cell immunotherapy is defined as the passive transfer of tumor-reactive T cells into the tumor-bearing host that results in the direct or indirect destruction of established tumors. Utilizing inbred strains of mice where transplantable tumors were established, investigators in the 1950s and 1960s were able to cause regression of established tumors by adoptively transferring lymphocytes derived from normal mice that were immunized with various tumor vaccine preparations. This provided the proof-of-principle that appropriately immunocompetent cells can mediate tumor regression upon transfer to a syngeneic host. The major obstacles to developing these therapies clinically was the ability to expand sufficient quantities of T cells ex vivo, and more importantly, being able to isolate tumor-reactive T cells from the tumor-bearing host.

The discovery of interleukin-2 (IL-2) in the mid-1970s as a T cell growth factor provided an opportunity to allow investigators to expand T cells in large quantities. In fact, one of the first large clinical trials of adoptive cellular immunotherapy in patients with advanced cancers that included melanoma, was the transfer of lymphokine-activated killer (LAK) cells administered in conjunction with IL-2 (1,2). LAK cells were generated by culturing lymphocytes in high concentrations of IL-2, which resulted in the differentiation of cytolytic cells that could lyse tumor cells nonspecifically. Through subsequent studies, it was found that the LAK cells combined with IL-2 therapy contributed minimally to the antitumor effects of IL-2 alone. Nevertheless, the LAK cell experience stimulated investigations into developing more effective tumor-specific adoptive cellular therapies (ACTs). This chapter will review some of the approaches that have been investigated in clinical trials.

Tumor-Infiltrating Lymphocytes

Adoptive cellular immunotherapy involves the passive transfer of large numbers of tumor-specific lymphocytes into a tumor-bearing host. One of the impediments to the wider application of this therapy is the difficulty in identifying and subsequently generating large numbers of tumor-reactive cells. While the clinical trial utilizing LAK cells failed to demonstrate a benefit when compared with IL-2 alone, it stimulated further interest in the development of tumor-specific cellular therapies. Subsequently, the majority of lymphocytes studies in ACTs have broadly focused on two lymphocyte groups: tumor-infiltrating lymphocytes (TIL) and tumor-specific, major histocompatibility complex (MHC) class I–restricted, cytotoxic T lymphocytes (CTL).

One of the challenges of targeting cellular-based therapies in cancer lies in the inherently poor immunogenicity of most solid tumors. Intuitively, TIL should demonstrate recognition of the associated tumors. However, the majority of solid human tumors rarely contain CTL that recognize autologous tumor. Two exceptions to this are melanoma and renal cell carcinoma. In particular, melanoma lesions yield a significant number of lymphocytes that recognize not only the primary tumor, but also human leukocyte antigen (HLA)-matched tumors as well. It has been reported that as many as 78% of TIL are tumor reactive (3). In preclinical models, TIL were found to mediate specific killing of the tumor from which they were derived. They also produced specific cytokine secretion when cocultivated with the autologous tumor (4). Adoptive transfer of TIL with the addition of IL-2 has been effective at treating established lung and liver metastases in a variety of murine models (5).

This promising preclinical data led to a pilot study in patients with metastatic solid tumors. Twelve patients, including six with melanoma, four with renal cell carcinoma, one with breast carcinoma, and one with colon carcinoma were treated with varying doses and combinations of TIL, IL-2, and cyclophosphamide. TIL were extracted from autologous tumors, expanded ex vivo, and re-administered into the patient. Two partial responses (PR) to therapy were observed. One patient with melanoma demonstrated regression of pulmonary and mediastinal masses and a patient with renal cell carcinoma demonstrated regression of a lymph node mass. One additional patient with breast cancer experienced a transient partial regression of disease in nodal and cutaneous sites with complete elimination of malignant cells from a pleural effusion. No toxic effects were directly attributable to TIL infusions. Unlike the nonspecific lytic activity characteristic of LAK cells, the TIL from five of six melanoma patients demonstrated lytic activity specific for the autologous tumor target by chromium-release assays (6).

In a series of 89 consecutive patients with metastatic melanoma, autologous TIL were administered with high-dose IL-2 with a 34% objective clinical response rate. Overall response rates for high-dose IL-2 are approximately 17% and therefore the additional response rate was inferred to be secondary to the addition of TIL. Predictors of clinical response were related to TIL age, rapidity of doubling times, and a higher production of tumor-specific cytokine secretion (7). Most of the responses, however, were transient and limited persistence of the transferred cells was observed (8). These results demonstrated that ACTs could mediate tumor regression of metastatic lesions and initiated further investigations to optimize therapies.

With these encouraging results, ACT has been performed in the adjuvant setting. In one trial, 88 patients with regional melanoma metastasis underwent lymphadenectomy. The patients were subsequently randomized to receive IL-2 alone or in combination with TIL. No statistically significant increase in relapse-free survival was observed after a median follow-up of 46.9 months. However, in subset analysis, patients with a single lymph node metastasis who received TIL plus IL-2 demonstrated improved relapse-free and overall survivals when compared with IL-2 alone ($p = 0.0285$ and $p = 0.039$, respectively) (9).

Further efforts have been directed at optimizing ACT in the setting of metastatic melanoma. Preclinical data suggest that the addition of chemotherapy to ACT potentiates antitumor effects in murine models (10). The most encouraging results of ACT have also been demonstrated in the setting of a preconditioning, nonmyeloablative chemotherapy. At the National Cancer Institute, 35 patients with refractory metastatic melanoma received a lymphodepleting but nonmyeloablative chemotherapy, consisting of cyclophosphamide and fludarabine, followed by the infusion of autologous ex vivo rapidly expanded TIL and high-dose IL-2 therapy (Fig. 1). This conditioning regimen resulted in a transient myelosuppression and a near-complete elimination of circulating lymphocytes for about a week. After cellular infusions, many of the patients had a dramatic lymphocytosis, with an almost clonal repopulation of the immune system with tumor-reactive TILs. These cells demonstrated the functional ability to secrete inflammatory cytokines and lyse HLA-matched tumors ex vivo and were also found to have trafficked to the tumor sites in patients postinfusion. Tumor biopsies obtained from responding patients demonstrated infiltration of the transferred cells. Ultimately, 18 of 35 (51%) patients experienced objective clinical responses. Three patients had complete responses (CR) and 15 had PR with a mean duration of 11.5 months (11). Some patients also exhibited symptoms of autoimmune melanocyte destruction including vitiligo or uveitis. Finally, persistence of the lymphocytes was observed in several patients up to 146 days posttransfer and was statistically related to objective clinical response (12).

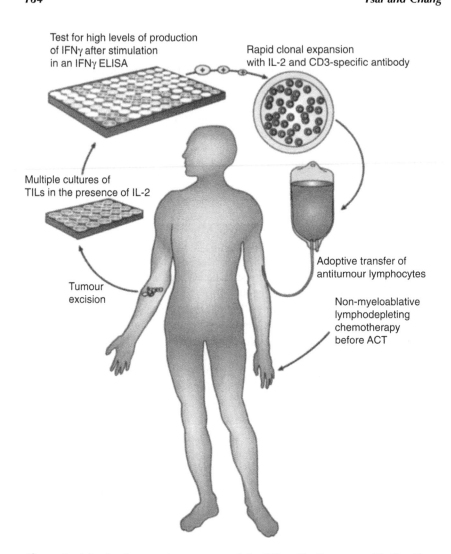

Test for high levels of production
of IFNγ after stimulation
in an IFNγ ELISA

Rapid clonal expansion
with IL-2 and CD3-specific antibody

Multiple cultures of
TILs in the presence of IL-2

Tumour
excision

Adoptive transfer of
antitumour lymphocytes

Non-myeloablative
lymphodepleting
chemotherapy
before ACT

Figure 1 Adoptive immunotherapy protocol for TIL cells. Tumor-specific T cells are isolated ex vivo from melanoma lesions using high concentrations of IL-2. TIL cells are screened for their ability to secrete high levels of IFN-γ when cultured with tumor antigen. The selected TIL cells are expanded using anti-CD3 antibody and expanded in IL-2. Prior to cell infusion, patients undergo chemotherapy to induce a lymphodepletion within the host. *Abbreviation*: ACT, adoptive cellular therapies. *Source*: From Ref. 59 (*See Color Insert*).

The addition of a lymphodepleting chemotherapy regimen has augmented antitumor responses beyond what had previously been observed with ACT of TIL and IL-2 alone, suggesting that the optimal ACT requires not only the selection of the ideal effector cell, but also may require manipulation of the host environment as well. An important regulatory cell type, which may be impaired by a lymphodepleting regimen, is the $CD4^+CD25^+$ T regulatory cell (T_{reg}). In murine models, T_{reg} cells have been shown to suppress the antitumor activities of adoptively transferred tumor-reactive T cells (13). Augmented antitumor responses were observed after ACT of $CD8^+$ T cells to $CD4^{-/-}$ but not $CD8^{-/-}$ mice, suggesting that $CD4^+$ cells are the regulatory component. Of $CD4^+$ cells, transfer of $CD4^+CD25^+$ cells abrogated the ACT, while $CD4^+CD25^-$ (T_{helper}) cells significantly augmented it. Furthermore, in melanoma patients, the T_{reg} population is twofold greater in metastatic lymph nodes than that seen in tumor-free lymph nodes and autologous peripheral blood mononuclear cells (PBMC) (14). Interestingly, treatment with high-dose IL-2 has been noted to promote expansion of the T_{reg} population in humans (15). Therefore, selective elimination of T_{reg} cells may augment the efficacy of ACT in the setting of lymphodepletion. It is also hypothesized that the depletion of T_{reg} cells may allow for expansion of T_{helper} cells and further bolster CTL activity. Ex vivo depletion of T_{reg} cells was performed in the setting of a nonmyeloablative chemotherapy and ACT. In five patients with metastatic melanoma, PBMCs underwent $CD25^+$ depletion and were readministered to patients after a lymphodepleting chemotherapy regimen, in combination with high-dose IL-2. No patient experienced an objective tumor response or autoimmunity. In addition, the T_{reg} population rapidly repopulated in the peripheral blood of treated patients with up to 63% of $CD4^+$ cells expressing FOXP3, a transcription factor associated with T_{reg} cells (16). Further modifications of ACT with alternative cytokines, such as IL-7 or IL-15, or cotransfer of T_{reg}-depleted antigen-specific T cells may be warranted.

Another mechanism by which lymphodepletion is thought to augment ACT is by the elimination of cytokine sinks. In the setting of lymphodepletion, transferred T cell populations can proliferate independent of MHC peptide presentation, but are dependent on cytokine secretion. Key cytokines crucial for the homeostatic proliferation of naïve and memory T cells are IL-7 and IL-15. In transgenic mice, the absence of these cytokines results in impaired proliferation of $CD8^+$ T cells (17), while the overexpression of IL-7 and IL-15 promotes preferential expansion of the memory $CD8^+CD44^{hi}$ T cells (18). In studies in $Rag^{-/-}$ mice, which lack endogenous B and T cells, tumor-specific $CD8^+$ T cell efficacy can be enhanced by IL-7 and IL-15 (19). This suggests that ACT may be augmented by the addition of exogenous cytokines, thus negating the competition for available endogenous cytokines. Furthermore, murine models suggest that a synergistic effect may be observed by the addition of a combination of cytokines (20). In current protocols of ACT, high-dose IL-2 is utilized in the rapid expansion of TIL and after cellular infusion. Although IL-2 is important for T cell expansion, it also supports the suppressive function of T_{reg} cells (21). In the future, ACT with IL-7 or IL-15 in vitro and in vivo expansion may be doubly beneficial by abrogating the effect of T_{reg} cells while simultaneously augmenting cytokine-driven proliferation of effector cells.

   The effects of lymphodepletion have been one area of intense investigation
in ACT. Another area of focus has been the effect of T cell differentiation and
effector function (Fig. 2). It is hypothesized that CD8$^+$ T cells undergo progressive differentiation through early, intermediate, and late effector stages.
With progressive differentiation, T cells lose the ability to home in on lymphoid
tissues, have impaired responses to homeostatic cytokines, and ultimately reach a
state of replicative senescence (22). Initially, late effectors were thought to be the
most effective cells because of their high in vitro cytotoxicity. However, in
murine models, late effector CD8$^+$ T cells are up to 100-fold less effective
in vivo than T cells at an early stage of differentiation (23). This has also been

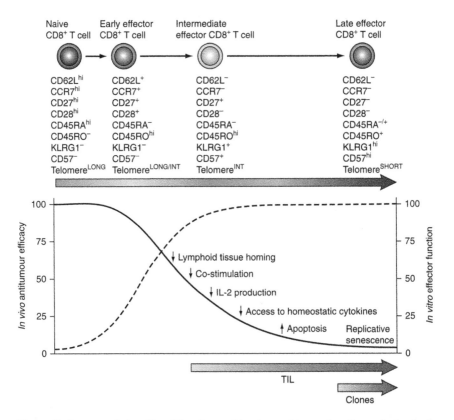

Figure 2 Inverse relationship of in vitro and in vivo antitumor functions of adoptively
transferred naïve and effector T cell subsets. At increasing strength of stimulation, naïve
CD8$^+$ T cells proliferate and progressively differentiate through early, intermediate, and
late effector stages. The phenotypic and functional changes that characterize this process
are illustrated as no expression (–), intermediate expression (+) and high expression (hi) of
the various markers. The progressive acquisition of full effector functions (*dashed line*) is
associated with a decreased ability of T cells to cause tumor regression after adoptive
transfer (*solid line*). *Source*: From Ref. 59 (*See Color Insert*).

demonstrated in clinical trials. Earlier attempts at generating T cell clones for ACT failed to demonstrate objective responses in either immunoreplete or immunodepleted patients (24,25). In current clinical ACT protocols, TIL are generated by undergoing several rounds of rapid expansion, which induces progressive CD8$^+$ T cell differentiation. This progressive differentiation of TIL may result in impaired effector function by several mechanisms. In the late effector state, T cells lose the expression of the lymphoid homing molecule CD62L. The homing of T cells to secondary lymphoid organs facilitates their interaction with antigen-presenting cells (APC). In murine models, the transfer of CD62L-deficient T cells demonstrated impaired antitumor efficacy when compared with CD62L$^+$ T cells (23). Not only do late-effector T cells demonstrate impaired homing to lymphoid organs, but the expression of costimulatory molecules is also downregulated. The interaction of CD28 with its corresponding costimulatory ligands on the surface of APC allows for amplification of cellular response. However, the expression of CD28 is progressively lost with further T cell differentiation, with early effector phenotypes demonstrating the highest levels of CD28. T cells that persisted in vivo following ACT were remarkable for high levels of CD28 (26). In addition, these T cells also demonstrated longer telomere lengths. Telomere erosion has been observed with T cell proliferation and late differentiation. The shortening of telomere length ultimately results in replicative senescence. In comparison to patient TIL prior to and after ACT, impaired telomerase activity was observed in the setting of clonal expansion, resulting in rapid telomere shortening (12). This suggests a survival advantage for transferred T cells with an early effector phenotype. Current criteria for selection of T cells for ACT focuses on in vitro selection by cytolysis and cytokine secretion; however, in the future, consideration of cellular phenotype and telomere length may improve antitumor efficacy and lasting response.

Genetically Modified T Cells

One limitation of TIL is the requirement of patients to have resectable lesions from which highly tumor-specific TIL can be generated. Approximately half of all patients chosen for ACT either do not have an adequate site of resectable disease or fail to produce TIL from their tumors. An alternative option for such patients is the transduction of high-affinity T cell receptors (TCR) into their peripheral blood lymphocytes (PBL). Most naturally occurring TCR do not demonstrate a high affinity for self/tumor antigens secondary to thymic deletion. However, high-affinity TCRs have been identified in populations of TIL that have demonstrated a significant in vivo antitumor response. At the National Cancer Institute (NCI), the genes for the α and β chains of a TCR against a melanoma antigen, MART-1, were isolated from T lymphocytes that mediated regression of tumor in patients with metastatic melanoma (27). These genes were cloned and inserted into retroviral vectors. Subsequent transduction of PBMC yielded functional T cells, which demonstrated recognition of peptide-pulsed

APCs and produced inflammatory cytokines. In the first clinical trial using this approach, PBL from patients with metastatic melanoma underwent retroviral transduction of a MART-1 TCR followed by ACT (28). Two of 17 patients demonstrated complete responses. Both responders had high circulating levels of the gene-transduced cells persistent one year after infusion. No toxicity was observed from this trial. This initial finding has stimulated further interest in the identification and transduction of other highly avid TCRs against target antigens, such as anti-NY-ESO-1 or p53. Genetically engineered lymphocytes have the potential for extending the application of ACT to a variety of malignancies that previously had not been amenable to immunotherapy.

Efforts to improve the response rate of ACT with genetically engineered lymphocytes have been directed at optimizing the gene transduction as well as identifying higher avidity TCR. Transduction of TCRs with retroviruses requires cellular proliferation and thus also promotes T cell differentiation. An alternative means of transduction is via a lentiviral vector. Lentiviruses are less dependent on active cell division and may allow the generation of a greater population of naïve lymphocytes. Furthermore, some evidence suggests that rapid expansion upregulates negative costimulatory molecules such as PD-1(29). Lentiviral transduction may circumvent the development of late-effector T cells as well as diminish any negative costimulatory signals.

Another obstacle to successful genetically engineered cells for ACT may be related to mispairing of the transduced α and β chains with the endogenous TCR subunits. In the MART-1 trial, a significant disparity was reported between the number of cells expressing the Vβ12 protein specific for the TCR and MART-1 tetramer-binding cells, suggesting mispairing of the subunit chains. The addition of a cysteine molecule on the α and β chains has been proposed as a potential solution to this problem. The additional cysteine has been reported to promote the formation of an additional interchain disulfide bond, stabilizing the receptor (30). Cysteine-modified receptors were more highly expressed than wild type on the surface of human lymphocytes and were able to mediate higher levels of cytokine secretion and specific lysis when cocultured with HLA-matched tumors. An alternative solution is the transduction of hematopoietic stem cells (HSC). HSC can be induced to differentiate into naïve CD8$^+$ T cells in vitro, which may repress the endogenous TCRβ expression (31). Finally, TCR transduction into $\gamma\delta$ T cells, which lack $\alpha\beta$TCR, has been reported (32).

The initial success of genetically engineered lymphocytes has stimulated efforts to further identify the optimal TCR for transduction. In studies of both viral infection and cell-mediated immunity against tumors, highly avid T cells have demonstrated superior function over low avidity T cells. It is postulated that improving TCR avidity may also augment the efficacy of genetically engineered lymphocytes. T cell clones reactive to MART-1 have been isolated from TIL obtained from tumors of five different melanoma patients who participated in clinical trials. Interestingly, the MART-1 TCR clone that has been characterized and utilized in the clinical trial was not the most avid TCR identified. An additional TCR clone was identified that demonstrated high avidity against MART-1 tumor in vitro and after RNA electroporation into donor T cells (33).

An alternative approach to engineering tumor-antigen-specific receptors has involved the use of "T bodies," which are chimeric receptors that have antibody-based external receptor structure and cytosolic signaling domains (34). Unlike TCR, T bodies identify tumor in a MHC-unrestricted manner, but are able to effect specific TCR function. Three studies utilizing T bodies have been reported in ovarian and renal cell carcinoma and neuroblastoma, with variable results. A pilot trial that tested T cells expressing a T body receptor specific for a folate-binding protein on the surface of ovarian carcinoma cells has demonstrated the approach to be safe; however, further optimization of T body expression and persistence is needed (35).

Vaccine-Primed Lymph Node Cells

An alternative source of effector T cells for adoptive immunotherapy is lymph nodes. Lymph nodes are important secondary lymphoid organs where dendritic cells interact with T cells to initiate a primary immune response (36). Our laboratory has characterized the effectiveness of either tumor-draining or vaccine-primed lymph node cells as effector cells in adoptive immunotherapy (37,38). The generation of effector T cells from tumor-draining lymph nodes (TDLN) or vaccine-primed lymph nodes (VPLN) is restricted by the immunogenicity of the tumor cells and the kinetics of response within the draining lymph nodes, and requires secondary activation ex vivo for differentiation and expansion of the lymphoid cells to become immunocompetent effector cells in adoptive immunotherapy.

Utilizing the poorly immunogenic B16-BL6 melanoma cell line, we have demonstrated in animal models the ability to generate effector T cells from TDLN that were capable of mediating the regression of both experimentally induced and spontaneous metastases (39). In those studies, the growth of B16-BL6 tumor cells inoculated intradermally did not elicit effector cells in the TDLN. It required the coadministration of an immune adjuvant, in this case, *Corynebacterium parvum,* to induce effector cells in the TDLN that could be activated secondarily by anti-CD3 monoclonal antibody and expanded in IL-2. These observations resulted in an early pilot study we conducted in patients with advanced melanoma and renal cell cancer who were vaccinated with irradiated autologous tumor cells admixed with the bacterial adjuvant bacillus Calmette Guèrin (BCG), and who went on to receive VPLN cells that were activated with anti-CD3/IL-2 (40). In that study, we were able to demonstrate the preferential expansion of CD8$^+$ T cells from the VPLN, which responded to autologous tumor cells in vitro with MHC class I–restricted secretion of IFN-γ and GM-CSF cytokines. In addition, clinical responses were noted in patients with either melanoma or renal cell cancer. A subsequent phase II trial of anti-CD3-activated VPLN cells was performed in patients with stage IV renal cell cancer (41).

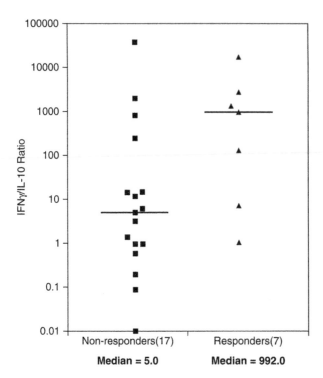

Figure 3 Ratio of IFN-γ to IL-10 cytokine release of vaccine-primed lymph node cells for responders and nonresponders after adoptive immunotherapy. Each dot represents a patient. Median values (*horizontal lines*) were significantly different at $p = 0.047$. *Source:* From Ref. 41.

Durable tumor responses were noted in 27% of the treated patients and were correlated with the cytokine profile released by the VPLN cells in response to autologous tumor cells. With a greater IFN-γ:IL-10 ratio, a higher likelihood of a response was observed (Fig. 3).

We have also examined alternative vaccine strategies to prime draining lymph nodes as a means of eliciting effector cells for adoptive immunotherapy. In a preclinical model utilizing the B16-BL6 melanoma, we examined the utility of genetically modifying tumor cells with different cytokine genes as a means of generating vaccines that could prime draining lymph nodes (42). We found that GM-CSF was superior to other cytokines in enhancing the immunogenicity of the melanoma tumor cell line. In an adoptive immunotherapy model, we demonstrated that B16-BL6 tumor cells transduced to secrete GM-CSF were superior to tumor cells admixed with a bacterial adjuvant in eliciting effector cells in VPLN (43). On the basis of these observations, we conducted a pilot study in patients with stage IV melanoma where autologous tumor cells were transduced retrovirally to secrete GM-CSF and were utilized as vaccines to generate VPLN cells for adoptive immunotherapy (44). In that study, we found that the local release of GM-CSF at the vaccine site resulted in a significant infiltration of dendritic cells into the microenvironment. One patient out of five went on to have a complete clinical response to therapy that has been durable.

Our laboratory has continued to optimize the culture conditions by which TDLN or VPLN cells can be activated and expanded ex vivo. It was apparent that effector cells that release a type 1 cytokine profile in response to tumor antigen were more capable of mediating tumor regression compared to effector cells that release a type 2 cytokine response (45,46). Furthermore, we have found that only a small subset of cells within primed lymph nodes constitute the "pre-effector" cell population that mediate the antitumor response. These are $CD8^+$ and $CD4^+$ cells that express P-selectin ligand^{high} ($Plig^{high}$) markers and release the greatest amount of IFN-γ in response to tumor antigen (47). The cultured $Plig^{high}$ TDLN were 10- to 20-fold more active against established pulmonary micrometastases than cultured unfractionated TDLN and greater than 30-fold more active than cultured TDLN cells depleted of the $Plig^{high}$ fraction before expansion.

Besides utilizing anti-CD3 monoclonal antibodies (mAb) to secondarily activate tumor-primed lymph node cells, we have investigated the addition of costimulatory signals to generate effector cells for adoptive immunotherapy. This has included the use of anti-CD28 mAb in addition to anti-CD3 to activate lymphoid cells. In preclinical animal studies, this has resulted in enhanced type 1 and type 2 cytokine responses of activated tumor-primed lymphoid cells in response to tumor antigen (48). $CD4^+$ cells are generated via this method, which was not the case with anti-CD3 activation alone. TDLN cells activated with anti-CD3 and anti-CD28 were therapeutically more effective than anti-CD3 activated cells in adoptive immunotherapy. We are currently conducting a clinical trial utilizing this method of activating VPLN cells for adoptive therapy. In other studies, we have also evaluated the effect of anti-4-1BB mAb in conjunction with anti-CD3/anti-CD28 mAb to activate tumor-primed lymph node cells. The addition of anti-4-1BB resulted in TDLN cells that polarized the cytokine release response of the activated cells to a type 1 response, which correlated with enhanced antitumor responses in adoptive immunotherapy (49). The enhanced in vivo efficacy of cells activated with anti-4-1BB may be related to improved survival and proliferation of the activated cells after adoptive transfer (50).

FUTURE PERSPECTIVES

To date, adoptive immunotherapy of properly sensitized T cells has been much more effective in mediating significant tumor responses compared with other forms of immunotherapies (i.e., vaccine therapies). There are areas where combinatorial therapies appear to be advantageous. A prime example is the use of chemotherapeutics to induce lymphopenia with the resulting homeostatic effects seen with subsequent transfer of T lymphocytes that appear to enhance the persistence or survival of the transferred cells (13,19). In this regard, the use of different cytokines to augment the persistence and function of adoptively transferred T cells may be more advantageous than the use of IL-2 that has significant toxicities associated with its use. These newer cytokines included IL-15 (51,52) and IL-21 (20,53).

Another area of increasing interest is the role of regulatory T cells in adoptive immunotherapy. These cells play a significant role in the modulation of the host immune response to tumor antigens (54,55). The administration of IL-2 has been shown to induce the proliferation and expansion of T_{reg} cells that can have immunosuppressive function (15). Hence, the use of IL-2 in adoptive immunotherapy may in part have a deleterious effect. The depletion of regulatory T cells has been shown in preclinical tumor models to enhance the therapeutic efficacy of adoptively transferred effector T cells (13,56,57).

It is clear that there is a dynamic balance within the immune system between the effector arm and the suppressor arm. Mediators of the effector arm include various cytokines and costimulatory signals that can magnify the immune response. On the other hand, there are cytokines and coinhibitory signals that suppress the immune response (58). The blockade of these latter factors may be useful therapeutically. In the future, adoptive cell therapies will involve treatments that will combine immune strategies to tip the balance in favor of the effector arm.

REFERENCES

1. Rosenberg SA, Lotze MT, Muul LM, et al. A progress report on the treatment of 157 patients with advanced cancer using lymphokine-activated killer cells and interleukin-2 or high-dose interleukin-2 alone. N Engl J Med 1987; 316(15):889–897.
2. Rosenberg SA, Lotze MT, Muul LM, et al. Observations on the systemic administration of autologous lymphokine-activated killer cells and recombinant interleukin-2 to patients with metastatic cancer. N Engl J Med 1985; 313(23):1485–1492.
3. Dudley ME, Wunderlich JR, Shelton TE, et al. Generation of tumor-infiltrating lymphocyte cultures for use in adoptive transfer therapy for melanoma patients. J Immunother 2003; 26(4):332–342.
4. Topalian SL, Solomon D, Rosenberg SA. Tumor-specific cytolysis by lymphocytes infiltrating human melanomas. J Immunol 1989; 142(10):3714–3725.
5. Rosenberg SA, Spiess P, Lafreniere R. A new approach to the adoptive immunotherapy of cancer with tumor-infiltrating lymphocytes. Science 1986; 233(4770): 1318–1321.
6. Topalian SL, Solomon D, Avis FP, et al. Immunotherapy of patients with advanced cancer using tumor-infiltrating lymphocytes and recombinant interleukin-2: a pilot study. J Clin Oncol 1988; 6(5):839–853.
7. Rosenberg SA, Yannelli JR, Yang JC, et al. Treatment of patients with metastatic melanoma with autologous tumor-infiltrating lymphocytes and interleukin 2. J Natl Cancer Inst 1994; 86(15):1159–1166.

8. Rosenberg SA, Aebersold P, Cornetta K, et al. Gene transfer into humans–immunotherapy of patients with advanced melanoma, using tumor-infiltrating lymphocytes modified by retroviral gene transduction. N Engl J Med 1990; 323(9):570–578.
9. Dreno B, Nguyen JM, Khammari A, et al. Randomized trial of adoptive transfer of melanoma tumor-infiltrating lymphocytes as adjuvant therapy for stage III melanoma. Cancer Immunol Immunother 2002; 51(10):539–546.
10. Cheever MA, Greenberg PD, Fefer A. Specificity of adoptive chemoimmunotherapy of established syngeneic tumors. J Immunol 1980; 125(2):711–714.
11. Dudley ME, Wunderlich JR, Yang JC, et al. Adoptive cell transfer therapy following non-myeloablative but lymphodepleting chemotherapy for the treatment of patients with refractory metastatic melanoma. J Clin Oncol 2005; 23(10):2346–2357.
12. Shen X, Zhou J, Hathcock KS, et al. Persistence of tumor infiltrating lymphocytes in adoptive immunotherapy correlates with telomere length. J Immunother 2007; 30(1):123–129.
13. Antony PA, Piccirillo CA, Akpinarli A, et al. CD8+ T cell immunity against a tumor/self-antigen is augmented by CD4+ T helper cells and hindered by naturally occurring T regulatory cells. J Immunol 2005; 174(5):2591–2601.
14. Viguier M, Lemaitre F, Verola O, et al. Foxp3 expressing CD4+CD25(high) regulatory T cells are overrepresented in human metastatic melanoma lymph nodes and inhibit the function of infiltrating T cells. J Immunol 2004; 173(2):1444–1453.
15. Ahmadzadeh M, Rosenberg SA. IL-2 administration increases CD4+ CD25(hi) Foxp3+ regulatory T cells in cancer patients. Blood 2006; 107(6):2409–2414.
16. Powell DJ Jr., de Vries CR, Allen T, et al. Inability to mediate prolonged reduction of regulatory T cells after transfer of autologous CD25-depleted PBMC and interleukin-2 after lymphodepleting chemotherapy. J Immunother 2007; 30(4): 438–447.
17. Ku CC, Murakami M, Sakamoto A, et al. Control of homeostasis of CD8+ memory T cells by opposing cytokines. Science 2000; 288(5466):675–678.
18. Kieper WC, Tan JT, Bondi-Boyd B, et al. Overexpression of interleukin (IL)-7 leads to IL-15-independent generation of memory phenotype CD8+ T cells. J Exp Med 2002; 195(12):1533–1539.
19. Gattinoni L, Finkelstein SE, Klebanoff CA, et al. Removal of homeostatic cytokine sinks by lymphodepletion enhances the efficacy of adoptively transferred tumor-specific CD8+ T cells. J Exp Med 2005; 202(7):907–912.
20. Zeng R, Spolski R, Finkelstein SE, et al. Synergy of IL-21 and IL-15 in regulating CD8+ T cell expansion and function. J Exp Med 2005; 201(1):139–148.
21. Antony PA, Paulos CM, Ahmadzadeh M, et al. Interleukin-2-dependent mechanisms of tolerance and immunity in vivo. J Immunol 2006; 176(9):5255–5266.
22. Appay V, Dunbar PR, Callan M, et al. Memory CD8+ T cells vary in differentiation phenotype in different persistent virus infections. Nat Med 2002; 8(4):379–385.
23. Gattinoni L, Klebanoff CA, Palmer DC, et al. Acquisition of full effector function in vitro paradoxically impairs the in vivo antitumor efficacy of adoptively transferred CD8+ T cells. J Clin Invest 2005; 115(6):1616–1626.
24. Yee C, Thompson JA, Byrd D, et al. Adoptive T cell therapy using antigen-specific CD8+ T cell clones for the treatment of patients with metastatic melanoma: in vivo persistence, migration, and antitumor effect of transferred T cells. Proc Natl Acad Sci USA 2002; 99(25):16168–16173.

25. Dudley ME, Wunderlich JR, Yang JC, et al. A phase I study of nonmyeloablative chemotherapy and adoptive transfer of autologous tumor antigen-specific T lymphocytes in patients with metastatic melanoma. J Immunother 2002; 25(3): 243–251.

26. Huang J, Khong HT, Dudley ME, et al. Survival, persistence, and progressive differentiation of adoptively transferred tumor-reactive T cells associated with tumor regression. J Immunother 2005; 28(3):258–267.

27. Hughes MS, Yu YY, Dudley ME, et al. Transfer of a TCR gene derived from a patient with a marked antitumor response conveys highly active T-cell effector functions. Hum Gene Ther 2005; 16(4):457–472.

28. Morgan RA, Dudley ME, Wunderlich JR, et al. Cancer regression in patients after transfer of genetically engineered lymphocytes. Science 2006; 314(5796):126–129.

29. Tsai S, Mixon A, Farid S, et al. Co-stimulatory signals upregulate PD-1 expression on human T lymphocytes: implications for cancer immunotherapy. J Am Coll Surg 2006; 203(3 suppl 1):S81.

30. Cohen CJ, Li YF, El-Gamil M, et al. Enhanced antitumor activity of T cells engineered to express T-cell receptors with a second disulfide bond. Cancer Res 2007; 67(8):3898–3903.

31. Schlissel MS. Regulating antigen-receptor gene assembly. Nat Rev Immunol 2003; 3(11):890–899.

32. Carding SR, Egan PJ. $\gamma\partial$ T cells: functional plasticity and heterogeneity. Nat Rev Immunol 2002; 2(5):336–345.

33. Johnson LA, Heemskerk B, Powell DJ Jr., et al. Gene transfer of tumor-reactive TCR confers both high avidity and tumor reactivity to nonreactive peripheral blood mononuclear cells and tumor-infiltrating lymphocytes. J Immunol 2006; 177(9): 6548–6559.

34. Eshhar Z, Waks T, Bendavid A, et al. Functional expression of chimeric receptor genes in human T cells. J Immunol Methods 2001; 248(1–2):67–76.

35. Kershaw MH, Westwood JA, Parker LL, et al. A phase I study on adoptive immunotherapy using gene-modified T cells for ovarian cancer. Clin Cancer Res 2006; 12(20 Pt 1):6106–6115.

36. Stephenson KR, Perry-Lalley D, Griffith KD, et al. Development of antitumor reactivity in regional draining lymph nodes from tumor-immunized and tumor-bearing murine hosts. Surgery 1989; 105(4):523–528.

37. Yoshizawa H, Chang AE, Shu S. Specific adoptive immunotherapy mediated by tumor-draining lymph node cells sequentially activated with anti-CD3 and IL-2. J Immunol 1991; 147(2):729–737.

38. Tanigawa K, Takeshita N, Eickhoff GA, et al. Antitumor reactivity of lymph node cells primed in vivo with dendritic cell-based vaccines. J Immunother 2001; 24(6): 493–501.

39. Geiger JD, Wagner PD, Cameron MJ, et al. Generation of T-cells reactive to the poorly immunogenic B16-BL6 melanoma with efficacy in the treatment of spontaneous metastases. J Immunother Emphasis Tumor Immunol 1993; 13(3): 153–165.

40. Chang AE, Aruga A, Cameron MJ, et al. Adoptive immunotherapy with vaccine-primed lymph node cells secondarily activated with anti-CD3 and interleukin-2. J Clin Oncol 1997; 15(2):796–807.

41. Chang AE, Li Q, Jiang G, et al. Phase II trial of autologous tumor vaccination, anti-CD3-activated vaccine-primed lymphocytes, and interleukin-2 in stage IV renal cell cancer. J Clin Oncol 2003; 21(5):884–890.

42. Strome SE, Krauss JC, Cameron MJ, et al. Immunobiologic effects of cytokine gene transfer of the B16-BL6 melanoma. Arch Otolaryngol Head Neck Surg 1993; 119(12): 1289–1295.

43. Arca MJ, Krauss JC, Aruga A, et al. Therapeutic efficacy of T cells derived from lymph nodes draining a poorly immunogenic tumor transduced to secrete granulocyte-macrophage colony-stimulating factor. Cancer Gene Ther 1996; 3(1):39–47.

44. Chang AE, Sondak VK, Bishop DK, et al. Adoptive immunotherapy of cancer with activated lymph node cells primed in vivo with autologous tumor cells transduced with the GM-CSF gene. Hum Gene Ther 1996; 7(6):773–792.

45. Aruga A, Shu S, Chang AE. Tumor-specific granulocyte/macrophage colony-stimulating factor and interferon gamma secretion is associated with in vivo therapeutic efficacy of activated tumor-draining lymph node cells. Cancer Immunol Immunother 1995; 41(5):317–324.

46. Aruga A, Aruga E, Tanigawa K, et al. Type 1 versus type 2 cytokine release by Vbeta T cell subpopulations determines in vivo antitumor reactivity: IL-10 mediates a suppressive role. J Immunol 1997; 159(2):664–673.

47. Tanigawa K, Takeshita N, Craig RA, et al. Tumor-specific responses in lymph nodes draining murine sarcomas are concentrated in cells expressing P-selectin binding sites. J Immunol 2001; 167(6):3089–3098.

48. Li Q, Yu B, Grover AC, et al. Therapeutic effects of tumor reactive CD4+ cells generated from tumor-primed lymph nodes using anti-CD3/anti-CD28 monoclonal antibodies. J Immunother 2002; 25(4):304–313.

49. Li Q, Carr A, Ito F, et al. Polarization effects of 4-1BB during CD28 costimulation in generating tumor-reactive T cells for cancer immunotherapy. Cancer Res 2003; 63(10):2546–2552.

50. Kroon HM, Li Q, Teitz-Tennenbaum S, et al. 4-1BB costimulation of effector T cells for adoptive immunotherapy of cancer: involvement of Bcl gene family members. J Immunother 2007; 30(4):406–416.

51. Roychowdhury S, May KF Jr., Tzou KS, et al. Failed adoptive immunotherapy with tumor-specific T cells: reversal with low-dose interleukin 15 but not low-dose interleukin 2. Cancer Res 2004; 64(21):8062–8067.

52. Teague RM, Sather BD, Sacks JA, et al. Interleukin-15 rescues tolerant CD8+ T cells for use in adoptive immunotherapy of established tumors. Nat Med 2006; 12(3): 335–341.

53. Moroz A, Eppolito C, Li Q, et al. IL-21 enhances and sustains CD8+ T cell responses to achieve durable tumor immunity: comparative evaluation of IL-2, IL-15, and IL-21. J Immunol 2004; 173(2):900–909.

54. Zou W. Regulatory T cells, tumour immunity and immunotherapy. Nat Rev Immunol 2006; 6(4):295–307.

55. Antony PA, Restifo NP. CD4+CD25+ T regulatory cells, immunotherapy of cancer, and interleukin-2. J Immunother 2005; 28(2):120–128.

56. Chen A, Liu S, Park D, et al. Depleting intratumoral CD4+CD25+ regulatory T cells via FasL protein transfer enhances the therapeutic efficacy of adoptive T cell transfer. Cancer Res 2007; 67(3):1291–1298.

57. Tanaka H, Tanaka J, Kjaergaard J, et al. Depletion of CD4+ CD25+ regulatory cells augments the generation of specific immune T cells in tumor-draining lymph nodes. J Immunother 2002; 25(3):207–217.
58. Chen L. Co-inhibitory molecules of the B7-CD28 family in the control of T-cell immunity. Nat Rev Immunol 2004; 4(5):336–347.
59. Gattinoni L, Powell DJ Jr., Rosenberg SA, et al. Adoptive immunotherapy for cancer: building on success. Nat Rev Immunol 2006; 6:383–393.

13

Procurement of Human Melanoma Specimens for Translational Research: Practical and Legal Considerations

Tyron C. Hoover

*World BioBank, Accelerated Community Oncology Research Network, Inc.,
Memphis, Tennessee, U.S.A.*

Jane L. Messina

*H. Lee Moffitt Cancer Center and the Department of Pathology and Cell
Biology, University of South Florida College of Medicine, Tampa, Florida, U.S.A.*

Shane A. Huntsman

H. Lee Moffitt Cancer Center, Tampa, Florida, U.S.A.

Vernon K. Sondak

*H. Lee Moffitt Cancer Center and the Departments of Oncologic
Sciences and Surgery, University of South Florida College of Medicine,
Tampa, Florida, U.S.A.*

INTRODUCTION

Translational research in melanoma has been hampered by limited access to tumor tissue, especially from primary melanomas. Most melanomas are diagnosed by shave, punch, or excisional biopsy, often in the office setting rather than in a hospital, and typically the entire lesion is removed for pathologic analysis. Therefore, much of the research performed on primary melanoma has relied on the use of formalin-fixed paraffin-embedded (FFPE) tissue. FFPE tissue from primary melanomas may be difficult to obtain; often the block is archived at a large reference dermatopathology laboratory not associated with an academic medical center. Even at academic centers there is often great reluctance to part with paraffin blocks because of medicolegal concerns. Tissue from precursor lesions, such as dysplastic or common melanocytic nevi, can be even more difficult to procure for research purposes. Reliance on FFPE tissue brings with it questions about the persistence of relevant proteins over time.

The rare melanoma that is diagnosed by incisional biopsy, and as such provides a source of residual primary tumor for banking, is often unrepresentative of "typical" primary melanoma. It is usually quite large, often nodular, and yet has not manifested widespread metastases. Frozen tissue from more typical primaries has been extremely elusive. The majority of melanoma tissue available for acquisition and cryostorage in tissue banks is from advanced-stage patients with bulky metastatic disease.

In this chapter, we will review the potential research uses of FFPE and fresh-frozen melanoma tissue, discuss the medicolegal issues that surround acquisition of primary melanomas and precursor lesions, and discuss our protocol for acquiring frozen tissue from primary melanomas for research purposes without compromising the diagnostic process.

USES OF FORMALIN-FIXED PARAFFIN-EMBEDDED TISSUE

The identification of successful techniques to analyze FFPE tissue is essential because there is such a vast repository of these specimens in clinical laboratories and hospitals, often with complete clinical annotation. The most common use of FFPE tissue from primary melanomas and precursor lesions is the investigation for the presence of a target antigen by immunohistochemical stains. The feasibility of staining may be limited by the amount of target antigen present in tissue. This type of research is also limited by the availability of appropriate antibodies that can bind successfully in formalin-fixed tissue. Optimal staining depends on prompt tissue fixation as well as adequate antigen retrieval techniques. Properly performed, there appears to be little or no significant decrease over time in the quality of immunohistochemical staining, even in decades-old archival tissue. As an example, one study evaluated the expression of five markers in bladder carcinoma tissue from 1932 to 2004 and concluded that if adequate antigen retrieval is performed, there is no decrease in the quality of staining in older specimens (1). However, immunohistochemical analysis on archival tissue is not free from problems with antigen loss. There is some evidence that staining performed on years-old tissue should be performed on sections freshly cut from the block, rather than stored unstained recut sections. In a study of 11 immuno-histochemical markers performed on recut sections from children aged 3 months to 10 years, there was significant alteration in staining results for 4 of 11 antigens tested, including markers of cytoplasmic membrane, cytoplasm, and nucleus. While most of the alterations were in archival recuts up to the age of 10 years, in the case of estrogen receptor, even recuts three months old were negatively affected (2). In this same study, vimentin staining was actually stronger in older slides, and the authors hypothesized that antigen alteration rather than degradation may be occurring in tissues stored in paraffin long term.

In retrospective large-scale immunohistochemical analyses, however, it may be difficult to obtain tissue blocks from laboratories that may be reluctant to part with their permanent record of the case. In such cases, recut slides are the only alternative for staining. It may be possible to mitigate the effects of long-term storage of recuts by storing them in a protected fashion. One group tested the effects of storing recuts under three conditions: ambient air, paraffin coating, or dessicating nitrogen chamber. Evaluation of staining results for cytokeratin, estrogen receptor protein, and Ki-67 revealed that the combination of paraffin coating and storage in nitrogen produced the best retention of antigenicity. Quantitation of staining of storage recuts compared with freshly made recuts revealed preservation of 72% to 99% of tissue antigenicity (3).

The recent development of the tissue microarray technique (TMA) has allowed researchers to utilize FFPE tissue from large numbers of specimens (either multiple specimens from the same patient or multiple patients' specimens or both) for high-throughput evaluation of immunohistochemical expression of various antigens. In this technique, first reported by Kononen and colleagues (4), tiny cylinders of tissue are extracted from primary tumor blocks and arrayed in a recipient paraffin block that can contain up to 1000 tissue samples. Slides cut from this recipient block can then be used for simultaneous analysis of DNA, RNA, or protein expression of all the arrayed specimens. Judicious sampling of primary tumor blocks for TMA can acquire small amounts of tissue from many tumors for fairly extensive testing. Even rare tumor types that must be collected from multiple centers over many years can be processed in a single TMA, allowing analyses that would be difficult or impossible to perform any other way. The recent explosion of automated image analyzers such as Ariol, Aperio, and AQUA allows high-throughput, quantitative analysis of stained sections cut from TMA blocks, adding greatly to the value of the technique (5).

In situ hybridization can be successfully performed on FFPE tissue to evaluate the presence of specific nucleic acid sequences, either DNA or mRNA, and is most commonly performed using fluorescent-labeled probes [fluorescence in situ hybridization (FISH)]. Several recent reports have investigated the frequency of copy number changes in genes of particular interest in melanoma, such as *BRAF, cyclin D1, MDM2*, and *c-MYC*, using this method (6–9). There are differences in the number of gene copies based on tumor site and epidemiology, with *cyclin D1* amplification more frequently found in acral and uveal melanomas and melanomas associated with chronic sun exposure, *MDM2* amplification in acral melanomas, and *c-MYC* amplification in uveal melanomas. Some studies suggest *BRAF* gene amplification, rather than mutation, may be the cause of BRAF activation in a subset of melanomas (7,10). Changes in copy number for *CDKN2A* and *c-MYC* have been linked to clinical outcome in melanoma, with nodular tumors demonstrating decreases in *CDKN2A* and increases in *c-MYC* having a significantly better outcome (8). FISH can be performed on slides cut from a tissue microarray, and a series of overlapping probes can be used to focus on a chromosome of particular interest, such as chromosome 20 in melanoma (11).

The use of FFPE tissue for analysis of DNA or RNA is limited by the formalin-mediated degradation and chemical alteration (cross-linking) of nucleotides. For example, a recent study analyzing the suitability of DNA extracted from FFPE tissue for polymerase chain reaction (PCR) found that amplification was only successful when using amplimers of more than 250 base pairs (bp) in length (12). The quality of extracted DNA also appears to be improved by shorter fixation times, specifically one day or less, but not affected by time of storage in paraffin, at least when comparing samples of one to five years (13). DNA extracted from FFPE tissues has been used successfully in a number of other applications in melanoma besides PCR. White et al. were able to successfully extract DNA and perform comparative genomic hybridization on 82 of 100 archival uveal melanoma specimens (14).

Analysis of mRNA expression is, of course, a central component in the molecular genetic profiling of melanoma. Utilization of RNA from FFPE tissue can be even more problematic than DNA, because of the small amounts of mRNA present in the tissue to begin with and its rapid degradation by RNases. A comparison of quantitative mRNA analysis on FFPE tissue and fresh-frozen tissue revealed that up to 99% of total mRNA could be lost in fixed tissue. However, this same study showed that up to 100-fold amplification could be achieved by amplifying short (<136 bp) rather than long amplimers, specifically demonstrated using primers for the *MART1* gene (15).

More recently, proteomic analysis of FFPE tissue has been touted as a method of discovering potential biomarkers and therapeutic targets. This technique involves laser microdissection of the tissue of interest, followed by protein extraction and quantitation of target proteins using liquid chromatography and mass spectroscopy (16). As yet, this technique has not had major application in melanoma, but there is no inherent reason why it could not be used in future research efforts.

USES OF FRESH-FROZEN TISSUE

While a significant amount of melanoma research has, by necessity, involved FFPE tissue, the advantages of studying fresh or fresh-frozen tissue are numerous. When promptly harvested and promptly cryopreserved, the quality of extracted DNA, RNA, and protein is far superior to that obtained from FFPE tissue. The quality of nucleic acid recovered from frozen tissue can be affected by storage temperature and uniformity of freezing, especially in larger tissue samples (17). The diverse methodologies used for this extraction may also cause variation among study results. This is especially important when tumor extracts are used for quantitative analysis of biomarkers related to patient prognosis or treatment. To this end, the European Organization for Research and Treatment of Cancer has proposed a standardized method for the preparation of nucleic acid extracts from human tumor tissue (18).

Fresh-frozen tissue can be thawed for use in conventional (metaphase) cytogenetics, which involves short-term, limited passage number tissue cultured for the generation of long-term cell lines. Small chunks of thawed frozen tumor tissue can be used for in vivo tumorigenicity and chemosensitivity assays by subcutaneous implantation into immunocompromised animals such as athymic nude mice, or under the renal capsule in immunocompetent mice. Fresh-frozen tissue can also be used to make an autologous tumor vaccine, for use after recovery from surgery or much later, at the time of development of distant metastatic disease (19).

Recognizing these advantages, there are important disadvantages and caveats when using cryopreserved tumor tissue. Freezing has to take place quickly or many of the benefits are lost, and artifacts are introduced. For optimal preservation, a dedicated tissue procurement specialist should be available to handle the specimen as soon as it is removed in the operating room or at the location where a biopsy is performed (increasingly in Radiology with the widespread use of image-guided biopsies). Freezing therefore must take place before the specimen has been entirely sampled for routine pathologic analysis, introducing the possibility of interference with the diagnostic process, and even allegations of negligence in the advent of a more adverse clinical outcome than expected based on the pathologic diagnosis. To address this concern, harvested frozen tissue should, if at all possible, be quarantined until diagnostic analysis has been completed satisfactorily before using it for research purposes.

One way to gain some of the advantages of freezing without some of the disadvantages is to place the specimen in an appropriate fixative that deactivates or at least strongly inhibits DNases and RNases. This offers far greater convenience than having a person standing by in the operating room or biopsy suite to immediately freeze the tissue or to transport it to the laboratory in liquid nitrogen. But currently, those fixatives are inadequate for histologic fixation, at least to the standards required for diagnostic pathology purposes.

Given the real and significant limitations of FFPE tissue for analyzing primary melanoma tumor tissue and the potential value that acquiring suitably preserved fresh tumor tissue has for increasing our understanding of the biology of this disease, increased efforts to procure primary melanoma specimens are clearly justified. But these efforts, as previously outlined, involve alterations to the normal handling and processing of clinical material for histopathologic analysis. These alterations introduce risks—risks to the patient stemming from incomplete or inaccurate pathologic evaluation and risks to the physicians of legal action alleging a violation of the standard of care that resulted in the direct cause of harm to the patient. We turn now to a comprehensive analysis of the extent of these medicolegal risks, some of which we feel have been overemphasized not only to the detriment of melanoma research but also to the disadvantage of patients afflicted with this disease.

MEDICOLEGAL CONSIDERATIONS IN PRIMARY MELANOMA TUMOR PROCUREMENT

A discussion of *potential* legal liability in procuring human melanoma tissues for research begins with several assumptions that will be implicit in the discussions that follow. First, it is assumed that physicians will be the persons selecting and harvesting this tissue or will directly supervise the process. Second, it is assumed that this tissue will be harvested from living donors (as opposed to cadaveric tissue procurement).[a] Third, it is assumed that the physicians harvesting the tissue have a physician-patient relationship with the donor, i.e., they are the donor's treating physician as well as part of the research team. Fourth, it is assumed that the donor has agreed to participate in a research project involving the procurement of their tissue prior to the actual procedure.[b] In short, for purposes of this brief discussion, it will be assumed that the research team is prospectively identifying melanoma patients, consenting them prior to tissue removal and then using their melanoma samples for research. This is, in fact, the case for our melanoma tissue banking efforts at Moffitt.

That being said, as far as legal analysis goes, there is nothing special or specific to melanoma procurement that demands a distinct legal assessment when compared with any other tumor type (although melanoma presents some unique situations owing to the scarcity of it as a tissue resource and the significance of the clinical decisions that are made on the basis of histopathologic analysis).[c] As such, much of what is discussed below may be equally applicable to other tissue types and situations.

NEGLIGENCE

The most common, and perhaps most feared, cause of action against physicians is a negligence cause of action. In fact, unless otherwise specified, when the term "medical malpractice" is used (even by attorneys) one means negligence. To the extent that a physician-patient relationship exists, a physician may be liable to a donor of melanoma tissue for injuries caused during or as a result of the procurement of tissue samples. To lose a negligence lawsuit, four elements must be proven and no viable defenses must exist. The four elements are (*i*) existence of duty to the patient, (*ii*) breach of that duty (via a breach of the standard of care), (*iii*) causation (actual cause and legal, or proximate, cause), and (*iv*) damages or injury.

---

[a] Mishandling of a corpse might entail its own legal pitfalls, but would not include those dependent on the physician-patient relationship such as negligence causes of action. See, e.g., *Colavito v. New York Organ Donor Network, Inc.*, 438 F.3d 214 (2d Cir. 2006) (discussing interest in a dead body as a quasi-property right), or *Jacobsen v. Marin Gen. Hosp.*, 192 F.3d 881 (9th Cir. 1999) (discussing the interest as an intentional infliction of emotional distress claim).

[b] As opposed to a research project that attempts to obtain informed consent after the procedure or which seeks to access tissue from clinical repositories, such as paraffin block archives in pathology departments utilizing a waiver of consent.

[c] See, e.g., *Dobran v. Francisco Med. Ctr.*, 806 N.E. 2d 537 (Ohio 2004) (where half of a histologically negative sentinel lymph node was lost in transit en route to a central research laboratory where PCR was to be performed as part of the Sunbelt Melanoma Trial, and a claim for negligent infliction of emotional distress as a result of fear of metastatic cancer was found not to be viable).

A duty to the participant patient exists when there is a physician-patient relationship. This is normally not a contested issue in a negligence lawsuit involving a physician. If one is caring for the patient, or simply diagnosing the patient, one has normally established a physician-patient relationship and subsequent duty to render standard of care treatment. In the context of a surgeon excising melanoma samples and a pathologist analyzing some or all of those samples as part of the clinical care of the patient, a duty certainly exists to deliver standard of care treatment to the patient.

A breach of duty implies a breach of the legal standard of care. It should be emphasized that the legal standard of care is not determined by physicians or health care providers. "Standard of care" is a specific legal term, not synonymous with the general medical concept, and it is only determined on a case-by-case basis by the judge or jury in a lawsuit. The guiding legal principle is that the standard of care is "what a reasonable physician with the same or similar training and experience would have done in the same or similar circumstances, given the facts that were known or reasonably should have been known at that time."[d] The question then is what would a reasonable surgeon have done in the same or similar situation: (*i*) in the removal of a melanoma sample for the clinical care of the patient (diagnostic and/or therapeutic) at the time of surgery and (*ii*) in the harvest of a melanoma sample for research purposes?

From a legal standpoint at least, there is not always a discernable line between what is done for the care of the patient and what is done for research purposes, particularly when there is only a single operative event. In fact, many courts do not make a clear distinction between the two, a fact that may be problematic if legal standards are inappropriately applied. Some courts may judge mishaps that occur under the guise of research against legal standards for medical negligence, while others may judge research mishaps under ordinary negligence standards. Few, if any, courts treat research mishaps under a separate legal standard (20). Thus, because it is not always clear what legal standards will be applied to a mishap in the procurement of tissues, it is prudent to ensure that clinical care of the patient is not compromised while also ensuring that all necessary institutional approvals and participant consent forms have been obtained for the research project in question.

In procuring melanoma samples for medical research, the standard practice is to procure only excess material for research. Standard care is given in the form of a standard operative excision and standard pathologic evaluation of the specimen. After both of these are complete, the pathologist determines what tissue may be deemed excess and made available for research. Tissue that is otherwise ultimately destined for the incinerator would certainly have some

---

[d] In essence this is similar to an ordinary negligence standard where the standard is what a reasonable person would have done in same or similar circumstances—the medical standard essentially just substitutes the "reasonable physician" for the "reasonable person."

value to advance medical science. This happens hundreds, if not thousands, of times per day in many academic and private pathology labs involved in research.[e]

Because the determination of when tissue becomes "excess" and hence available for research is, in most cases, the duty of the pathologist and because many pathologists are hesitant to relinquish any part of submitted pigmented or melanotic lesion for research for fear of losing a piece that would alter diagnosis or therapy, melanoma samples are historically difficult to come by for researchers.[f] With the method we have implemented at Moffitt, we have incorporated the surgeon in the operating theater into the process of determining what tissue from excised melanoma samples becomes available for research.[g]

We have been able to do this because our surgeons and our dermatopathologists have jointly agreed to participate in this arrangement. Without buy-in from both specialists and ongoing outstanding communication, it would be unwise to attempt this type of arrangement. However, that is not to say that this arrangement does not meet the required clinical standard of care. The surgeon elects and performs the surgery exactly as they otherwise would absent a research project. Excised tissue is still examined by the pathologist in keeping with standard practices and institutional policies. The only thing that has been altered is that the surgeon indicates the part to be submitted for research rather than leaving the pathologists to make this determination entirely on their own[h]. Clinical care is not compromised in this scenario. Instead, some of the burden is

---

[e] One could argue that the standard for pathologists may under certain circumstances be to keep all unused tissue in a formalin bucket and then dispose of it without giving any to research (in the event it may be needed for special studies or additional examination in the future). But one could effectively argue that providing tissue for research instead of incinerating it in the end is an accepted standard of care owing to its frequency.

[f] It should be noted that however well founded the fears of prematurely giving a piece of diagnostic tissue away are, no tissues, including those submitted and evaluated in their entirety, are ever completely examined. Tissue is lost in the mere preparation of slides, and with virtually every slide prepared and examined, there is always tissue retained in the block that is not examined.

[g] As described subsequently, the surgeon essentially earmarks the part(s) of the specimen that they would like to go for research in the OR. However, per institutional policy all parts of the specimen, including that marked for research still flow through the pathology gross room for evaluation. There, the pathologist always has a full opportunity to reverse the surgeon's call and submit the piece for histopathologic evaluation if it is deemed necessary, or retrieve it from "quarantine" if evaluation of the initially submitted material later identifies concerns.

[h] Surgeons and pathologists commonly interact regarding the evaluation of excised tissues as an important aspect of quality care. For example, surgeons commonly indicate areas of interest to pathologists to guide them in the sampling of excised tissues and/or the evaluation of margins most at risk of tumor involvement. They also commonly indicate that certain excised specimens are to be evaluated grossly only and not examined microscopically. Another common practice is for surgeons to indicate a specimen to be sent to an outside laboratory for ancillary testing. In all of these cases, which occur every day in pathology laboratories, the surgeon guides the pathologist. Yet, the pathologist can, of course, override this guidance at their discretion.

removed from the pathologist's shoulders and carried by the surgeon, who guides the pathologist in selecting tissue that is unlikely to be needed for care of the patient. Regardless of who identifies the tissue for research, any research specimen is quarantined and not available for actual use until issuance of the final surgical pathology report; it can be recalled from the tissue bank for pathologic evaluation if needed[i].

Hence, we believe that our practice of mutual involvement of surgeon and pathologist in the designation of research tissue fully complies with the standard of care of what a "reasonable" academic surgical oncologist and dermatopathologist would do in handling surgical specimens. If an alleged breach of duty/standard of care can be proven, it must be a causative factor in a subsequent injury to the patient. Simplistically, it is a "no harm, no foul" situation. Injury does not necessarily have to be a physical injury; other types of injury including economic and other noneconomic injuries may suffice. However, by jointly involving surgeon and pathologist, awareness of the clinical requirements are enhanced. Consider, as an example, a case where the surgeon samples a primary melanoma after an initial punch biopsy diagnosed the tumor to be 1.2-mm thick but inadvertently removes the only area that is thicker—2.5 mm in thickness. There is no clinical significance to the restaging of the tumor as T3 (2.01-4.00 mm) versus T2 (1.01-2.00 mm) once a margin-negative-wide excision and appropriate staging of the regional nodes have taken place. If the allegation is that the tumor was actually T4 (>4.00 mm thick), the likelihood of a small sampling of the tumor for research purposes would somehow remove the only evidence that such a dramatic change in thickness must be considered quite small—certainly below the "more likely than not" threshold usually applied in malpractice actions. Plus, the consequence of such a dramatic but unlikely difference would also be considered quite small: It could be alleged that the patient was deprived the opportunity to receive adjuvant high-dose interferon for a T4N0 primary, but most such patients decline therapy and the incremental survival advantage of interferon in this setting is extremely small. Of course, if the tumor were node positive, the issue is moot because decision making regarding interferon is then similar for any primary thickness. The plaintiff's burden to prove that the research sampling resulted in substandard evaluation of the primary tumor and that this breach caused the patient to suffer harm would be great indeed. Recall that if all four elements of a negligence cause of action (existence of a duty to the patient, breach of the standard of care, causation, and damages or injury) cannot be proven, then the defendant physician wins.

---

[i] This second safety net (the first being thorough gross evaluation by the pathologist of all excised tissue, whether intended for research use or not) has been proven to work thus far without adverse incident in our experience.

INFORMED CONSENT

The other potential legal cause of action that might be leveled against a physician researcher in procuring melanoma specimens is one for lack of informed consent. In the medical setting, lack of informed consent is also known as battery, and the two terms may be used interchangeably.[j] Some courts equate informed consent for clinical procedures with informed consent for research (20), but they are different enough that they are wisely separated in time and space in most institutions.[k] Even though many agree that informed consent should be viewed as an ongoing process and not merely an event or a piece of paper signed by the patient/participant, that signed document will often be presumptive evidence of what was agreed to by the patient/participant and the researcher. In many respects there are contractual elements present, and courts may actually choose to interpret informed consents under laws of contract rather than tort law in some cases.[l] The informed consent sets the limits of what will and what will not be done and delineates risks to both sides. Like a contract, it should be entered into voluntarily and without duress or coercion.[m]

Claims of this sort are always very fact dependent as one can never be entirely sure that consent is truly informed for the mere fact that one can never be sure just what the patient/participant understood. Nevertheless, the goal of any contract is to attain a "meeting of the minds" between the researcher and the participant. Prior to procuring primary melanoma tissue for research, it is appropriate and prudent that an Institutional Review Board (IRB)-approved informed consent be signed in addition to the informed consent for the clinical procedure itself.[n] For our tissue-banking project at Moffitt, under which melanoma samples as well as samples of other primary and metastatic cancers are collected, we offer (multilingual) written and video informed consent processes, which have been approved by several different IRBs. While the extent of the informed consent process is one we are justifiably proud of, we note that simpler written consent forms would suffice just as well under the applicable regulations.

---

[j] Battery only requires an intentional offensive or harmful contact. See, e.g., *Boggess v. Roper*, 2006 U.S. Dist. LEXIS 63057 (D.N.C. 2006). "Offensive" may be interpreted very broadly: Even if the contact is beneficial, it may still be battery.

[k] And they have different, if similar, legal foundations. See, e.g., 45 C.F.R.§46.116 (2005) (the Code of Federal Regulation's general requirements for informed consent for human research subjects) or, TEX. CIV. PRAC. & REM. CODE ANN. §74.104–07 (2003) (outlining duties, manner, and effect of disclosure of risks and hazards associated with a proposed procedure).

[l] See, e.g., *Gray v. Grunagle*, 223 A.2d 663 (Pa. 1996) (characterizing informed consent for surgery as a contract—any deviation from that contract treads in the realm of battery).

[m] 45 C.F.R. §46.116(a) (2005).

[n] In contrast, informed consent after the fact or even waiver of informed consent may be appropriate when fully analyzed tissues, such as paraffin-embedded blocks or analyzed microscope slides, are obtained for research without involvement of the researchers in the tumor procurement process.

PROPERTY-BASED CAUSES OF ACTION

Property-based causes of action, though less common than the above causes of action, may be alleged in certain instances. Though uncommon, it might be expected that these types of claims will increase in the future as human tissue becomes increasingly valuable to researchers and industry. As an example, Andrews and Nelkin cite a 1998 New York Times article that placed the value of a 1998 barrel of crude oil at $40, while the equivalent volume of human blood products would have been $67,000 (21). The seminal case involving property rights to excised tissue is *Moore v. Regents of the University of California*. In that case, Moore, a man from Seattle was treated with a splenectomy for hairy cell leukemia. After that curative surgery, the man was instructed to periodically return to University of California at Los Angeles (UCLA) for harvest of various types of tissues from his body. It was alleged (and never contested) that these additional procedures were carried out under the pretense of necessary medical treatment that the patient could not receive in Seattle. This went on for a period of years. When Moore became suspicious, he hired an attorney, who discovered that researchers (including Moore's treating physician) at UCLA had developed and were attempting to commercialize a cell line developed from Moore's cells without his knowledge or approval.[o]

Among other things, Moore claimed in his subsequent lawsuit that UCLA and the researcher had 'stolen' his property—his tissues—under the legal doctrine of conversion. Under that doctrine, UCLA only had to intend to do what it did with the cells; that is, it did not have to have an evil intent or intend to do any wrong at all to Moore. All Moore had to establish was that the tissue taken from his body, here without consent, was his property. The California court would not go that far—the cells were deemed to not be his property. Reasons given by that court were that if a property interest in the tissue were recognized for Moore, there would be a chilling effect on research progress and there might potentially be a flood of similar litigation.

Though *Moore* may not be binding precedent on courts outside of that district in California, courts in other jurisdictions, which have considered the issue, have followed *Moore*'s reasoning to arrive at similar conclusions. *Moore* was decided in 1990. There are few, if any, similar reported cases subsequent to *Moore* until 2003, when a case with similar ownership issues to excised human tissue was decided in Florida. In that case, research participants (or their parents), sued Miami Children's Hospital and an investigator for unjust enrichment (among other things), claiming that the investigator had used tissue and resources provided by the plaintiffs in patenting discoveries to his financial and professional benefit. The facts of this case were fairly unique. The unjust enrichment claim was allowed because the participants were more than merely

---

[o] The researchers even named the cell line after Moore. See *Moore v. Regents of the Univ. of Cal.,* 793 P.2d 479 (Cal. 1990)

donors; they had expended time, money and, effort (as well as tissue) in financing the research effort. Other claims levied against the hospital and investigator were breach of informed consent, breach of fiduciary duty, fraudulent concealment, conversion and misappropriation of trade secrets. These claims were all dismissed by the court.[p]

Then, in June 2007, the 8th Circuit Court of Appeals decided the *Catalona* case. There the legal question was who owned tissues submitted for research.[q] Relying heavily on the wording of the informed consent as evidence of the participants' intent at the time of donation, it was determined that the tissue belonged to the University, not the researcher or the research participants. The court relied on relevant State law in its analysis of whether or not the participants completed an inter vivos gift, i.e., a gift given while still alive. It found that they had intended to deliver the tissue to the University as a gift, where the informed consent characterized it as a "donation" and other related materials presented to potential participants characterized the property transfers as "free and generous gift(s) to research."

Even given the apparent inclination of courts to find that research participants have no real property interest in excised tissues, the prudent course of action is to clearly delineate these property issues in the informed consent document(s) and in the research protocol. The consent and protocol documents should be clear as to what rights, if any, the participant has regarding excised tissue and its derivatives. A right participants should retain regarding their tissue is the right to withdraw consent for its further use if they decide to stop participating in the research protocol.[r] Retaining this right does not legally seem to equate to owning the tissue or maintaining a right to control its use, as the above cases illustrate. But if the researchers purport to give property rights to the participant and spell these out in the informed consent, courts might well enforce them.

THE TEAM APPROACH TO MELANOMA TUMOR PROCUREMENT

As noted above, we have found that successful melanoma tissue procurement efforts require close cooperation between surgeons and pathologists, and a well-established infrastructure above and beyond "routine" institutional efforts at tumor procurement. Also key is a good working relationship between community dermatologists and dermatopathologists and those at the research center. In all these areas, our institution has worked to develop highly productive and collaborative relationships that enhance the ability to collect and study primary melanoma tumor tissue. Together, we have developed a protocol for the

---

[p] *Greenberg v. Miami Children's Hosp.*, 264 F.Supp. 2d 1064 (S.D. Fla. 2003).

[q] A departing investigator sought a declaratory judgment that prostate cancer tissues could be controlled by the donors and directed to him, while the university sought a declaratory ruling that the tissues were owned by it. *Wash. Univ. v. Catalona*, 2007 U.S. App. LEXIS 14442 (8th Cir. 2007).

[r] The right to withdraw from participation in research is codified at 45 C.F.R.§46.116(a) (8) (2005).

procurement of melanoma specimens that requires interaction between surgeons, pathologists, and tissue procurement personnel. All patients from whom fresh tumor is to be procured must have signed a written informed consent document, approved by the institutional IRB, prior to surgery. This consent is obtained in a noncoercive manner by an individual not directly part of the surgical team, either in the outpatient clinic or in the Preanesthesia Evaluation Center.

Once consent is obtained and the patient is taken to the operating room, a well-established protocol is followed for submission of the most representative, best quality tumor tissue to the tissue procurement laboratory, without compromise of the surgical pathology specimen. Our institutional procedure for procuring tumor from primary melanomas or abnormal lymph nodes or distant metastases (but not from clinically normal ''sentinel'' lymph nodes) is as follows:

1. The surgeon identifies the area of the specimen to be designated for research intraoperatively, selecting an area that is not expected to interfere with margin assessment.

2. As soon as practical after the tumor-containing tissue is removed from the patient, the surgeon physically separates the area for research from the rest of the specimen by punch biopsy or limited excision on the back table, secluded from the surgical instrumentation used for the procedure. The size of the tissue to be submitted depends on the clinical situation. This is usually a 3- or 4-mm punch from a primary melanoma or a larger section cut from palpable metastatic disease in such a way as not to impair the assessment of tumor size or extent of invasion.

3. The specimen to be submitted for research is placed by the surgeon in a separate container marked ''For Tumor Bank.'' It is sent along with the diagnostic (clinical) specimen to pathology for evaluation. The surgeon then discards the instruments used for tumor procurement and changes gloves before returning to the operative field.

4. The research specimen is evaluated in conjunction with the diagnostic specimen in the gross room by the pathologist and/or pathology assistant. At this time, the gross appearance of both the research and diagnostic specimens are evaluated, providing the first level of assurance that procurement of tissue for research will not interfere with standard diagnostic evaluation. The gross description is dictated, documenting and recording that the research tissue is submitted entirely to the Tissue Procurement Core.

5. The designated research specimen is snap-frozen in its entirety but quarantined within the Tissue Core's cryostorage facility. Thus segregated, the sample cannot be used for research purposes until the microscopic analysis of the diagnostic specimen has been completed.

6. If for any reason the pathologist considers the diagnostic specimen incomplete or compromised in any way, or finds that the submitted specimen does not contain tumor, the research specimen is retrieved and processed for standard diagnostic pathology (Fig. 1)

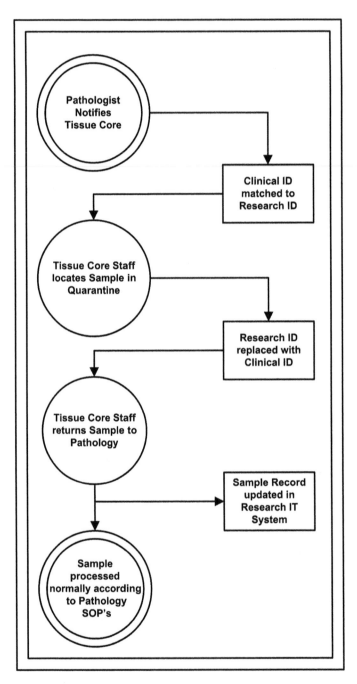

Figure 1 Flowchart outlining Tissue Core handling of melanoma research samples when the pathologist requests return of the research tissue to complete the diagnostic evaluation.

In the first year this protocol for melanoma tumor tissue acquisition was in place, nearly all the patients approached elected to participate in the procurement protocol and signed the informed consent document. Over 140 specimens were banked, and approximately 50 of these were from cutaneous primary tumors. The rate of "callback" by the pathologist was extremely low. Specifically, four cases were retrieved of the initial 140 specimens: three from enlarged lymph nodes suspected to contain melanoma and one from a large, irregular pigmented lesion suspected to represent a second primary melanoma. In these four cases, no tumor was found in the specimen submitted for pathology. The research specimen was promptly retrieved from quarantine and submitted in its entirety for diagnostic evaluation. In all the four cases, there was no evidence of melanoma in the research specimen either. In our remaining cases, we have seen no evidence whatsoever that the submission of a research specimen interfered with the evaluation of any standard pathologic parameter (Fig. 2). There was also no

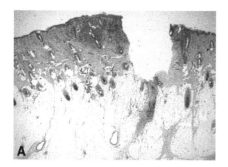

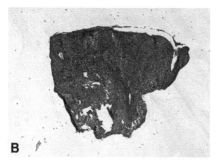

Figure 2 (**A**) Photomicrograph of diagnostic pathology slide made from primary melanoma-wide local excision after harvesting of tumor for research purposes by means of a 4-mm punch biopsy (12.5 × magnification, H&E stained). The defect from the tissue procurement punch biopsy is clearly visible. The diagnosis on initial incisional biopsy (not shown) was malignant melanoma, 1.27 mm in maximum depth. This wide local excision specimen demonstrated residual tumor, grossly measuring 1.1 × 0.6 cm and microscopically measuring 1.28 mm in depth. (**B**) Corresponding frozen section of procured specimen (25 × magnification, H&E stained). The procured specimen revealed melanoma, which did not extend to the previously measured maximum depth, and thus tumor procurement did not alter the final pathology results in any fashion. *Abbreviation*: H&E, hematoxylin and eosin (*See Color Insert*).

evidence of any compromise of clinical decision making for patients whose tumor was procured in part for research purposes.

Procurement of fresh tissue from clinically normal lymph nodes, particularly sentinel lymph nodes, poses unique challenges. Investigators frequently seek fresh tissue from normal-appearing sentinel nodes in melanoma patients for detection of submicroscopic tumor deposits using reverse-transcriptase PCR (RT-PCR) or for immunologic analyses of these tumor-draining nodes. Routine histopathologic processing of sentinel nodes is more rigorous than the standard examination of most lymph nodes, and involves serially sectioning the sentinel node along its long axis, generally cutting the node into multiple approximately 3-mm thick sections (22). Each section is then embedded in paraffin and stained with hematoxylin and eosin (H&E) and immunohistochemical stains as appropriate. It is well established that this more rigorous examination detects small tumor deposits at a greater rate than standard approaches that split the lymph node into two halves (23,24). Although the extent to which the sentinel sections need to be evaluated and the clinical significance of the small foci of metastatic melanoma detected by these extended examination approaches continues to be debated, there is at least some evidence that long-term prognosis is worse for patients with even tiny micrometastases in the sentinel node compared with node-negative patients (25). Pathologic misclassification of a tumor-positive sentinel node as tumor negative therefore might have potential impact on patient outcomes and, of course, might have an impact on research results as well. For these reasons, we propose a modified approach to procurement of sentinel lymph node tissue for research purposes, differing slightly from the algorithm outlined above for primary tumors or obviously tumor-containing lymph nodes. While not yet tested as extensively as our primary tumor procurement algorithm, we believe the following approach to harvesting fresh specimens from sentinel lymph nodes will adequately meet the needs of researchers and provide for adequate pathologic analysis of patient specimens.

1. The surgeon submits the sentinel node in its entirety for immediate pathologic assessment and tissue procurement. As soon as practical after the node is removed from the patient, the entire node is brought to pathology for evaluation.
2. The sentinel node specimen is evaluated in standard diagnostic fashion in the gross room by the pathologist and/or pathology assistant. The lymph node is cut into 3-mm sections along its long axis, any areas grossly suspicious for malignancy are identified and the gross description is dictated. Any indicated immediate pathologic evaluation, such as frozen-section analysis or touch preparation cytology is carried out in routine fashion. One grossly normal-appearing section from at or near the periphery of the node is selected for further sampling for research purposes (since nodal metastases are frequently clustered along the "equator" of the lymph node), while the other sections are processed in standard diagnostic

fashion. Touch preparation cytology slides are prepared from both edges of the cut section, and the cut section is divided again along its long axis. One half or less is submitted for research, while the remainder is processed in standard diagnostic fashion. Using this approach, 90% or more of the sentinel node should be submitted for diagnostic processing, and both cytologic and histologic evidence is available to document the tumor status of the node as a whole and of the portion procured for research.

3. The designated research specimen is snap-frozen and quarantined within the Tissue Core's cryostorage facility, just as for any procured specimen. The algorithm then continues as outlined previously and, as before, the procured sample cannot be used for research purposes until the microscopic analysis of the diagnostic sentinel node specimen has been completed.

HANDLING OF TISSUE BY THE TISSUE PROCUREMENT CORE

Once the procured tumor leaves the operating room and is examined in the pathology department, it comes under the auspices of the Tissue Procurement Core. The procedure for handling this tissue after this is as follows (Fig. 3):

1. The specimen is transported from the pathology gross room to the Tissue Procurement Core in liquid nitrogen by Tissue Core staff, to maintain specimen integrity and chain of custody.
2. Collection data are entered into the research specimen inventory system of record by Tissue Core staff. At this point, a unique specimen identifier is created and a protected link established between the patient's identifying information and the sample(s) collected. Specimens in the Tissue Core are labeled with the new unique identifier; this ID is then used to reference the now de-identified sample for all subsequent processes.
3. Specimens are transferred to a "working" temporary storage area in the Tissue Core Histology section, consisting of a dedicated ultralow temperature freezer ($-80°C$). Samples are removed from this temporary storage unit only in small working batches and are placed on dry ice to maintain the necessary low specimen temperature.
4. Representative frozen sections are cut and stained using standard H&E protocols (identical in process to clinical intraoperative consultation slides, Fig. 2). Of note is that all histologic handling is approached with specimen volume preservation as a primary concern. The specimen remaining after sectioning, still surrounded by frozen optimal cutting temperature (OCT) media, is returned to the "working" temporary storage unit.
5. The stained slides are brought to a research surgical pathologist for evaluation: confirmation of malignancy and assessment of tumor cellularity, viability, pigmentation, and "contaminating" elements such as normal tissue and stroma. These sample composition data are annotated in the

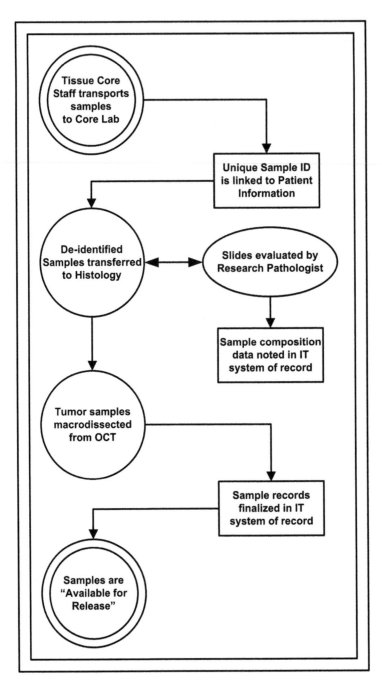

Figure 3 Flowchart outlining Tissue Core processing of melanoma samples for research from initial receipt in the pathology department to ultimate availability for release to researchers conducting IRB-approved research projects.

research specimen inventory system of record. Each slide is marked by the pathologist to allow the slide to act as a ''map'' for the scalpel macro-dissection process outlined below.

6. Tissue Core staff removes the OCT-surrounded tissues from temporary storage and places the samples on dry ice. Along with the H&E slide map, a scalpel is used to remove the viable representative tumor from the OCT. The tumor tissue is then placed into a prechilled cryostorage vial, weighed, and returned to long-term cryostorage in a vapor-phase nitrogen unit. Of note here is that all the processes involving the handling of frozen tissues are conducted while maintaining the frozen state of these samples.

7. The sample record is finalized with the necessary remaining data elements: mass, storage location, and clinical data (immunohistochemical testing and treatment information). At this point, the sample is considered ''available for release'' to qualified researchers for use in IRB-approved research projects.

RELEASE OF SPECIMENS FROM THE TISSUE PROCUREMENT CORE

The Tissue Procurement Core functions as part of Moffitt's Honest Broker System, which is charged with ensuring the safety and security of research participant privacy and maintaining their confidential information. The Honest Broker System involves certain aspects of Research Information Technology at Moffitt necessarily, as much of this information is stored electronically. All reasonable physical and electronic measures are taken to ensure the integrity of samples. Storage facilities are under lock and key, have authorized-access only, are monitored, and have appropriate backup systems. Electronic data are firewall protected, encrypted, and accessible only to authorized users at prespecified levels of access.

As an Honest Broker, the Tissue Procurement Core is authorized to receive identified specimens from within or outside Moffitt. All specimens received are stripped of identifiers (including Protected Health Information as defined by the Health Insurance Portability and Accountability Act (HIPAA) prior to storage and release. A link is maintained between the de-identified specimen and the identifying information. Only the Honest Broker and the Tissue Procurement Core have access to the link and can reassociate identifying information with a given sample as needed. This applies regardless of the state of the specimen, whether it be fresh, frozen, formalin fixed, or paraffin embedded—all are de-identified by the Core.

The Core's policy is to release only completely de-identified samples to investigators, except when written evidence from the institutional IRB has been received to document that other information may be released along with the sample. In that event, information is released only to the extent necessary and approved.

FUTURE DIRECTIONS IN PRIMARY MELANOMA TUMOR PROCUREMENT

Furtherance of our scientific understanding of the basic biology of melanoma and its precursor lesions will require additional enhancements to our ability to procure and utilize tumor and tissue specimens from a variety of sources. Enhanced ability to extract nucleic acids from FFPE tissue is absolutely essential, because only through the use of FFPE tissue can we conduct long-term, retrospective studies with clinical annotation, including prolonged follow-up information and disease-specific survival information. Advances are occurring in this arena, and the commercialization of a PCR-based predictive assay for hormone-receptor positive, lymph-node negative breast cancer (the so-called Oncotype DX assay) illustrates the potential for future development in melanoma. Our knowledge needs to increase regarding how much high-quality DNA and RNA can be extracted from samples of small primary tumors embedded in paraffin for many years, since at least 20-year follow-up would be necessary to determine whether a patient with a T1N0 melanoma was truly cured of his/her disease.

New preservatives that can preserve tissue for diagnostic quality H&E staining as well as immunohistochemical analysis while also preserving adequate DNA and RNA for modern genetic and epigenetic testing would clearly go a long way to increasing our ability to study and understand melanoma biology. How close we are to the development and commercialization of such preservatives remains to be seen. Until then, an alternative approach that bears increased attention is improved noninvasive diagnosis of melanocytic lesions. Dermoscopy and confocal microscopy are two new techniques that, in experienced hands, have a high predictive value for distinguishing straightforward primary melanomas (even melanoma in situ) from banal compound nevi and from atypical but not malignant nevi (26,27). Judiciously applied, these noninvasive diagnostic tools—and others still in development—have the potential to allow immediate referral of the patient to a melanoma center for primary tumor removal, pathologic evaluation, and tumor procurement.

Tumor procurement from primary melanomas and melanoma precursors presents major challenges to the entire melanoma research team and requires the involvement of the entire team—but especially melanoma surgeons and pathologists—for optimal results. We strongly feel that a properly structured tissue procurement program does not compromise patient safety nor does it expose surgeons or pathologists to risks of litigation beyond those that, unfortunately, we have all come to associate with the day-to-day practice of modern medicine.

REFERENCES

1. Litlekalsoy J, Vatne V, Hostmark JG, et al. Immunohistochemical markers in urinary bladder carcinomas from paraffin-embedded archival tissue after storage for 5–70 years. BJU Int 2007; 99:1013–1019.

2. Bertheau P, Cazals-Hatem D, Meignin V, et al. Variability of immunohistochemical reactivity on stored paraffin slides. J Clin Pathol 1998; 51;370–374.
3. DiVito KA, Charette LA, Rimm DL, et al. Long-term preservation of antigenicity on tissue microarrays. Lab Invest 2004; 84:1071–1078.
4. Kononen J, Bubendorf L, Kallioniemi A, et al. Tissue microarrays for high-throughput molecular profiling of tumor specimens. Nat Med 1998; 4:844–847.
5. Cregger M, Berger AJ, Rimm DL. Immunohistochemistry and quantitative analysis of protein expression. Arch Pathol Lab Med 2006; 130:1026–1030.
6. Glatz-Krieger K, Pache M, Tapia C, et al. Anatomic site-specific patterns of gene copy number gains in skin, mucosal, and uveal melanomas detected by fluorescence in situ hybridization. Virchows Arch 2006;449:328–333.
7. Willmore-Payne C, Holden JA, Hirschowitz S, et al. BRAF and c-kit gene copy number in mutation-positive malignant melanoma. Hum Pathol 2006; 37:520–527.
8. Berger AJ, Camp RL, Divito KA, et al. Automated quantitated analysis of HDM2 expression in malignant melanoma shows an association with early-stage disease and improved outcome. Cancer Res 2004; 64:8767–8792.
9. Koynova D, Jordanova E, Kukutsch N, et al. Increased C-MYC copy numbers on the background of CDKN2A loss is associated with improved survival in nodular melanoma. J Cancer Res Clin Oncol 2007; 133:117–123.
10. Stark M, Hayward N. Genome-wide loss of heterozygosity and copy number analysis in melanoma using high-density single-nucleotide polymorphism arrays. Cancer Res 2007; 67:2632–2642.
11. Koynova DK, Jordanova ES, Milev AD, et al. Gene-specific fluorescence in-situ hybridization analysis on tissue microarray to refine the region of chromosome 20q amplification in melanoma. Melanoma Res 2007; 17:37–41.
12. Dedhia P, Tarale S, Dhongde G, et al. Evaluation of DNA extraction methods and real time PCR optimization on formalin-fixed paraffin-embedded tissues. Asian Pac J Cancer Prev 2007; 8:55–59.
13. Inoue T, Nabeshima K, Kataoka H, et al. Feasibility of archival non-buffered formalin-fixed and paraffin-embedded tissues for PCR amplification: an analysis of resected gastric carcinoma. Pathol Int 1996; 12:997–1004.
14. White JS, McLean IW, Becker RL, et al. Correlation of comparative genomic hybridization results of 100 archival uveal melanomas with patient survival. Cancer Genet Cytogenet 2006; 170:29–39.
15. Abrahamsen HN, Steiniche T, Nexo E, et al. Towards quantitative mRNA analysis in paraffin-embedded tissues using real-time reverse transcriptase-polymerase chain reaction: a methodological study on lymph nodes from melanoma patients. J Mol Diagn 2003; 5:34–41.
16. Crockett DK, Lin Z, Vaughn CP, et al. Identification of proteins from formalin-fixed paraffin-embedded cells by LC-MS/MS. Lab Invest 2005; 85:1405–1415.
17. Farkas DH, Drevon AM, Kiechle FL, et al. Specimen stability for DNA-based diagnostic testing. Diagn Mol Pathol 1996; 5:227–235.
18. Schmitta M, Mengelea K, Schuerena E, et al. European Organisation for Research and Treatment of Cancer (EORTC) Pathobiology Group standard operating procedure for the preparation of human tumour tissue extracts suited for the quantitative analysis of tissue-associated biomarkers. Eur J Cancer 2007; 43:835–844.
19. Sondak VK, Sabel MS, Mulé JJ. Allogeneic and autologous melanoma vaccines: where have we been and where are we going? Clin Cancer Res 2006; 12:S2337–S2340.

20. Morreim EH. Medical research litigation and malpractice tort doctrines: courts on a learning curve. Houst J Health Law Policy 2003;4:1–86.
21. Andrews L, Nelkin D. Biocommerce: the people in the body. In: Body Bazaar: The Market for Human Tissue in the Biotechnology Age. New York, NY: Crown Publishers, 2001: 25–26.
22. Messina JL, Glass LF, Cruse CW, et al. Pathologic examination of the sentinel lymph node in malignant melanoma. Am J Surg Pathol 1999; 23:686–690.
23. Karimipour DJ, Lowe L, Su L, et al. Standard immunostains for melanoma in sentinel lymph node specimens: which ones are most useful? J Am Acad Dermatol 2004; 50:759–764.
24. Cook MG, Green MA, Anderson B, et al. The development of optimal pathological assessment of sentinel lymph nodes for melanoma. J Pathol 2003; 200:314–319.
25. Scheri RP, Essner R, Turner RR, et al. Isolated tumor cells in the sentinel node affect long term prognosis of patients with melanoma. Ann Surg Oncol 2007; 14:2861–2866.
26. Garbe C, Eigentler TK. Diagnosis and treatment of cutaneous melanoma: state of the art 2006. Melanoma Res 2007; 17:117–127.
27. Pellacani G, Cesinaro AM, Seidenari S. In vivo confocal reflectance microscopy for the characterization of melanocytic nests and correlation with dermoscopy and histology. Br J Dermatol 2005; 152:384–386.

Glossary

Adjuvant Therapy: The use of additional treatment, usually chemotherapy, immuno-therapy, or radiation, after complete surgical resection to decrease recurrence rates and/or enhance survival rates by eradicating clinically undetectable residual microscopic disease.

Adoptive T Cell Immunotherapy: An investigational approach to cancer therapy that involves the transfer of tumor-specific T cells, usually developed and expanded ex vivo, into a tumor-bearing host. This is intended to result in the direct destruction of tumors by the transferred T cells themselves via lytic processes or cytokine secretion or in the indirect destruction of tumors by augmenting the preexisting antitumor immunity of the host.

Anoikis: A form of programmed cell death that occurs when a cell is deprived of its usual interactions with other cells or extracellular matrix proteins. From the Greek word for "homelessness," successful transformation of a normal cell to a cancerous cell requires evasion of this process. (See **apoptosis**)

Apoptosis (also known as Programmed Cell Death):   The cellular process, mediated by carefully regulated sets of pro- and antiapoptotic proteins and enzymes, by which a cell dies without any resulting tissue inflammation or damage to surrounding cells.

BCG (Bacillus Calmette Guèrin):   A live, attenuated mycobacterium that induces a potent inflammatory reaction at the site of injection. Still currently in use in some countries as a tuberculosis vaccine, it has been administered by direct injection into superficial tumors and used in several antitumor vaccine trials as an immunologic adjuvant to augment the immune response of the recipient to the vaccine therapy. It is also used in the intravesicle therapy of superficial bladder cancer.

Basic Helix-Loop-Helix Leucine Zipper: A characteristic sequence of amino acids within a regulatory protein that confers the ability to homodimerize, bind to DNA, and alter the expression of target genes.

Bevacizumab (also known as Avastin^{TM}): A monoclonal antibody that inhibits vascular endothelial-derived growth factor. It is used in the clinical setting of cancer therapy in order to inhibit tumor-induced angiogenesis, either administered alone or along with chemotherapy or other agents. It is FDA approved for colorectal cancer therapy in combination with chemotherapy.

Breslow Thickness (also known as Breslow Depth): The microscopic measurement of the depth of melanoma invasion from the granular layer of the epidermis, or the base of the ulcer if the epidermis is ulcerated, to the deepest contiguous underlying tumor cell. This two-dimensional measurement is a surrogate for tumor volume and is directly proportional to the propensity for the melanoma to metastasize and correlates well with overall prognosis. Melanomas less than or equal to 1 mm in thickness are considered "thin" melanomas and have a favorable prognosis, while those greater than 4 mm are considered "thick" and have a relatively poor prognosis.

Caspase: A class of intracellular enzymes that, when activated, induce the process of apoptosis or programmed cell death.

cDNA Microarray Technology: An automated, high-throughput technique that quantitates the expression of thousands of genes within a specific cell type. The process involves extraction of RNA from cells of interest, reverse transcription to convert to cDNA, and hybridization to a gene chip. The gene chip contains spots of thousands of short DNA sequences from normal tissue (see definition of **oligomer**) corresponding to known genes. The degree of hybridization is taken to be directly proportional to the intensity of expression. By comparing the gene expression of neoplastic cells with their nonneoplastic counterparts, patterns of gene expression can be identified that may have significant implications for studies of the etiology, prognosis and treatment of cancer. See also **gene expression profiling**.

Chaperone Protein: A cytoplasmic protein that aids in the conformational folding of other proteins to ensure proper posttranslational functioning.

Chemoprevention: The use of therapeutic agents (including chemotherapy drugs, targeted agents, hormones, or drugs such as statins or nonsteroidal anti-inflammatory drugs used for nonneoplastic disorders) in order to reduce the incidence of a particular cancer, typically in a high-risk population prior to the development of the disease or in patients successfully treated for an early stage cancer but considered at high risk for development of a second primary malignancy.

Comparative Genomic Hybridization (CGH): A method of screening tumor cells for genetic changes by comparing them to cells from normal tissue. The alterations are classified as chromosomal gains and losses, or, in the case of array CGH, specific genetic sequence changes, and can reveal a characteristic pattern of mutations at chromosomal and sub-chromosomal levels for a particular tumor type.

Costimulatory Molecules: Membrane-bound ligands and their corresponding receptors found on antigen-presenting cells (APCs) and immune effector cells whose signaling is required, in addition to antigen presentation, in order to elicit optimal activation of effector cells. The lack of appropriate costimulatory molecule function is thought to contribute to the relatively poor efficacy of tumor vaccine therapy.

Cytokine: A diverse class of regulatory molecules, generally secreted by immune cells, which function in immunomodulatory pathways. Cytokines can be pro- or anti-inflammatory, depending upon the individual molecule. Examples include tumor necrosis factor, interleukins, interferons, and hematopoietic growth factors.

Cytotoxic T Lymphocyte (CTL): A subtype of T cell that, when activated by antigen via its specific T cell receptor, directly lyses target cells in an antibody-independent manner. Part of the adaptive immune system, meaning the cells can recognize their targets more effectively after prior exposure to them. Most CTL express the CD8 molecule.

Dendritic Cell (DC): A specific type of antigen-presenting cell (APC), typically found in skin, mucosal surfaces, and lymphoid tissue, that is considered one of the most potent APCs for activating naïve T lymphocytes. It is widely used in studies investigating immune responses to tumor.

Desmoplastic Melanoma: A variant of melanoma that is histologically characterized by growth of malignant spindled melanocytes, surrounded by desmoplastic stromal change. Commonly found on the head and neck of older patients and often relatively thick at diagnosis, this variant frequently lacks visible pigmentation and exhibits a relatively higher rate of perineural invasion but seems to have a lower incidence of lymph node metastases.

Epigenetic Event: A process by which gene expression is altered, thereby changing the phenotype of a cell, but which does not involve changing the genotype of a cell (i.e., no mutation of DNA sequence). The process can involve DNA methylation, DNA or histone acetylation, or changes to chromatin folding. In addition to DNA mutation, epigenetic changes are another mechanism thought to be important in tumor initiation and promotion.

Eumelanin: One of the two subtypes of human melanin pigment; predominant in brown and black skin and hair. See also **pheomelanin.**

Expressed Sequence Tag (EST): A short DNA sequence that represents a small portion of a transcribed gene. ESTs can be used to identify the full gene sequence in genomic DNA by matching base pairs in published genome databases.

Fluorescence In Situ Hybridization (FISH): A technique that involves hybridization of a fluorescent-labeled DNA probe to its corresponding complementary sequence on chromosomal DNA, either metaphase spreads or interphase nuclei. This technique allows the detection of chromosomal gains, losses, or translocation in neoplastic tissue, including paraffin-embedded formalin-fixed pathology specimens.

Gene Expression Profiling: A technique that quantitates global patterns of messenger RNA expression in a specific cell, tissue, or tumor type. Frequently performed using **cDNA microarrray technology** or **SAGE** (see also **serial analysis of gene expression**). This technique has also been applied in the clinical setting to identify subgroups of tumor types to predict response to a specific treatment and overall prognosis.

Immunohistochemistry (IHC): A histopathologic technique that involves the detection of specific antigens within a tissue section. Performed on either frozen or formalin-fixed tissue, the process involves permeabilizing the cells and incubating the tissue with an antibody directed against a specific antigen of interest. A second, labeled antibody detects the first and is visualized with a chromogenic reaction.

Immunoproteosome: An intracellular vesicle found in APCs, which breaks down and processes nonself proteins into short peptides to be used in the presentation of antigen to effector cells.

In Situ Hybridization: A technique that involves the detection of specific RNA or DNA sequences within a tissue section, either frozen or formalin-fixed on a slide. The process involves permeabilizing the cells of excised tissue and hybridizing with a fluorescent-labeled DNA probe that is complementary to the RNA or DNA sequence of interest.

Interferons: A family of secreted regulatory molecules that function in immuno-modulatory pathways. Originally identified on the basis of their ability to "interfere" with viral replication, the interferons represent a subset of cytokines that are typically pro-inflammatory. Recombinant interferon alpha (referred to by the generic name interferon α-2b) is widely used in the adjuvant therapy of high-risk melanoma, but toxicity is high and the survival impact modest at best.

Interleukins: A family of secreted regulatory molecules that function in immuno-modulatory pathways. They represent a subset of cytokines that can exhibit pro- and anti-inflammatory effects. Recombinant interleukin 2 (sometimes referred to by its generic name aldesleukin) is approved for use in the treatment of metastatic melanoma; but its toxicity is very high, limiting its use to highly selected patients treated in experienced centers.

Human Leukocyte Antigen (HLA): A type of cell surface antigen that allows the immune system to differentiate between self and nonself. These antigens are coded by genes in the major histocompatibility complex (MHC). Different classes of HLA antigens are expressed by different cells; for example, HLA class II molecules are typically expressed only on white blood cells and APCs like dendritic cells. HLA molecules bind protein antigens in the form of peptide fragments and display them on the cell surface, where they are recognized by the immune system "in context." Any given protein may contain various peptide fragments that can only be presented by certain specific HLA antigens; these peptides are referred to as HLA-restricted (or MHC-restricted) antigens.

Kinase: An enzyme that catalyzes the addition of a phosphate group to a protein, resulting in a change in protein function or stability. The "kinome" is the set of all kinases existing within a given tissue, tumor, or whole organism. See also **phosphorylation.**

Knockdown: The process of inhibiting expression of a specific gene, usually involving interference with the translation of messenger RNA. See also **RNAi.**

Knockout: The elimination of expression of a specific gene, often done by genetically engineering mice.

Lymphokine-Activated Killer (LAK) Cells: A class of lymphocytes that, when activated ex vivo by cytokines such as IL-2, can lyse cells resistant to natural killer (NK) cells. Part of the innate immune system, meaning the cells can recognize their targets without prior exposure.

Lymphokine: A class of regulatory molecules specifically secreted by lymphocytes, which function in immunomodulatory pathways. Many cytokines, such as IL-2 and interferon, are secreted by activated lymphocytes and hence are also by definition lymphokines.

Melanosome: A membrane-bound intracellular granule containing melanin that originates in melanocytes and is transferred to keratinocytes, as part of skin coloration and/or the protective response to ultraviolet radiation.

Melanotropin: A hormone secreted by the pituitary that promotes the synthesis of melanin by melanocytes, also known as melanocyte-stimulating hormone (MSH).

Microarray Technology: A collection of techniques involving assembly of many specimens in a small area, such as a glass slide or silicone chip, which affords the ability to assay multiple specimens in a time- and cost-efficient manner. See also **cDNA microarray technology** and **tissue microarray.**

microRNA (miRNA): A naturally occurring short, single-stranded RNA molecule that regulates gene expression by inhibiting translation of an RNA transcript in a sequence-dependent manner; fewer than 1000 such sequences have been shown to exist in mammalian cells.

Molecular Signature: A constellation of characteristic changes in gene expression, usually of a particular tumor type in comparison with the corresponding normal tissue of origin. Other "signatures" may characterize tumors of varying degrees of aggressiveness or responsiveness to a given therapy.

Natural Killer (NK) Cells: A subtype of lymphocyte that can lyse nonself, virally infected, or neoplastic cells. Part of the innate immune system, meaning the cells can recognize their targets without prior exposure.

Objective Response Rate: The calculated frequency of improvement in a disease state involving a group of treated patients that can be measured by an unbiased method, typically radiographically or histopathologically. In cancer clinical trials, the objective response rate is the percentage of patients enrolled in the trial having either a partial or a complete response to therapy. According to World Health Organization (WHO) criteria, for patients with a solid, measurable tumor, partial response is defined as at least a 50% reduction in the product of longest tumor diameter and the corresponding orthogonal length and no evidence of new lesions or progression of any other existing lesion. Complete response is defined as complete disappearance of all known tumor and no evidence of new lesions or progression of any other existing lesion. More recently, the RECIST (Response Evaluation Criteria in Solid Tumors) criteria have been used in cancer therapy trials to define partial response: a 30% reduction in the sum of the maximal diameters of targeted lesions without the development of new lesions. However, for targeted therapies (such as the use of imatinib for gastrointestinal stromal tumors), neither WHO nor RECIST criteria accurately identify all patients responding to therapy.

Oligomer: A short sequence of nucleotides typically synthesized to correspond to a portion of a gene of interest so that it can uniquely identify that gene.

Peripheral Blood Mononuclear Cells (PBMC): Circulating white blood cells with round, uniform nuclei (i.e., monocytes and lymphocytes, but not neutrophils), which are typically studied when investigating the adaptive immune system.

Phase I Clinical Trial: The initial study of an investigational therapy in either afflicted patients or normal volunteers, which typically involves dose escalation in order to determine dose-related and dose-limiting toxicity (the maximally tolerated dose), as well as pharmacokinetics. Efficacy (e.g., objective response rate) is not a primary endpoint of a phase I trial.

Phase II Clinical Trial: The subsequent study after phase I involving afflicted patients treated at or near the maximally tolerated dose to determine whether an investigational therapy has documentable efficacy in a particular disease state and to further quantitate the toxicity profile.

Phase III Clinical Trial: A study performed after phase II trials document efficacy and acceptable toxicity in which patients are treated to determine whether an investigational therapy is superior to existing standard therapy. The study is typically performed in a randomized fashion.

Pheomelanin: One of the two subtypes of human melanin; predominant in red-headed and fair-complexioned individuals. See also **eumelanin.**

Phosphorylation: The enzymatic addition of a phosphate group to a protein that results in a conformational change, which typically affects protein function or stability. See also **kinase.**

Real-Time PCR (Polymerase Chain Reaction):   Also known as quantitative PCR, the method used to quantitate the amount of DNA of a specific sequence within a particular sample. The method uses a pair of primers, each about 20 nucleotides in length, that are complementary to a defined sequence on each of the two DNA strands. These primers are extended by a DNA polymerase so that a copy of the sequence is generated. The procedure is repeated multiple times, resulting in logarithmic amplification of the desired sequence. This method is frequently combined with reverse transcription in order to determine the quantity of transcribed RNA in a particular sample.

Regulatory T Cell (T_{reg}):   A subset of T lymphocytes that typically suppresses the function of effector T cells. T_{reg} function is thought to prevent autoimmunity but also contributes to the relatively poor efficacy of tumor vaccine therapy. Regulatory T cells can be present naturally or induced by exposure to cytokines like TGF-β.

Relapse-Free Survival: The length of time following the institution of a particular therapy (or in the case of a clinical trial, the date of enrollment onto that trial) that a group of patients survives without evidence of recurrence of disease. This applies particularly to **adjuvant therapy,** where patients are treated in the absence of known disease. When therapy is administered to patients with clinically evident tumor, progression-free survival is the length of time from institution of therapy or trial enrollment to the first evidence of development of new tumors or progression of existing disease. Cancer progression is measured using the same criteria used to define **objective response rate,** such as the WHO or RECIST criteria. Although patients may value relapse-free (or progression-free) survival highly, most clinical trials are designed with overall survival (time from study entry until death from any cause) as the primary endpoint.

Response Element: A DNA sequence typically found upstream of or within the promoter region of a gene, which binds to proteins responsible for regulating gene expression.

RNA Interference (RNAi):   The inhibition of gene expression using small RNA molecules that are complementary in sequence to a portion of the target gene. See also **knockdown** and **siRNA.**

SAGE: See **serial analysis of gene expression.**

Senescence: The absence of cellular proliferation; ''aging'' in a group of cells that is the result of the natural limit of mitotic events. Neoplasms avoid this limitation because of mutations in genes that mediate this homeostatic process.

Serial Analysis of Gene Expression (SAGE):   An alternative method to cDNA microarray analysis that also quantitates gene expression in a group of cells. Rather than hybridization, this technique involves direct sequencing of short segments of transcribed genes and therefore is considered to be more labor-intensive than microarray analysis. However, SAGE generates an absolute count of mRNA transcripts within a cell, so this technique has less lab-to-lab variation than microarray analysis, and libraries made years apart can be accurately compared.

Short Hairpin RNA (shRNA): Synthetic RNA that is engineered to cause the inhibition of gene expression in a sequence-specific manner. shRNA molecules are designed to contain a sense portion, an antisense portion, and a short noncomplementary sequence in the middle, forming a hairpin loop. shRNA molecules are thought to be more stable and efficient in inhibiting gene expression compared with linear, nonlooped siRNA.

Single Nucleotide Polymorphism (SNP): Naturally occurring variations in DNA sequences involving a single base position. While most of these polymorphisms have little or no biological significance, many have physiologic effects on the gene of interest, and specific SNPs have been reported in various databases that can predict how patients develop disease and/or respond to therapeutic interventions.

Small Interfering RNA (siRNA): Small pieces of RNA that cause the inhibition of gene expression in a sequence-specific manner by binding to complementary transcribed messenger RNA. This technique has been applied in the laboratory setting to reduce the expression of genes potentially important for homeostasis and metastasis of neoplastic cells for investigative purposes. See also **knockdown** and **RNAi.**

Spitz Nevus: A benign melanocytic neoplasm most commonly observed in children and young adults, which can be difficult to differentiate from malignant melanoma histopathologically.

Spitzoid Melanoma: A rare form of melanoma that histologically appears similar to benign Spitz nevus. As a variant of melanoma, its clinical behavior, including metastatic potential, is similar to that of conventional melanoma.

Stem Cell: A type of undifferentiated cell that is capable of unlimited mitosis, but in addition is capable of terminally differentiating into specialized cell types.

SUMOylation: A form of posttranslational modification of proteins that involves the addition of SUMO, a small ubiquitin-like modifier, which can alter the function, stability, or localization of the protein. See also **ubiquitination.**

T$_{reg}$: See **regulatory T cell.**

Targeted Therapy: A type of pharmacologic therapy rationally designed to inhibit a specific protein or function of a cancer cell that is generally not present in or not critical to the survival of normal cells.

Therapeutic Index: The ratio of the lowest dose of therapy causing toxicity to the lowest dose of therapy resulting in benefit. This ratio is used to estimate the safety of a particular therapy; many antineoplastic drugs have a low therapeutic index.

Tissue Microarray (TMA): A method of utilizing multiple samples of tissue, typically tumor specimens, from conventional paraffin blocks so that tissue from multiple patients or blocks can be seen on the same slide. This is done by using a needle to biopsy the donor block and placing the core into an array on a recipient paraffin block. The recipient TMA block can be cut into multiple sections and stained, allowing for quality-controlled, high-throughput analysis of protein expression using **immunohistochemistry.**

Transgenic Murine Model: An experimental system in which the genome of a mouse embryo is altered in order to change gene expression. The mouse is then studied in order to elucidate the function of the gene of interest, the "transgene."

Ubiquitination: A form of posttranslational modification of proteins that comprises the initial process of protein degradation in which ubiquitin, a short peptide, is covalently attached to a target protein. The addition of ubiquitin targets the protein for degradation. See also **SUMOylation.**

Vitiligo: A condition in which immune-mediated destruction of melanocytes causes the absence of pigmentation in skin and other pigment-bearing tissues. Technically, the term vitiligo applies to a spontaneous autoimmune phenomenon in otherwise normal individuals, but this immune-mediated depigmentation can also occur in patients with melanoma, spontaneously or following the use of immunotherapy or other treatments. In these cases, it is thought to be associated with a favorable clinical outcome.

Xenograft: A transplant of tissue from one species to another, such as the implantation of human tumor tissue into an immunodeficient ("nude") mouse.

Index

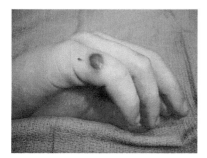

Figure 3.1 Symmetrical, dome-shaped brown papule on finger of five-year-old male. Clinically consistent with either a Spitz nevus or a Spitzoid melanoma, this lesion proved to be a benign Spitz nevus (Fig. 3.2) (*see page 29*).

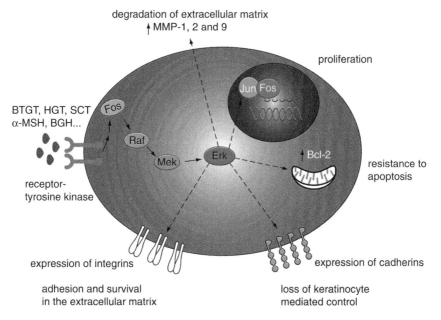

Figure 5.1 The RAS-MAPK signal transduction pathway. RAF kinases are serine/threonine protein kinases that initiate the mitogenic kinase cascade that ultimately modulates gene expression by way of the phosphorylation of transcription factors such as Jun, Elk1, c-Ets1/2, STAT 1/3, or Myc. *Source*: From Ref. 33 (*see page 58*).

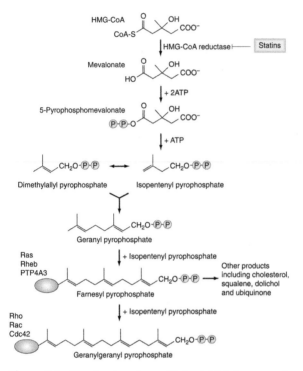

Figure 5.2 Mevalonate pathway. Statins inhibit the conversion of HMG-CoA to mevalonate. Molecules of ATP are then used to phosphorylate mevalonate to pyrophosphomevalonate, which is then converted to IPP. IPP can be reversibly converted to DMAPP. IPP and DMAPP can then be combined to form the 10-carbon isoprenoid GPP. Additional IPPs can be added to produce FPP, the 15-carbon isoprenoid, and GGPP, the 20-carbon isoprenoid. Inhibition of this pathway by statins prevents the formation of both mevalonate and its downstream product IPP. This inhibition can be reversed completely with mevalonate. Supplementation with FPP will restore farnesylation but not geranylgeranylation, as IPP is not available to convert FPP into GGPP. Supplementation with GGPP will only restore geranylgeranylation. Several other branches of this pathway can convert FPP into various other products, including cholesterol. In general, FPP helps prenylate proteins in the RAS, Rheb, and PTP4A3 families, whereas GGPP helps prenylate proteins in the Rho, Rac, and Cdc42 families. A few G-proteins (including RHOB and NRAS) can be either farnesylated or geranylgeranylated. *Abbreviations*: HMG-CoA, 3-hydroxy-3-methylglutaryl coenzyme A; ATP, adenotriphosphate; IPP, isopentenyl pyrophosphate; DMAPP, dimethylallyl pyrophosphate; GPP, geranyl pyrophosphate; FPP, farnesyl pyrophosphate; GGPP, geranylgeranyl pyrophosphate. *Source*: From Ref. 45 (*see page 60*).

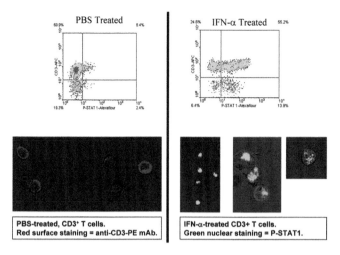

Figure 9.2 Flow cytometric analysis and fluorescent microscopy of phosphorylated STAT1 (P-STAT1) in peripheral blood mononuclear cells treated with PBS (vehicle; *Left Panel*) or IFN-α (10^4 U/mL; 15 minutes; *Right Panel*). Cells were also costained with an antibody targeting CD3. *Abbreviations*: STAT, signal transducer and activator of transcription; PBS, phosphate buffer solution (*see page 121*).

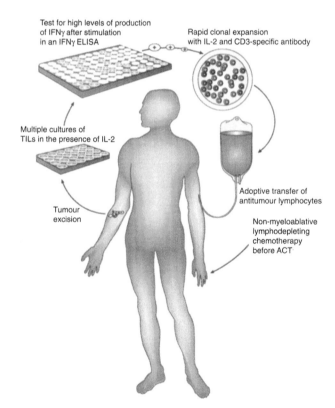

Figure 12.1 Adoptive immunotherapy protocol for TIL cells. Tumor-specific T cells are isolated ex vivo from melanoma lesions using high concentrations of IL-2. TIL cells are screened for their ability to secrete high levels of IFN-γ when cultured with tumor antigen. The selected TIL cells are expanded using anti-CD3 antibody and expanded in IL-2. Prior to cell infusion, patients undergo chemotherapy to induce a lymphodepletion within the host. *Abbreviation*: ACT, adoptive cellular therapies. *Source*: From Ref. 59 (*see page 164*).

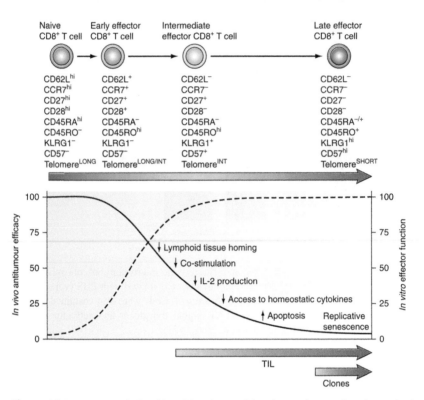

Figure 12.2 Inverse relationship of in vitro and in vivo antitumor functions of adoptively transferred naïve and effector T cell subsets. At increasing strength of stimulation, naïve CD8⁺ T cells proliferate and progressively differentiate through early, intermediate, and late effector stages. The phenotypic and functional changes that characterize this process are illustrated as no expression (–), intermediate expression (+) and high expression (hi) of the various markers. The progressive acquisition of full effector functions (*dashed line*) is associated with a decreased ability of T cells to cause tumor regression after adoptive transfer (*solid line*). *Source*: From Ref. 60 (*see page 166*).

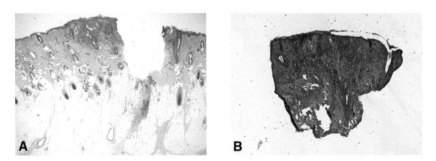

Figure 13.2 (A) Photomicrograph of diagnostic pathology slide made from primary melanoma-wide local excision after harvesting of tumor for research purposes by means of a 4-mm punch biopsy (12.5 × magnification, H&E stained). The defect from the tissue procurement punch biopsy is clearly visible. The diagnosis on initial incisional biopsy (not shown) was malignant melanoma, 1.27 mm in maximum depth. This wide local excision specimen demonstrated residual tumor, grossly measuring 1.1 × 0.6 cm and microscopically measuring 1.28 mm in depth. (B) Corresponding frozen section of procured specimen (25 × magnification, H&E stained). The procured specimen revealed melanoma, which did not extend to the previously measured maximum depth, and thus tumor procurement did not alter the final pathology results in any fashion. *Abbreviation*: H&E, hematoxylin and eosin (*see page 191*).

Printed and bound by CPI Group (UK) Ltd, Croydon, CR0 4YY

23/10/2024

01778227-0002